COGNITIVE-BEHAVIORAL THERAPY FOR PTSD

MINDSPACE
RECOVERY COLLEGE

Return Date

Please return book by date stamped

MINDSPACE
RECOVERY COLLEGE

27 JUN

Guides to Individualized Evidence-Based Treatment

Jacqueline B. Persons, *Series Editor*

Providing evidence-based roadmaps for managing real-world cases, volumes in this series help the clinician develop treatment plans using interventions of proven effectiveness. With an emphasis on systematic yet flexible case formulation, these hands-on guides provide powerful alternatives to one-size-fits-all approaches. Each book addresses a particular disorder or presents cutting-edge intervention strategies that can be used across a range of clinical problems.

Cognitive Therapy of Schizophrenia
David G. Kingdon and Douglas Turkington

Treating Bipolar Disorder: A Clinician's Guide to Interpersonal
and Social Rhythm Therapy
Ellen Frank

Modular Cognitive-Behavioral Therapy for Childhood Anxiety Disorders
Bruce F. Chorpita

Cognitive-Behavioral Therapy for PTSD: A Case Formulation Approach
Claudia Zayfert and Carolyn Black Becker

Cognitive-Behavioral Therapy for PTSD

A CASE FORMULATION APPROACH

Claudia Zayfert
Carolyn Black Becker

Series Editor's Note by Jacqueline B. Persons

THE GUILFORD PRESS
New York   London

© 2007 The Guilford Press
A Division of Guilford Publications, Inc.
72 Spring Street, New York, NY 10012
www.guilford.com

Paperback edition 2008

Printed in the United States of America

This book is printed on acid-free paper.

Last digit is print number: 9 8 7 6 5 4

Library of Congress Cataloging-in-Publication Data
Zayfert, Claudia.
    Cognitive-behavioral therapy for PTSD : a case formulation approach /
Claudia Zayfert, Carolyn Black Becker.
        p. ; cm. — (Guides to individualized evidence-based treatment)
    Includes bibliographical references and index.
    ISBN: 978-1-59385-369-3 (hardcover: alk. paper)
    ISBN: 978-1-60623-031-2 (paperback: alk. paper)
    1. Post-traumatic stress disorder—Treatment.   2. Cognitive
therapy. I. Becker, Carolyn Black.   II. Title.   III. Series.
    [DNLM: 1. Stress Disorders, Post-Traumatic—therapy.   2. Cognitive
Therapy—methods.   3. Stress Disorders, Post-Traumatic—
psychology.   WM 170 Z39c 2007]
    RC552.P67C644 2007
    616.85′21—dc22
                                                            2006027917

In memory of Sami

    —C. Z.

In memory of Sue

    —C. B. B.

About the Authors

Claudia Zayfert, PhD, a clinical psychologist and an Associate Professor of Psychiatry at Dartmouth Medical School, has been involved in treatment, research, and training related to posttraumatic stress disorder (PTSD) for over 15 years. She completed her doctoral degree at West Virginia University and was a Research Associate at the National Center for PTSD. She is Director of the Anxiety Disorders Service and the Posttraumatic Stress Disorder Treatment Program in the Department of Psychiatry at Dartmouth Hitchcock Medical Center. Dr. Zayfert's primary interests have been the treatment of PTSD with comorbid conditions. Her current research is focused on treatment of posttraumatic insomnia. Dr. Zayfert has published extensively and has presented at national and international conferences to promote the use of empirically supported treatments for anxiety disorders in clinical practice. She routinely provides training and consultation regarding cognitive-behavioral treatments for complicated PTSD.

Carolyn Black Becker, PhD, is an Associate Professor of Psychology at Trinity University, San Antonio. Trained at Rutgers University, Dr. Becker is a practicing clinical psychologist who specializes in the treatment of PTSD, anxiety disorders, and eating disorders. She has over 14 years of experience with cognitive-behavioral treatments for a variety of anxiety disorders, including PTSD. The primary focus of her teaching, research, and clinical work is the implementation of scientifically supported prevention and treatment interventions in clinical settings. In addition to numerous publications on these topics, Dr. Becker regularly presents at national and international conferences and provides training and consultation to clinicians.

Series Editor's Note

The person who has posttraumatic stress disorder (PTSD) typically has a host of problems. In addition to PTSD, the person generally has several co-occurring disorders and difficulties, such as bulimia nervosa, borderline personality disorder, substance abuse, chaotic and abusive relationships, financial problems, and more. Although the traumas that caused the PTSD are long past—and in part because they are so long past and have not been treated—these individuals' lives are often shattered, and they experience significant suffering and extensive disability.

The good news is that several effective treatments for PTSD have been developed. Ironically, the development of these effective treatments for PTSD is also the bad news (Strosahl, 1998) because of all the questions they raise. The fact that multiple, similar cognitive-behavioral treatments are available can lead to confusion for the treatment provider, who has difficulty sorting through these therapies to determine which are effective. Are some more effective than others? How do they differ? Which one should I use to treat the patient who is in my office right now? Your difficulties are compounded when you focus on your patient's multiple, co-occurring disorders and difficulties, which raise the following questions: Should I treat the patient's various disorders and problems sequentially? If so, in what order? Or should I treat them simultaneously? Is the answer to this question different for different patients? What strategy can I use to determine the answer to this question?

Claudia Zayfert and Carolyn Black Becker answer all of these questions in this book. To answer the questions about the treatment of PTSD itself, the authors describe the various evidence-based cognitive-behavioral models of PTSD and distill from them their essential ingredients. The authors describe both conditioning and cognitive views of the acquisition and maintenance of PTSD symptoms, and they describe cognitive-behavioral views of fear, panic, anxiety, and the many other emotions that commonly occur in PTSD (e.g., anger, shame, guilt, and hopelessness). The authors provide for the clinician reader a sophisticated understanding of cognitive-behavioral conceptualizations of PTSD at the level of general principles rather than at the level of the procedural details of the currently available treatment protocols. Zayfert and Becker propose that two basic interventions, exposure and cognitive restructuring, are at the heart of effective cognitive-behavioral therapy for PTSD, and they describe those interventions in detail, both at the theoretical level and at the here-and-now, clinical level, with many case examples and details.

As is typical of the books in this series, Guides to Individualized Evidence-Based Treatment, Zayfert and Becker show the reader how to use the cognitive-behavioral view of PTSD and its treatment as the foundation for an individualized case formulation and treatment plan that addresses the unique details of each patient's PTSD symptoms, along with his or her comorbid problems and disorders. They show the therapist how to use the individualized case formulation and cognitive-behavioral principles to guide clinical decision making, including creative methods for blending and sequencing treatments for the multiple-problem patient. The strategy here is not to eliminate the need for clinical decision making by providing a detailed manual (cf. Wilson, 1997), but to provide the clinician with a systematic approach to making clinical decisions.

This book describes both the theoretical underpinnings and the nitty-gritty details of therapeutic work. The therapeutic relationship receives detailed attention, as do underdiscussed topics such as therapists' and patients' reluctance to undertake exposure. In a feature that is particularly important in view of recent evidence demonstrating that outcome monitoring at every session can improve treatment outcomes (Lambert, Hansen, & Finch, 2001), the authors provide specific methods for tracking weekly patient progress, and show how to use the progress data and the case formulation to guide treatment, including making changes in the case formulation and treatment plan when the patient does not improve as expected.

The authors' extensive experience working with PTSD is evident on every page. In addition, they convey a striking compassion for these patients, who are not always easy to work well with or to like. This book is ideal for the sophisticated and thoughtful clinician who wishes to provide top-quality care for this challenging patient population.

JACQUELINE B. PERSONS, PhD
San Francisco Bay Area Center
for Cognitive Therapy

Preface

We wrote this book for mental health clinicians who want to enhance their ability to help traumatized adults recover from posttraumatic stress disorder (PTSD) and live more satisfying lives. Research indicates that cognitive-behavioral therapy (CBT) for PTSD significantly reduces symptoms of PTSD. Despite this, you may wonder whether CBT for PTSD is appropriate for your clinical practice patients with PTSD, who likely present with a complicated array of symptoms and problems.

Two schools of thought have emerged regarding the usefulness of CBT for PTSD in clinical practice (Kilpatrick, 2005). One school contends that you should use evidence-based interventions, such as manualized CBT, as your first-line approach when treating just about any patient with PTSD. The other school argues that research trials are flawed, that clinical practice patients with PTSD differ from those in research trials, and that manualized treatments such as CBT inappropriately limit your creativity and flexibility. According to this school, CBT may *not* be the best approach for your complicated patients. This perspective may underlie the finding that cognitive-behavioral PTSD treatment methods are underutilized in clinical practice (Becker, Zayfert, & Anderson, 2004; Rosen et al., 2004)

Our aim in this book is to find the common ground between these two schools of thought. Based on both research findings and our own experiences, we contend that CBT is a powerful treatment that can significantly improve the lives of many patients with PTSD who are treated in clinical practice. Yet we also recognize that implementing CBT for PTSD on a daily basis in clinical practice often is daunting. Patients with PTSD frequently present with a complex clinical picture, including significant comorbidity, and manualized treatments such as CBT for PTSD typically target a single disorder. As such, they include limited advice regarding strategies for managing comorbid conditions or other problems. Likewise, cognitive-behavioral formulations of psychopathology often focus on models for understanding specific disorders such as PTSD or panic disorder. Yet if you want to integrate multiple models to better conceptualize complicated patients, you will find limited guidance in the CBT literature.

Our goal is to show how CBT for PTSD can be implemented in a *flexible* manner that addresses the varying needs of your unique and complicated patients. We demonstrate how you can combine various CBT models in a creative, hypothesis-testing manner to conceptualize the individual problems faced by a particular patient. We also offer a variety of troubleshooting suggestions for making CBT work for complicated patients, and recommend some other skill sets that you as a CBT practitioner may find helpful in treating such patients. We hope that this information will help you master the *art* of implementing CBT for PTSD, while staying true to its scientific roots.

This book relies heavily on our experiences implementing CBT for PTSD on a daily basis in a rural medical center anxiety clinic. We treat a civilian population, most of whom have experienced multiple traumatic events, typically including at least one childhood event. Many of our patients face various life problems and must negotiate logistical barriers to treatment such as having to travel a significant distance for therapy. One-third of our patients are unemployed, and half meet criteria for two or more comorbid disorders. Many are referred by medical clinics and have co-occurring health problems, such as migraine headaches, fibromyalgia, or sleep disorders. Our patients also often are unaware that they have PTSD when they are referred, and many are surprised that trauma treatment is indicated. Treatment in this clinic is not supported by research grants, but rather by a mix of third-party payers, including private insurance. Each of us has experience carrying a full-time clinical caseload in this setting. In summary, much of this book is based on our experience implementing CBT for PTSD in a setting that poses typical clinical practice challenges.

We use the term "complicated PTSD" in the book to reflect the array of challenges presented by this clinical population. We deliberately avoid the term "complex PTSD" because it has been used to connote a specific constellation of problems with emotion regulation and interpersonal dysfunction emerging from childhood trauma that is akin to borderline personality disorder. The approach described in this book *can* be applied to many patients with PTSD who have these problems. Yet we do not wish to imply that we are offering a treatment that is explicitly aimed at the deficits conceptualized as "complex PTSD."

This book is ultimately a hands-on guide designed to teach the clinician how to use the case formulation approach espoused by Persons (2005) to administer CBT for PTSD to individual patients on a case-by-case basis. We first review the necessary background needed to assess and treat PTSD from a cognitive-behavioral perspective (Chapters 1–2). We then discuss assessment and the case formulation approach (Chapter 3). The remaining chapters (Chapters 4–10) are largely devoted to the intricacies of weaving the core components of CBT into an individualized treatment using the case formulation approach.

Whether you are new to PTSD treatment or a seasoned clinician, treating PTSD will inevitably present emotional challenges for you as a therapist. First, clinicians implementing CBT for PTSD must be ready to administer an intervention that may produce some temporary exacerbation of discomfort. In the same way that a person with a broken bone knows that, although painful, setting the bone is necessary for proper healing, recovering from trauma inevitably involves accessing unpleasant emotions to learn new ways of coping with reactions to horrific events. Rather than being solely a source of soothing, as a therapist you must simultaneously be resource, coach, and catalyst for acquisition of new skills. Second, a unique challenge of doing CBT for PTSD relative to other anxiety disorders is that it requires the therapist to be immersed, along with the patient, in traumatic stimuli, memories, and thoughts. Compared to other forms of therapy for PTSD, CBT also requires you to explore a level of trauma detail that is somewhat uncommon. In writing this book we have used realistic clinical material, much of which is based on actual patients and their stories. As a result, you may find some of the vignettes in this book unpleasant and graphic. Our aim in this approach is to provide a realistic clinical context for understanding the concepts presented and *also* to help prepare you, the therapist, for hearing this detail in your sessions. In addition, we have sought to demonstrate the full range of problems, and the degree of trauma, that can successfully be treated using CBT for PTSD.

Acknowledgments

We are grateful to many people who have contributed both directly and indirectly to this project. First and foremost, we thank our patients, who not only trusted us with their problems but also influenced our thinking about PTSD and its treatment. Many patients also actively supported the writing of this book by agreeing to have their case material included. We truly appreciate this additional contribution, and their desire to help others who struggle with PTSD.

Several teachers and mentors have profoundly contributed to our professional development, and this project would never have been possible without their guidance over the years. In particular, we are very grateful to Tim Ahles, the late Connie Dancu, Barry Edelstein, Georg Eifert, Edna Foa, Rick Gross, Matt Friedman, Mark Hegel, Lib Hembre, Kevin Larkin, Kim Mueser, Donn Posner, Ray Rosen, Paula Schnurr, Liz Simpson, and Terry Wilson. We also would like to thank several colleagues from the Association for Behavioral and Cognitive Therapies, our professional home, and from the International Society for Traumatic Stress Studies, which has been an influential professional resource. We thank the following for their contributions to our thinking and/or their support and encouragement: Jim Carter, Jason DeViva, Rob Ferguson, Marty Franklin, David Foy, Allison Harvey, Stefan Hofmann, Amy Ikelheimer, Brett Litz, Marsha Linehan, Mike Otto, Irene Powch, Barbara Rothbaum, Joe Scotti, Merv Smucker, Beth Stamm, Gail Steketee, Amy Wagner, Maureen Whittal, and Jerome Yoman. We also are grateful to all of the clinicians who provided both feedback and encouragement at workshops and to our trainees from whom we are always learning. A number of colleagues graciously donated their time to read chapters and provide feedback. We thank Wendy Bayles-Dazet, Jason Goodson, Kristin Oliver, Kay Watt, and Brenda Vale for their insightful comments on the manuscript. We would be remiss in failing to note that this project never would have come about without the support of Series Editor Jackie Persons and Guilford Executive Editor Kitty Moore. We thank them for their patience, their wonderful feedback and editing, and, above all, their endless encouragement. We are very grateful for all of the time and energy they contributed.

Finally, we would like to thank Brent Becker for being a backbone of support during our years of collaboration. We also thank our families and our friends for, quite simply, everything.

Contents

COGNITIVE-BEHAVIORAL THERAPY FOR PTSD

ONE

Cognitive-Behavioral Therapy for PTSD
Overview and Empirical Foundation

Bonnie, a 35-year-old homemaker referred by her doctor, reports loss of interest in her daily activities and feeling "wound up" most of the time. She spends a good portion of each day cleaning and only goes out to shop at night, when the stores are less crowded. During the assessment, Bonnie reports that although she has always been quite anxious, her anxiety became a more serious problem a few years ago, when her oldest daughter turned 12. She notes that between ages 12 and 14 she was sexually abused by her uncle. Currently she suffers from regular nightmares and frequent flashbacks. In addition, she avoids any reminders of her sexual abuse, including family photos, men who remind her of her uncle, and the soap that he used. She also acknowledges "losing time" during the day, although she has learned to hide this from her family. She tried psychotherapy in the past, but always dropped out because she has difficulty trusting anyone other than her husband and daughter. She also had difficulty in therapy because of losing time during therapy sessions, and she has been afraid to share this information because she feared she would be labeled "crazy." Bonnie meets diagnostic criteria for posttraumatic stress disorder (PTSD), generalized anxiety disorder, and major depressive disorder. She also has a history of binge eating and alcohol abuse, although she currently drinks little alcohol and has not had an eating binge for the past year. Bonnie has "had it with feeling so anxious and depressed all of the time" and wants to "feel better" as quickly as possible. Her physician told her that you could help her achieve her goals, and she is willing to give treatment a "real try this time."

The best treatment for patients with multiple problems like Bonnie is one that has as much empirical support as possible. For Bonnie, cognitive-behavioral therapy (CBT) offers the best possibility for resolution of her PTSD and associated difficulties. In this chapter, we lay the groundwork necessary to implement CBT for PTSD. We first provide an overview of CBT in general, then outline the core components of CBT for PTSD. We also provide a summary of the research supporting CBT for PTSD. It is important for you to be informed about the research so that you can answer patients' questions about the evidence and convey the appropriate level of confidence in the interventions. Our review of the research is written with this aim in mind. Finally, we address possible questions about other interventions with some empirical support, such as eye movement desensitization and reprocessing therapy and stress inoculation therapy.

WHAT IS CBT?

CBT is a structured form of psychotherapy resulting from a marriage between behavior modification strategies, which are rooted in behavioral science (or "behavior analysis"), and cognitive therapy, which is linked to cognitive models of psychopathology. The main premise supporting CBT is that emotional problems or disorders such as PTSD result from learned responses and can be altered by new learning. Thus, by teaching patients like Bonnie to change overt behavior and covert thought processes, you can effect changes in their problem emotions and behaviors. Although the specifics of CBT may vary when you implement it with different patients, several defining features remain constant. These include (1) reliance on hypothesis testing, goal setting, and data collection; (2) formation of a collaborative alliance; (3) emphasis on learning new responses to life situations (i.e., skills); (4) focus on concrete and observable goals; and (5) focus on changing current and future reactions.

These common features reflect both the role of empiricism as a foundation underlying CBT and a reliance on the "scientist-practitioner" model. CBT scientists influence practice by formulating specific models, with specific hypotheses, about the etiology and maintenance of particular disorders, and by developing new interventions based on these models. They also test these interventions with groups of individuals. CBT interventions ideally are studied in randomized controlled trials (RCTs), which are considered the gold standard for scientific testing of interventions.

As a CBT practitioner, you will function as a scientist by formulating and testing hypotheses on a case-by-case basis and blending results from research trials with systematic observations of individual clients. This scientific approach to the individual patient has received little attention, however, in treatment development efforts. Thus, few treatments offer specific guidance regarding how to integrate research findings systematically with individual patient information. Instead, this guidance has been provided through supervision, expertise that has not been available to all clinicians. One of our goals in this book is to offer this kind of supervision with respect to CBT for PTSD.

One additional defining feature of CBT is its structure. CBT tends to be more structured than many other forms of therapy. This structure stems from CBT's emphasis on learning new behaviors, which often is best accomplished through goal setting and practicing specific activities. Structure helps both you and your patients proceed through treatment goals logically and consistently, and it is critical to CBT's efficacy. As Linehan (1993a) noted, however, therapy involves a balance between structure and flexibility. An approach that is too rigid may fail to address your patients' present concerns and lead to problems such as increased dropout (Hembree, Foa et al., 2003). Yet an approach that is too flexible may facilitate avoidance of challenging or unpleasant, but necessary, therapy tasks. For example, if Bonnie often comes to sessions distraught about arguments with her daughter, you may be led away from doing what is needed to help Bonnie achieve her treatment goals. In deciding how to respond, you have to weigh Bonnie's desire to discuss the arguments with your knowledge that Bonnie may be afraid of treatment components that are critical to reducing her distressing symptoms in a timely fashion. In summary, implementation of CBT involves balancing structure with appropriate flexibility.

WHAT IS CBT FOR PTSD?

CBT for PTSD aims to modify the behaviors and cognitions that developed in response to trauma and are presumed to maintain PTSD. It emphasizes a collaborative alliance; therefore, it routinely begins with education about the cognitive-behavioral model and an in-depth treatment rationale, so that patients can be educated participants in treatment. Treatment also typically targets avoidance behavior and unrealistic or unhelpful thinking, which according to the CBT model are key factors that maintain PTSD. A number of variants of CBT for PTSD have been developed. Different forms can be labeled by their core components (e.g., cognitive restructuring or exposure), or they may be referred to by specific names such as cognitive processing therapy (Resick & Schnicke, 1993) or prolonged exposure (Foa & Rothbaum, 1998). Yet most forms of CBT for PTSD consist of three core components emphasized to varying degrees: psychoeducation, exposure, and cognitive restructuring. Each holds true to the defining characteristics listed earlier. In this book, we will teach you how to use each of these core components to treat PTSD.

Briefly stated, psychoeducation provides patients with information about the cognitive behavioral formulation of PTSD. It facilitates patients' understanding of the treatment rationale, which is necessary if patients are to make informed therapy decisions. Establishing a shared understanding of PTSD also helps you build a collaborative relationship with your patients. You will rely on the persuasive rationale (discussed in Chapter 5) and collaborative relationship to help patients tolerate the challenging moments in trauma-focused therapy.

Exposure targets avoidance and involves encouraging patients to approach feared stimuli, so that they learn that safe (but feared) stimuli need not be avoided. During exposure, your patients will approach stimuli (1) for prolonged periods of time to bring about an immediate decrease in fear (i.e., within-session habituation) and (2) over repeated trials to promote more enduring fear reduction (i.e., between-session habituation). Exposure can take several forms. During imaginal exposure, patients repeatedly recount trauma memories, whereas during *in vivo* (live) exposure, patients confront specific situations or stimuli in real life. Finally, interoceptive exposure involves experiencing avoided physical sensations. Exposure may involve presenting stimuli in either a graduated or concentrated manner.

Cognitive restructuring teaches trauma survivors to become aware of and modify unhelpful thoughts. Your patients will learn to observe their thoughts, to identify and systematically challenge maladaptive thinking, and to formulate adaptive responses. Cognitive restructuring for PTSD sometimes is organized around specific trauma-related themes, as in cognitive processing therapy (Resick & Schnicke, 1993). It also may be applied to all distressing thoughts that result from traumatic experiences.

SUMMARY OF RESEARCH ON CBT FOR PTSD

Many therapies have been developed to assist trauma survivors. CBT for PTSD, however, has accumulated the most evidence in support of its efficacy not only for treatment of PTSD but also for common co-occurring problems. CBT for PTSD is challenging because you must convince patients to come face-to-face with their trauma memories, something they often have avoided for extended periods of time. Helping patients complete aversive tasks is easier, however, when the research indicates that the task will help. The research offers much evidence to support the rationale for treatment, which should increase your confidence in CBT for PTSD. This evidence also provides patients some reassurance that, despite their fear, treatment is worth trying.

Evidence Supporting CBT for PTSD

Several main conclusions emerge from a careful review of the research on CBT for PTSD.

   1. *For a variety trauma populations, CBT, consisting of some form of exposure and/or cognitive restructuring, appears to be more effective than no treatment or supportive counseling.* These populations include sexual assault survivors (Foa et al., 1999; Foa, Rothbaum, Riggs, & Murdock, 1991; Resick, Nishith, Weaver, Astin, & Feuer, 2002), childhood abuse survivors (Cloitre, Koenen, Cohen, & Han, 2002; McDonagh et al., 2005), motor vehicle accident survivors (Blanchard et al., 2003; Ehlers et al., 2003), veterans (Boudewyns & Hyer, 1990; Cooper & Clum, 1989; Keane, Fairbank, Caddell, & Zimering, 1989), and survivors of various traumatic events (Bryant, Moulds, Guthrie, Dang, & Nixon, 2003). For example, Resick et al. (2002) compared CBT with a strong cognitive restructuring focus (i.e., cognitive processing therapy) to CBT with a strong exposure focus (i.e., prolonged exposure) and to waiting-list control in rape survivors. Both therapies were superior to the waiting list. Approximately 80% of patients who completed either form of CBT no longer met criteria for PTSD, and most showed marked improvement in depression. As a clinician, you also may be interested in a more conservative analysis that includes all the patients randomized to a treatment rather than only those who complete treatment. This gives you an estimate that is more akin to what you can expect when you implement the treatment in clinical practice. In the Resick et al. study, approximately half of the women who began either therapy no longer met diagnostic criteria for PTSD following treatment and at follow-up. In contrast only 2% in the waiting-list group had lost the PTSD diagnosis. Bryant et al. (2003) had similar results in an RCT that compared exposure alone, exposure plus cognitive restructuring, and supportive counseling in civilians with PTSD resulting from various traumatic events. At follow-up, 65–80% of participants who completed either form of CBT were free of PTSD diagnosis, compared to less than 40% of those who completed supportive counseling. Similarly, 50–60% of CBT participants who began treatment were diagnosis-free compared to approximately 20% of those who began supportive counseling.
   2. *There is no clear evidence that any form of CBT is superior to other forms.* For example, although Foa et al. (1999) found that exposure alone was superior to exposure plus

stress management skills training in sexual assault survivors, Bryant et al. (2003) reported finding that imaginal exposure plus cognitive restructuring was superior to imaginal exposure alone. Similarly, whereas Marks et al. (1998) found that exposure (either alone or with cognitive restructuring) was superior to cognitive restructuring alone in a mixed civilian trauma sample, several other investigators found that exposure and cognitive restructuring did not differ in efficacy (Tarrier et al., 1999; Resick et al., 2002; Paunovic & Ost, 2001).

3. *CBT that includes exposure has amassed the greatest amount of empirical support across different trauma populations* (Foa, Rothbaum, & Furr, 2003). For this reason, exposure has been the cornerstone of treatment in our clinic, and it provides the foundation for treatment as described in this book.

In summary, the literature offers convincing support for the efficacy of CBT based on exposure, cognitive restructuring, or both. As a whole, the research suggests that CBT is associated with substantially greater likelihood of ending treatment without a diagnosis of PTSD compared with no treatment or supportive counseling.

Translating Research into Practice: Exposure Alone, in Combination, or Not at All?

Experts currently are divided regarding the relative merits of treatment that emphasizes exposure, cognitive restructuring, or both. Thus, we recommend that clinicians learn both sets of skills and actively consider *both* strategies when formulating a PTSD treatment plan.

Why Should I Consider Both Exposure and Cognitive Restructuring Instead of Exposure Alone?

Exposure is an extremely potent means of altering dysfunctional cognitions, and many patients can be successfully treated using exposure alone. In some cases, however, PTSD is not eliminated by exposure alone. Patients with PTSD also often present with many other problems that can be obstacles to using exposure, such as intense anger or profound shame, and exposure may not be the best intervention for these problems. Thus, you must be prepared to address distress and obstacles in nonresponsive patients. Using an alternative technique with strong empirical support, such as cognitive restructuring, makes sense in such cases.

Another important consideration is research that suggests exposure and cognitive restructuring may differ in their power to address various emotions. For example, exposure may be more effective for modifying anxiety and beliefs about danger, whereas cognitive restructuring may be more effective at modifying guilt and thoughts about responsibility (Resick et al., 2002; Smucker, Grunert, & Weis, 2003). Likewise, cognitive restructuring may be more effective when PTSD is predominantly characterized by shame or anger rather than fear (Smucker et al., 2003). Therefore, you should consider cognitive restructuring in patients who exhibit intense guilt, shame, or anger, or when response to exposure alone is suboptimal.

As noted earlier, research also does not clearly support the efficacy of one variant of CBT for PTSD over another. Thus, we believe that the important clinical question is not *whether* to use exposure or cognitive restructuring, but rather how much of each should be included in the treatment of a given individual, and when each should be presented.

Finally, individual patients vary in their ability to use each method, and it is difficult to predict who will respond to which intervention. Whereas some individuals find cognitive restructuring too complex and confusing, others find it difficult to engage with their emotions during exposure. Thus, having both tools available enhances your ability to treat PTSD effectively. In summary, the "art" of CBT is implementing exposure and cognitive restructuring as suited for individual patients, such as Bonnie, using cognitive-behavioral models of PTSD as a guide.

Is In Vivo Exposure Necessary?

Some clinicians working with trauma survivors focus on imaginal exposure (i.e., exposure to trauma memories) to the exclusion of *in vivo* exposure (i.e., exposure to real-life situations or stimuli). Available data suggest, however, that imaginal exposure combined with *in vivo* exposure generally is more effective than imaginal exposure alone (Devilly & Foa, 2001; Bryant et al., 2003; Tarrier et al., 1999).

Combined exposure may be more effective, because PTSD often involves fears of real-life situations, as well as fears of memories. *In vivo* exposure provides the opportunity for exposure to such situational cues. For example, a survivor of a motor vehicle accident who reduces his distress while recalling the accident during imaginal exposure will nonetheless remain functionally impaired if he continues to avoid riding in a car. In addition, including *in vivo* exposure might also promote durability of fear reduction by broadening the contextual cues under which fear reduction occurs (Bouton & Nelson, 1998). This may be particularly true when imaginal exposure and *in vivo* exposure are combined (e.g., if Bonnie practices imaginal exposure in a bedroom similar to where she was assaulted). Thus, including *in vivo* exposure is likely to promote generalization and durability of fear reduction, as well as the greatest reduction in PTSD symptoms (Foa et al., 2003).

Aren't There Other Forms of CBT with Some Research Support?

Two other forms of CBT also have garnered some empirical support. The first, stress inoculation training (SIT), involves teaching patients various skills for managing stress, such as relaxation, thought stopping, assertive communication, and guided self-dialogue. The rationale is that after practicing these skills in lower stress situations, individuals will be able to deploy them to manage higher levels of stress and anxiety. The second form of CBT with some empirical support is eye movement desensitization and reprocessing therapy (EMDR), which aims to facilitate the processing of traumatic memories by having patients focus on external stimuli, such as a moving visual object (e.g., finger moving back and forth), while they revisit traumatic memories. EMDR also includes some cognitive restructuring. We discuss these forms of CBT separately, because we do not recommend either as a first-line treatment for PTSD.

Why Shouldn't SIT Be My First-Line Treatment Strategy If It Is Supported by Research?

Some anxiety management approaches (e.g., SIT; Meichenbaum, 1985) have some empirical support in the treatment of PTSD (Foa et al., 2003). Despite this, we do not recommend the use of SIT as a first-line strategy for several reasons. First, research suggests that the magnitude of treatment gains for SIT is not as great as that for exposure (e.g., Foa et al., 1999), and SIT does not have the range of studies supporting its efficacy.

Second, the theoretical rationale behind SIT does not readily fit with other CBT techniques (e.g., exposure) or with cognitive-behavioral models of PTSD (see Chapter 2), which emphasize the role of avoidance in maintaining PTSD (Foa, Steketee, & Rothbaum, 1989; Keane & Barlow, 2002). For example, thought stopping is a SIT technique in which patients distract themselves from distressing thoughts by mentally shouting "Stop." By discouraging engagement with distressing thoughts and emotions, SIT techniques, such as thought stopping and relaxation conflict with exposure instructions to engage with traumatic memories. Thus, although SIT has demonstrated efficacy for learning to manage daily life stressors, it does not appear as suitable and conceptually sound a method as exposure or cognitive restructuring for resolving traumatic stress.

Third, SIT is a more cumbersome treatment than either exposure or cognitive restructuring. For example, the SIT protocol evaluated in research (Foa et al., 1991, 1999) consists of nine sessions in which patients are taught a wide variety of different skills. In contrast, patients completing exposure only have to learn one primary skill, and patients completing exposure plus cognitive restructuring only have to learn two skills. There seems little reason to use a more complicated treatment when a more simple treatment will suffice.

Some SIT strategies, however, may be very appropriate for associated problems that accompany PTSD, and we frequently use such strategies when they are helpful. For example, we regularly use assertive communication training when patients have profound difficulties communicating their needs to others. We also use breathing retraining as a relaxation technique in patients with PTSD who present with extreme arousal symptoms.

What about EMDR?

We do not include EMDR (Shapiro, 1995) in our treatment, because it has less empirical support and appears to be less effective compared to CBT (Devilly & Spence, 1999). For example, in an RCT comparing CBT to EMDR, only 25% of those who began EMDR lost their PTSD diagnosis, in contrast to over 60% of patients who began CBT (Devilly & Spence, 1999). Studies that contradicted the Devilly and Spence study (i.e., Ironson, Freud, Strauss, & Williams, 2002; Lee, Gavriel, Drummond, Richards, & Greenwald, 2002) suffered from methodological problems. In a study with improved methodology, Taylor et al. (2003) found that patients who completed CBT reported a greater reduction in reexperiencing symptoms and avoidance than patients who completed EMDR, although those who started EMDR were as likely to be free of the PTSD diagnosis. In summary, the research support for EMDR is less robust than that for straightforward CBT.

Some researchers also have suggested that EMDR may make exposure and memory processing more tolerable to patients. Research, however, has not supported this conclusion (Devilly & Spence, 1999). Furthermore, no data support inclusion of eye movements as a critical therapy ingredient to achieve anxiety reduction (Chemtob, Tolin, van der Kolk, & Pitman, 2000; Hembree, Cahill, & Foa, 2003; Hembree & Foa, 2003).

Thus, although some clinicians report finding EMDR very useful, given the lack of evidence for the superiority of EMDR over CBT, we believe EMDR should be used only when standard CBT fails and/or when there are good reasons to think that the patient might find EMDR more useful. When patients request EMDR, we review with them the relevant research to facilitate their decision making about which treatment they wish to receive. If, after this discussion, a patient decides that he or she would prefer EMDR, we refer the patient to an appropriately trained provider.

CONCLUSION

The last 20 years have seen significant advances in treatments for PTSD, and by far the most efficacious intervention among new developments is CBT. As a result, a disorder that for many would have been a chronic condition, with very poor long-term psychosocial outcome, often can now be significantly altered within a few months time. Familiarity with the compelling evidence that CBT for PTSD can produce improvements in PTSD, however, will help you implement CBT with your patients on a case-by-case basis.

TWO

Cognitive-Behavioral Conceptualization of PTSD

This chapter provides an overview of the cognitive-behavioral conceptualization of PTSD. We start by briefly discussing why it is important to understand cognitive-behavioral principles when conducting CBT. We then review the critical components of the cognitive-behavioral conceptualization of PTSD, and briefly discuss why the models point to exposure and cognitive restructuring as key techniques in PTSD treatment.

RATIONALE FOR LEARNING TO "THINK" COGNITIVE-BEHAVIORALLY

When you set out to learn CBT, you may have envisioned that you would learn a set of procedures to follow in a cookbook-like fashion. Indeed, if you are like many clinicians, this expectation may have dampened your interest in CBT. Being an effective CBT therapist, however, requires much more than following a "cookbook." In fact, straightforward CBT may be likened to making a cheesecake. Even this uncomplicated dessert requires knowledge not explicitly described in the steps of the recipe. For example, if you do not know what "just set" means, you will not know when to stop baking the cake. As anyone who cannot cook will tell you, cooking, even with well-tested recipes, is an art.

More often, however, CBT is akin to cooking for a dinner party when you are informed that several attendees are vegetarian, others keep kosher, and still others do not eat dairy. Suddenly, your recipes need modification, and you have to improvise a meal that will suit everyone. Meeting diverse needs in one meal will require you to cook according to principles. For example, you may need to replace particular ingredients in certain recipes. It would be impossible to do this effectively if you did not have an understanding of the overarching principles of cooking. Similarly, although many patients respond to skilled application of relatively rote treatment procedures (equivalent to a skilled cook working with a solid recipe), other patients may require you to modify the treatment based on the overarching *principles* of CBT. Your ability to think like a

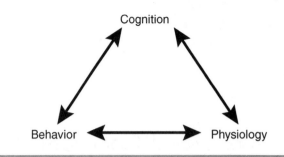

FIGURE 2.1. Cognition–physiology–behavior triangle.

cognitive-behaviorist will determine your ability to respond flexibly to the varying needs of your clientele. Thus, we encourage you to adopt the entire cognitive-behavioral approach, including the theoretical models upon which the techniques are built, rather than just borrowing cognitive-behavioral techniques. This chapter will help you understand cognitive-behavioral principles that underlie CBT for PTSD.

CONCEPTUALIZATION OF PTSD

Shared Basic Assumptions

Cognitive-behavioral models rest on several shared assumptions. First, models typically view PTSD as an anxiety disorder that is associated with nonanxiety symptoms.[1] According to such models, anxiety and fear consist of cognitive (e.g., fearful thoughts), behavioral (e.g., avoidance behaviors), and physiological features (e.g., autonomic arousal; see Figure 2.1). Each factor influences the others. For example, Susan is afraid of heights. When she starts to climb a ladder to change a light bulb in a chandelier hanging from a vaulted ceiling, she experiences fearful thoughts (e.g., "Climbing this ladder is dangerous; I could fall and break my neck"), physiological arousal (e.g., pounding heart, rapid breathing, trembling), and avoidance behaviors (e.g., getting off the ladder after climbing only two rungs and asking someone else to do the task for her). Thus, changing fearful thoughts about a situation (e.g., "I've seen Karen do this a million times without any problems; the ladder is strong and very stable; I can do this even though I feel anxious") may decrease avoidance and arousal. Similarly, by approaching instead of avoiding a feared situation or object, the individual's perception of the danger may diminish (e.g., after successfully climbing the ladder, Susan concludes that climbing the ladder was safer than she originally thought).

Second, cognitive-behavioral models assume that mechanisms involved in the development of adaptive fear also operate in the development of maladaptive fear. For example, it is widely recognized that humans are born fearing only a few situations (e.g., loud noises and falling; O'Leary & Wilson, 1987). CBT practitioners assume that all remaining fears, both adaptive and maladaptive, are learned. The adaptive function

---

[1]Although the terms "anxiety" and "fear" can sometimes be used interchangeably, "anxiety" refers to a state of apprehension or anticipation of a future negative event, whereas "fear" typically denotes the "fight–flight" response to a specific stimulus.

of anxiety is to encourage us to avoid (and escape from) objectively dangerous situations. For example, anxiety keeps us from going swimming with crocodiles and signals us to get out of the water when we notice a crocodile. Anxiety about situations that are not objectively dangerous (e.g., avoidance of swimming in a pool) can be learned, and therefore unlearned, by similar processes.

Behavioral and Conditioning Factors

Mowrer's (1947) behavioral two-factor conceptualization of anxiety is the foundation of the CBT conceptualization of PTSD presented here. Mowrer proposed that two types of learning, "classical" and "operant" conditioning, are involved in development of fears. He suggested that anxiety initially develops via classical conditioning, when a neutral stimulus is paired with a fear-producing stimulus. This is akin to the experience of Pavlov's dogs learning to salivate in response to a tone after it was repeatedly paired with food. Similarly, a neutral stimulus, such as a baseball bat, often after only one such pairing with a fear-producing situation, such as being beaten with a bat while being mugged, can evoke fear.

Rules of classical conditioning suggest that conditioned fear reactions should dissipate over time ("extinguish") if the feared object is not truly dangerous—much like Pavlov's dogs no longer salivating when they repeatedly experience the tone without being fed. The fact that many "irrational" fears of objects or situations that are not dangerous persist, however, suggested to Mowrer that something else must account for the maintenance of fears. Mowrer reasoned that a second factor, operant conditioning, might be responsible for the perpetuation of fear. "Operant conditioning" is learning that is based on the result that follows a behavior. Behavior that produces a favorable result (i.e., is "reinforced") tends to recur and increase in frequency, whereas behavior that produces an undesirable result (i.e., is "punished") tends not to be repeated. Mowrer reasoned that escape behavior is reinforced by a rapid decrease in fear when a person moves away from the feared object or situation; thus, it tends to recur and increase in frequency. He also proposed that fear is maintained over time because escape and avoidance behavior persist and prevent extinction. In summary, fear is initially learned via classical conditioning and maintained by operant conditioning.

For example, James developed a pronounced fear of large dogs after being bitten by a Labrador retriever. After the attack, James discovered that his anxiety rapidly diminished when he escaped because the dog's owner took it away, or because he himself left the situation. As a result, his escape behavior was reinforced and therefore increased. He started by crossing the street whenever he saw a dog coming toward him and eventually limited his activity outside his home to avoid any possible contact with dogs. According to Mowrer, escape and avoidance behaviors, by limiting the time James spent with dogs without being harmed, prevented James's anxiety from diminishing naturally. Thus, James failed to learn that his anxiety was unnecessary around most dogs, because the presence of a dog does not reliably predict being bitten.

Mowrer's theory is directly applicable to patients with PTSD, who after experiencing a traumatic event, typically avoid objects or situations closely associated with the event, and report (like James) extreme anxiety if forced into contact with such situations or objects. In addition, many trauma survivors attempt to block trauma memories, which may produce an effect similar to that of behavioral avoidance of real-life stimuli (Keane, Fairbank, Caddell, Zimering, & Bender, 1985). In other words, trauma survivors may fail to extinguish conditioned fears because they avoid trauma reminders both behaviorally and cognitively. For example, Sandra, who was beaten with a baseball bat during a mugging, coped with the fear evoked by bats and her memories of the mugging by giving up softball (i.e., avoiding bats) and avoiding thoughts about the mugging. Thus, she failed to learn that neither bats nor her traumatic memory could hurt her.

One noteworthy feature of PTSD in comparison to other anxiety disorders, such as specific phobia, is the wide range of fears that trauma survivors develop. Two fundamental principles of conditioning, higher-order conditioning and stimulus generalization, may account for the wide range of feared stimuli (Keane et al., 1985). Higher-order conditioning occurs when a previously neutral stimulus triggers a conditioned response by being paired with a conditioned stimulus; for example, James began to fear streets in the neighborhood where he encountered large dogs, and Sandra began to fear softball games. Neither the streets nor the softball games were ever paired with their assaults (the unconditioned stimuli), but both were associated with conditioned stimuli (dogs and bats). Stimulus generalization occurs when the individual responds to stimuli that resemble the conditioned stimulus; for example, James began to fear small dogs, and Sandra began to fear field hockey sticks. It is easy to see how higher-order conditioning and stimulus generalization rapidly expand the array of feared stimuli and lead to fears that "don't make sense."

Studies have shown that Mowrer's original theory suffers from several problems. In particular, it is clear that pathological anxiety can develop without classical conditioning. For example, fears can be acquired via information (e.g., you read about barracudas shortly before your Caribbean vacation and then fear swimming in the ocean) or vicariously (e.g., you observe your friend get stung by a dangerous jellyfish and come to fear ocean swimming; Rachman, 1977). Moreover, Mowrer's original theory does not easily account for nonanxiety symptoms associated with PTSD, such as shame.

Nonetheless, conditioning models explain many core features of PTSD, such as the wide range of stimuli that trigger traumatic memories, and the physiological and emotional arousal generated by these stimuli (Brewin & Holmes, 2003), and the model makes sense to patients. For example, Elizabeth, who had been repeatedly raped by her mother's boyfriend, reported experiencing a panic attack whenever she saw a wall clock. A clock hung over the bed in which she was raped and Elizabeth always stared at it while waiting for the rape to end. Using Mowrer's two-factor theory, we can hypothesize that Elizabeth's fear of wall clocks did not extinguish after the rapes stopped, because she avoided the room with the wall clock and averted her gaze whenever she encountered a wall clock. Elizabeth reported feeling "crazy," because she did not understand *why* something harmless that was associated with her rape would produce fear. The two-factor conceptualization helped her understand why and how she had come to fear wall clocks. She then reported that she no longer felt quite so crazy, because the model made sense and pointed to specific solutions.

One disadvantage is that the two-factor model does not account for individual factors, such as childhood experiences that predate the traumatic experience and may influence whether a trauma survivor develops PTSD. Addressing this weakness, Keane and Barlow (2002) developed a more detailed learning model of the etiology of PTSD. Figure 2.2 is a graphical depiction of the model.

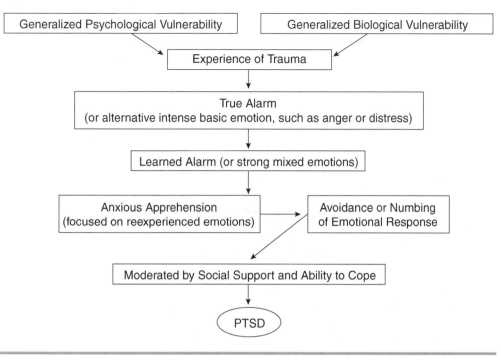

FIGURE 2.2. Keane and Barlow's (2002) model of the etiology of PTSD. From Keane and Barlow (2002, p. 429). Copyright 2002 by The Guilford Press. Reprinted by permission.

As illustrated at the top of the model, Keane and Barlow (2002) argue that both genetic and psychological factors can predispose an individual to develop PTSD after a traumatic event. "Generalized biological vulnerability" refers to a person's genetically based predisposition to develop any psychopathology after a traumatic event, *if* his or her early environment did not permit prediction or control of reinforcement and punishment (Barlow, 2002). Such early life experiences represent a generalized psychological vulnerability. Other factors, such as the nature of the trauma and repeated traumatic experiences, also can increase risk of developing PTSD by increasing the individual's generalized psychological vulnerability (Keane & Barlow, 2002).

Moving down the model, we see that during the actual traumatic event, the trauma survivor experiences a "true alarm," which has an evolutionary basis (Barlow, 2002). Our ancestors undoubtedly experienced true alarms when faced with dangerous animals (e.g., lions, wolves, snakes) or people and natural hazards. True alarms are fear reactions to actual dangerous situations. The adaptive function of a true alarm is to promote survival by activating a rapid response to physical threat. Much as firefighters fly into action in response to an alarm that alerts them about a real fire, true alarms mobilize our physical and cognitive resources to respond to threatening situations. Although most of us will not encounter dangerous animals such as lions, in today's world, true alarms can be activated in response to modern threats posed by explosions, car accidents, natural disasters, and dangerous people.

The mobilization of resources during a true alarm is usually referred to as the "fight–flight" response, although a more accurate name might be the "flight–fight–

freeze" response (Beck, Emery, & Greenberg, 1985). Our natural reaction to dangerous situations is to flee if possible. If we cannot flee, we tend to fight back. If both options are ruled out (as is often the case in sexual assaults and many other types of trauma), we fall back on an alternate response, which is to freeze—like a deer freezing in the woods so as not to be seen by a predator.

The physiological responses associated with the fight–flight system are numerous, well documented, and commonly observed in individuals with anxiety disorders. Heart rate increases and blood is redirected from hands and feet to major muscle groups to facilitate fleeing and fighting. In addition, peripheral areas of the body, which are most likely to be injured, will be less likely to bleed excessively if cut. A secondary result is that these parts of the body may appear pale and cold. Breathing also deepens and becomes more rapid to increase oxygen intake, which is needed for sudden bursts of activity. As we commonly note to patients, when faced with a snarling lion, one cannot typically ask for a 5-minute warmup period. Thus, the sympathetic branch of the autonomic nervous system, which is largely responsible for the fight–flight response, is "hard-wired" to enable instantaneous preparation for intense physical exertion. When the brain detects threat, it directs the body to release adrenaline, which immediately produces involuntary changes in physical functions that enable short-term survival activities. Many of the sensations reported by individuals experiencing a fight–flight response, such as dry mouth and queasiness, occur because long-term survival needs, such as digestion of food, are put on hold. Other symptoms, such as dizziness, are thought to be secondary effects caused by a lack of physical exertion. In other words, because there is no lion, the individual does not fight or flee. This produces a cascade of secondary effects (e.g., overoxygenated blood results in constriction of blood vessels in the brain) that result in additional symptoms (e.g., feeling lightheaded).

Keane and Barlow (2002) suggest that during the traumatic event, individuals associate a variety of stimuli (e.g., as in Elizabeth's case, the wall clock) with the experience of a "true alarm" and as result develop learned alarms via classical conditioning. Learned alarms are subsequently triggered by situations that resemble or contain features of the traumatic experience. They may also be triggered by situations that symbolize the event, such as anniversaries. Learned alarms produce the same response as a true alarm, but differ because of the absence of objective danger. A learned alarm is equivalent to a false fire alarm. Firefighters still fly into action, but there is no fire to fight. During the initial weeks after a traumatic event, it is common for most people to experience recurring distress in reaction to reminders of the event and to relive the event in memories, dreams, and flashbacks (North, Smith, McCool, & Lightcap, 1989; Riggs, Rothbaum, & Foa, 1995; Rothbaum, Foa, Riggs, Murdock, & Walsh, 1992). These early posttrauma learned alarms, however, usually fade over time.

Because traumatic events, in addition to fear, can also evoke intense emotions such as shame and guilt, these emotions may also be elicited by the same stimuli that produce learned alarms (Keane & Barlow, 2002). For example, Elizabeth reported that feelings of shame usually accompanied fear when she was exposed to wall clocks. In some cases, these emotions may be the predominant learned experience when individuals encounter stimuli that remind them of the traumatic event.[2] Regardless, because all of these emotional states (i.e., fear, anger, guilt, sadness, and shame) are unpleasant, survi-

---

[2]Often referred to as trauma "triggers" or "cues."

vors develop anxiety (i.e., "anxious apprehension") about encountering triggers and the emotional responses associated with them. This anxiety motivates trauma survivors to avoid trauma-related stimuli, and they may also seek to avoid their emotions altogether via emotional numbing.

Interestingly, Keane and Barlow (2002) argue that development of PTSD is not yet a *fait accompli*. Rather, whether the initial learned alarms become a persistent problem and snowball into full-blown PTSD depends on the trauma survivor's coping style and resources, and the accessibility of social support. For example, after returning from Afghanistan, Paul realized that no one wanted to hear about the horrible things he witnessed during combat. Rather, they wanted him to "just put it behind him." Thus, he adopted a coping strategy of avoiding thoughts about Afghanistan and situations that reminded him of combat; this coping strategy increased his risk for PTSD. What began as learned alarms snowballed via stimulus generalization and higher-order conditioning into more generalized fears and intensified efforts to avoid unpleasant emotions. In contrast, Steve, also a veteran, coped by turning to his support network, talking about what happened (even though he also had urges to avoid), and exposing himself to situations that reminded him of his combat experiences. Thus, he was less likely to develop PTSD.

All models of PTSD, including that of Keane and Barlow, point to avoidance as a critical factor in the development and maintenance of the disorder. Thus, trauma survivors who are exposed to triggers of learned alarms soon after the event are less likely to experience persistent distress (Wirtz & Harrell, 1987), which explains why distress dissipates for the majority of trauma survivors. Likewise, people whose posttrauma reactions have persisted over time can extinguish their conditioned responses by systematically exposing themselves to trauma triggers. This is one of the mechanisms of action presumed to underlie exposure. Considerable research supports both of these suppositions (Keane & Barlow, 2002), and conditioning models are very helpful in understanding many aspects of PTSD, particularly those related to anxiety. Yet they do not fully explain nonanxiety symptoms.

Cognitive Factors

Multiple cognitive models have been developed (Chemtob, Roitblat, Hamada, Carlson, & Twentyman, 1988; Ehlers & Clark, 2000; Foa et al., 1989; Resick & Schnicke, 1992). Cognitive models share a number of features, including a focus on the need to "process" or make sense of traumatic events as a part of adaptive coping, and an assumption that PTSD results from a *failure* to organize traumatic experiences successfully. Although there are differences between the models, all generally point to the need to reduce avoidance behaviors in a systematic manner and to process traumatic events so that they may be understood in an accurate and realistic way.

Cognitive Processing of Traumatic Events

Our brains like things to "make sense," to fit together in logically coherent ways. Therefore, after experiencing a trauma, it is natural to want to think things through—to organize and understand what happened. Consider, for example, how your mind works after you watch a movie with a twisting plot in which the loose ends come together in the final minutes of the film. As you leave the theater, you may find yourself reviewing the entire story from start to finish to make sense of the details in light of the new information. If there is incompatible or missing information, you may continue for the rest of the evening to review it, trying to fit all the pieces together. You may even dream about it that night.

The inclination to process our personal experiences is even stronger for emotionally charged ones than for less personally relevant ones, such as a movie. For example, imagine having been in a serious car accident. No one died, but several cars were wrecked. When you arrived home to family or friends, what would you do? Most people say "I would tell them what happened." Would you tell one person or many people? Would you simply say, "I was in a car accident," and leave it at that? Or would you describe the event in greater detail? For an event such as this, most people respond that they would tell several people what had happened in great detail. Clinically, this is often referred to as "telling the story" or "making sense of the story." Thus, clinical observation supports what has been tested by research: People seem to have an inclination to discuss difficult events, and discussing these events helps us to understand or "process" them. Studies of how people cope immediately after traumatic events also indicate that people who mentally disconnect from events and inhibit their emotional reactions tend to be at greater risk for developing PTSD (Ozer, Best, Lipsey, & Weiss, 2003).

A variety of factors can interfere with adequate processing of a traumatic experience. For example, the extreme nature of some traumatic events can disrupt memory and attention, and thereby impede processing of the event (Foa & Rothbaum, 1998; Foa et al., 1989). For example, during a mugging at gunpoint, Susan was only vaguely aware of what was happening to her boyfriend, because she was unable to pull her attention away from the gun pointed at her. Thus, she had difficulty making sense of the entire mugging event, which involved her boyfriend being extensively beaten. In our experience, this type of difficulty may be particularly true for childhood abuse survivors, possibly because children do not have fully developed cognitive abilities.

In addition, because traumatic events are typically characterized by a lack of predictability and control, individuals who hold beliefs about the importance of being able to predict and control events in their lives face an inherently challenging cognitive task when the traumatic event strongly contradicts these beliefs. For example, Evelyn believed that "everyone makes choices and is in control of what happens to them" and that "when bad things happen to you, it is because you made bad choices." As a result, she experienced significant shame about being raped by a stranger and blamed herself, even though there was little evidence that she could have prevented the event. Evelyn had difficulty reconciling her prior beliefs and evidence that the rape was not her fault.

When initial processing of the event is incomplete, disorganized, or inaccurate, a variety of strategies, such as exposure and cognitive restructuring, may be used to promote "reprocessing" of the event. "Reprocessing" simply refers to a meaningful reexamination and reorganization of the event aimed at promoting more successful, accurate, and realistic understanding. Most forms of trauma-focused treatment involve the patient communicating, at some point, the details of the traumatic event to the therapist and potentially others (e.g., group therapy members). The importance of reprocessing traumatic events has been recognized by various schools of therapy; trauma-focused treatment is not the exclusive domain of CBT. Nonetheless, for some clinicians, encouraging patients to revisit highly distressing events, such as rape, torture, and witnessing death, seems counterintuitive, particularly for highly distressed patients who may seem too fragile or lack coping skills. This, in general, has been the rationale for staged treatment of PTSD. Although some patients need to develop a base of skills before proceeding with exposure (see Chapter 9), it is important to note that many patients who appear fragile can tolerate and substantially benefit from processing their traumatic experiences.

Incomplete Processing and the Development of PTSD Pathological Fear

Cognitive models suggest that pathological fear develops when, as a result of a traumatic event(s), an individual (1) begins to label incorrectly benign stimuli as dangerous due to mistaken associations and interpretations, then (2) fails to learn corrective information. Thus, Elizabeth labeled the clock as dangerous and failed (because she avoided clocks when she encountered them) to learn that it was not. According to cognitive models, trauma-related information is organized in the mind of the trauma survivor in a "fear network" (Foa & Kozak, 1986; Foa et al., 1989; Lang, Levin, Miller, & Kozak, 1983). Fear networks link specific details regarding the event (including stimuli and memories), responses to the event (e.g., behaviors, thoughts, and sensations), and meanings/interpretations of the event. Fear networks can be thought of as programs we use to promote survival when faced with life-threatening danger.

When fear networks incorrectly link stimuli or contain flawed assumptions, the individual fears safe situations and objects. For example, cognitive models suggest that when encoding and storing the experience of being raped, Elizabeth associated wall clocks with danger. Thus, wall clocks activate her fear network, which contains the emotional experience of fear (including heightened arousal) and memories of the rape, as well as interpretations of the world (e.g., "All men are dangerous"). Elizabeth also experiences the urge to avoid both memories and the actual stimuli (wall clocks). In addition, because associations formed during dangerous situations are particularly strong, wall clocks now activate the fear network rather than previous, positive experiences with wall clocks. Yet wall clocks are not in themselves dangerous, nor are they accurate signals of danger.

Maladaptive conclusions (e.g., that wall clocks predict danger) result when trauma survivors trauma survivors interrupt processing before they incorporate corrective information that would allow them to draw more helpful conclusions. Two conditions are necessary to complete processing and reduce unhelpful fears (Foa et al., 1989). First, the fear network must be activated; that is, the individual must experience fear elicited by trauma cues and memories. Second, corrective information must be available at the same time to promote new learning. For example, Elizabeth avoided her fear by avoiding wall clocks and other danger cues associated with the rape, which prevented her from drawing more accurate conclusions about them. To reduce her fear of wall clocks, Elizabeth must experience the fear triggered by seeing a wall clock, *and* she must realize that she is safe—even though she is looking at a wall clock and feeling fear. Avoidance behaviors interfere with both activating the fear network and integrating corrective information about safety. In summary, Elizabeth's fear of wall clocks would diminish were she to conclude that wall clocks do not always signal danger.

GUILT, SHAME, AND ANGER

Nonanxiety-related emotions such as anger, guilt, and shame play a prominent role in many cases of PTSD. In some cases, nonanxiety emotions such as shame and anger, along with related beliefs, influence the degree to which trauma survivors are willing or able to process the event either through verbal disclosure or by mental review. For example, many people in our society are uncomfortable with the topic of rape, making it difficult for many rape survivors to talk about their experiences. In addition, survivors often want to protect family and friends from the details of their experiences. For example, Adele reported that after being raped, she did not tell her family what had happened, because she did not want them to realize that she was now "damaged." She also noted that when she finally told her best friend, she left out most of the details: "What was I going to say? You don't talk about the blow-by-blow details of being raped. You just don't."

Negative reactions from others also can exacerbate the shame of trauma. For example, veterans of the Vietnam War often perceived themselves as unwelcome by their fellow Americans, and feeling shame upon homecoming from Vietnam was associated with greater risk for PTSD among such veterans (Johnson et al., 1997). Similarly, disbelief, disapproval, or other negative reactions to disclosure of sexual assault or abuse have been associated with greater posttraumatic symptoms (Everill & Waller, 1995; Ullman, 1996). Shame the survivor experiences when the social environment is unsupportive of his or her disclosure can lead to increased avoidance of thinking about the event, which thus disrupts processing. Thus, negative emotional reactions can play a central role in maintaining PTSD and be the cause of substantial suffering in their own right. Therefore, they warrant attention in treatment. Many patients benefit from interventions specifically directed at reducing these emotions, particularly when they are not reduced by exposure (Resick et al., 2002; Smucker et al., 2003).

THE ROLE OF PREEXISTING BELIEFS

Cognitive models typically assume that individuals who experience traumatic events hold preexisting beliefs that are challenged by the event (Brewin, Dalgleish, & Joseph, 1996). Thus, after the traumatic event, individuals must resolve conflicts between what they believed about the world and themselves prior to the event and what the traumatic experience tells them. For example, Elizabeth believed that she was generally safe in the world as long as she took certain precautions that she could control. Being assaulted in her home, an environment that she assumed was safe, provided experiential evidence that refuted her belief that she was "safe unless proven otherwise." According to Resick and Schnicke (1992) there are three main cognitive solutions to this conflict. First, Elizabeth may alter her interpretation of the experience to fit with her belief system (e.g., "I made him want to rape me by wearing sexy clothes, because I thought he was good looking; women don't get randomly raped in their own house by friends" or "It wasn't really a rape, because I liked him and let him do it"). Second, Elizabeth might radically alter her belief system in a maladaptive way (e.g., "No place is safe anymore; I will never be safe"). Third, she might alter, or accommodate, her belief system in a more moderate, productive manner ("Although I liked him, I didn't ask him to rape me. Some men are dangerous, but many are not. I am still mostly safe as long as I am reasonably careful"). PTSD is associated with the first two cognitive solutions.

In Elizabeth's case, the new evidence led her to conclude that "no place is safe." Because it is extremely important for our survival to avoid danger, we, like Elizabeth, may be prone to err on the side of safety and assume danger even where none exists. Resick and Schnicke (1992) refer to conclusions such as "no place is safe" as "stuck points." Stuck points are trauma-related thoughts that contribute to negative posttraumatic reactions. In addition to focusing on danger, stuck points may focus on issues such as lack of trust, guilt, or other negative emotional reactions. Stuck points are often associated with reconciling previous beliefs and the traumatic event. As in Elizabeth's case they also may arise as a result of blaming comments by people she expected to be supportive (e.g., "Why did you tempt him by dressing provocatively?"), or because she is so avoidant that she refuses to think about anything unpleasant, and, therefore, cannot make sense of what happened to her. Finally, if Elizabeth has no relevant beliefs to help her make sense of the rape (e.g., if the traumatic event happened early in life), she may lack the tools to understand the event at all.

SECONDARY REACTIONS, AVOIDANCE, AND INCOMPLETE PROCESSING

Avoidance may be motivated by emotional reactions (e.g., fear and shame) to the reexperiencing symptoms themselves (Ehlers & Steil, 1995), and these secondary reactions can play a prominent role in driving the avoidance that maintains the disorder. For example, Betsy was assaulted at knifepoint in the parking lot of her workplace. After the assault, she found that she was flooded with memories of the assault when she anticipated going to the parking garage at the end of her workday. These memories often seemed so real that she felt compelled to check her office to make sure no one was there. Betsy began to fear these memories, because they disrupted her ability to work, and she did not want to lose her job. Thus, she struggled to suppress the memories. Yet the harder she tried to focus, the less control she seemed to have, and coworkers noticed her "acting weird." Betsy worried that she was "going crazy," because she could not dismiss her memories and was having "paranoid" thoughts. In summary, her emotional reaction (fear) to the intrusive memories (rather than her reaction to the assault itself) was her greatest source of distress and led to increased efforts to avoid the memories.

Such secondary emotional reactions also can involve feelings of shame (e.g., "The fact that I can't get over it means I'm weak"), hopelessness (e.g., "The fact that I'm still having these intrusive thoughts after all this time means I'm a failure") or anger (e.g., "It's not fair that I'm still suffering from what he did to me and he's just going about his life as if nothing happened"). By motivating further avoidance of processing the trauma, secondary emotional reactions themselves can not only play a significant role in maintaining PTSD but also cause substantial suffering.

EXPOSURE AND COGNITIVE RESTRUCTURING

Both conditioning and cognitive models point to the need to reduce avoidance behaviors, and this reduction in avoidance is presumed to underlie the efficacy of both exposure and cognitive restructuring. We discuss the presumed mechanisms of action for exposure in greater detail in Chapter 6. Briefly, however, during exposure, patients learn that trauma-related stimuli and memories are in fact not objectively dangerous in the present. Thus, patients learn to better discriminate between cues that reliably predict danger and cues that predict safety. According to cognitive models, exposure also facilitates reprocessing, which can lead to more accurate conclusions about the meaning of the event, thereby reducing a broad range of negative emotions associated with PTSD.

Cognitive restructuring also reduces avoidance by requiring patients to carefully examine trauma-related thoughts, and to review the event so as to gather evidence for and against specific conclusions. In addition, cognitive restructuring teaches patients to systematically explore their thinking, with the goal of helping them to understand (i.e., "process") the traumatic event better. Finally, cognitive restructuring helps patients become aware of and challenge stuck points.

CONCLUSION

In this chapter we have described a cognitive-behavioral conceptualization of PTSD and its treatment. This conceptualization was derived by distilling clinically relevant features of various cognitive-behavioral models (e.g., Brewin et al., 1996; Keane & Barlow, 2002; Mowrer, 1947; Foa et al., 1989; Resick & Schnicke, 1992); because different cognitive-behavioral models focus on different aspects of the disorder, we rely on several models to conceptualize our approach to treatment. The cognitive-behavioral conceptualization of PTSD directly points to specific treatment strategies; thus, relying on this model will help you implement CBT in a manner tailored for individual patients.

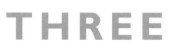

THREE

Assessment, Case Conceptualization, and Treatment Planning

Sophie, a 50-year-old African American woman living with her third husband, was referred by a therapist who was leaving the area. Her departure was a convenient point to transition Sophie toward PTSD treatment, a move she had been reluctant to make because of difficulties "trusting someone new." Her primary complaints were reluctance to travel far from home, paranoia, irritability, mood swings, and loneliness. Although she met criteria for PTSD due to physical abuse by her first husband and other, unspecified events in childhood, she declined to disclose these events, because she did not trust her new therapist. Instead she made vague allusions to "things that happened that I can't tell anyone." Sophie also met criteria for social phobia and borderline personality disorder. She reported passive suicidal ideation but had no history of suicidal behavior. Sophie admitted in the first session that she did not "have any idea what PTSD is." She also did not think the label applied to her, or that PTSD treatment would help her. Although she was unhappy with her emotional reactivity, she only agreed to the appointment because the previous therapist, whom she had come to trust after several months, had recommended it, and she knew she needed help.

Morgan, a 29-year-old single woman residing with a female roommate, initially sought treatment for an eating disorder. Morgan significantly restricted her food intake, vomited on average four to eight times per day, and binge ate two to three times per week. Her eating disorder symptoms began at age 14, after a family friend commented that she had "plumped up." Morgan's reported history of traumatic events included being raped at age 16 and having a coworker die in the World Trade Center collapse. She met criteria for bulimia nervosa, generalized anxiety disorder, and depression at intake, and she had some symptoms of PTSD, including pronounced avoidance symptoms related to both traumatic events.

One of the most difficult aspects of treating PTSD is the complexity of clinical presentations that frequently accompanies this disorder. As a result, it can be particularly challenging to tailor structured cognitive-behavioral treatments for PTSD to the needs of individual patients with PTSD. Such adaptation requires comprehensive assessment of patients' problems and a system for integrating individual patient information with CBT models of PTSD and co-occurring disorders.

In Chapter 2 we provided an overview of the cognitive-behavioral formulation of PTSD, which represents the "nomothetic" (i.e., general) formulation that underlies the CBT approach. In this chapter we show you how to use the case formulation approach (Persons, 2005) to select and tailor interventions to fit the individual needs of your patients. We discuss how to conduct a comprehensive assessment of patients with PTSD, then illustrate how to integrate the idiographic (i.e., individualized) analysis of your patients' problems with evidenced-based nomothetic formulations. We use Sophie and Morgan to demonstrate the case formulation approach. Both cases present with multiple problems, yet they challenge the therapist in different ways. In Sophie's case, the therapist integrated comorbid anxiety and Axis II symptoms into a case conceptualization that centers around PTSD. Morgan's case illustrates how to approach treatment with a patient who presents with another disorder as the primary concern, though you suspect that PTSD may underlie the presenting problem.

ASSESSMENT OF PTSD

Comprehensive treatment of PTSD requires thorough and ongoing assessment. Assessment organizes patients' stories, names their problems, and validates their experience. In rare instances, assessment also may be the cure, because processing of the trauma memory can occur during assessment.

Your goal during assessment is (1) to build rapport, (2) to assess PTSD and other associated problems comprehensively, so that you can generate a thorough problem list, (3) to determine and validate your patients' perceptions of their problems, and (4) to avoid overwhelming yourself with information that is not helpful. Given the importance of assessment, we offer a brief overview of important areas of assessment, a recommended assessment procedure, and a discussion of ongoing assessment during treatment.

Important Areas of Assessment: Trauma History, PTSD, Comorbidity, Physical Status, and Complicating Factors

Gathering basic information about patients' trauma histories is a core component of PTSD assessment. Unless your patient is one of the rare individuals whose symptoms improve after telling the story once, trauma history assessment involves walking a fine line. You need to gather enough information to develop a basic understanding of your patients' trauma histories without digging so deep that you inadvertently start exposing patients to their memories before it is therapeutic to do so. Patients who become overwhelmed by the assessment may not return. Yet underassessment of trauma history may leave you without enough information to generate an accurate case formulation and treatment plan. Also, some patients identify traumatic events that do not meet the following DSM-IV traumatic event criteria: (1) "The person experienced, witnessed, or was confronted with an event or events that involved actual or threatened death or serious injury, or a threat to physical integrity of self or others," and (2) "The person's response involved intense fear, helplessness, or horror" (American Psychiatric Association, 1994, p. 428). Determining whether an incident meets criteria for a traumatic event is important, because formulations for patients who have experienced traumatic events typically differ from those who are distressed by events that do not meet criteria for a traumatic event. Assessing the trauma history is not sufficient, however. You also need to determine whether patients actually meet criteria for PTSD, because case formulations for patients who meet criteria for PTSD differ from those who do not, even if both have experienced trauma.

We find that the best tool for assessing PTSD is the Clinician-Administered PTSD Scale (CAPS; Weathers & Litz, 1994), a structured clinical interview designed to assess PTSD and associated features, such as guilt and dissociation. The CAPS provides carefully developed questions aimed at eliciting the information needed to determine whether your patients have suffered a DSM-defined trauma and meet criteria for PTSD. You can purchase a CD-ROM (www.ntis.gov/products/pages/caps.asp) that provides guidance in administering the CAPS. You also can request a copy of the CAPS from the National Center for PTSD by going to their website (www.ncptsd.va.gov/publications/assessment/).

It is also important to assess comorbid disorders and associated problems, especially other anxiety disorders, mood disorders, hypochondriasis, eating disorders, and substance use, as well as Axis II disorders. Assessing these conditions will help you create your case formulation and may help you clarify a patient's readiness for trauma-focused treatment. For example, many patients with comorbidity, including Axis II disorders such as borderline personality disorder (BPD), can benefit from CBT. However, patients with especially severe Axis II disorders (e.g., those who severely self-injure, are highly suicidal, and/or are prone to extreme dissociation) may benefit from dialectical behavior therapy (DBT; Linehan, 1993a) or from limited, DBT-based skills training prior to starting trauma-focused treatment. DBT, a variant of CBT designed to address emotion regulation and destructive behaviors associated with BPD (Linehan, 1993a), differs from standard CBT in a variety of ways, particularly with respect to its emphasis on validation, mindfulness, and the dialectic of acceptance and change (see Chapters 4 and 9 for more information on DBT).

Our preferred measure for assessing comorbid problems is a structured interview, the Anxiety Disorders Interview Schedule for DSM-IV (ADIS-IV; Brown, DiNardo, & Barlow, 1994). The ADIS-IV takes a time to administer. To reduce its length, you can selectively focus on the questions most relevant for the case at hand. For example, if you assess PTSD using the CAPS, skip the ADIS-IV PTSD section. Also, many sections of the ADIS-IV ask patients if they began regularly using any drugs or developed a physical problem prior to the onset of the assessed psychological problem. If a patient does not take drugs or have any physical problems, you can skip these questions. You can order an ADIS-IV kit from Oxford University Press. If you choose to order online, go to www.oup.com/us and search for anxiety disorders.

The ADIS-IV assesses the primary comorbid conditions that commonly present with PTSD, including mood and substance use disorders. We supplement the ADIS-IV with an assessment of eating disorders (e.g., the Eating Attitudes Test; see below) in female patients, because eating disorders are not assessed by the ADIS-IV. Our research indicates that a meaningful number of female PTSD patients have eating disorders, and that clinicians do not always detect these eating disorders if they rely exclusively on the ADIS-IV (Becker, DeViva, & Zayfert, 2004).

It is essential to assess patients' physical status. Common health problems include headaches, irritable bowel syndrome, and chronic pain. Many of these problems interact with anxiety and/or may have a strong underlying anxiety basis. For example, Stuart, who developed PTSD after losing his hand in an industrial accident, reported chronic pain. His pain worsened markedly during his exposure sessions, then gradually improved over the course of treatment. Stuart's therapist used cognitive restructuring to challenge Stuart's belief: "If treating my PTSD makes my pain go away, it means that my pain was 'all in my head.' " The therapist was alert to the possibility of such beliefs, because he knew about Stuart's chronic pain and had developed a case formulation that hypothesized a relationship between Stuart's PTSD and his chronic pain.

Finally, it is important to assess factors that can either complicate or facilitate treatment. For example, assess for ongoing abusive relationships, life problems (e.g., marital, legal, housing, financial, work problems), and life demands (job, children, elderly parents, etc.), along with support systems and resources. Having a good understanding of both the stresses and strengths that patients bring to treatment helps you structure your treatment and troubleshoot when you encounter obstacles.

Why Structured Clinical Interviews Are Helpful in Clinical Practice

Structured clinical interviews such as the ADIS-IV and CAPS are not commonly used in clinical practice. If you are not accustomed to structured interviews, you may feel awkward using them at first. Nonetheless, accurate assessment sets the stage for a good case formulation, and these instruments can increase your assessment accuracy. Moreover, they help you avoid becoming so distracted by your patients' stories that you fail to assess everything that needs assessment.

If you are not familiar with the ADIS-IV and CAPS, it can be helpful to administer them to colleagues or other nonpatients to gain skill using them. The more comfortable you are with the phrasing of the questions, the easier it will be to remain empathic and build rapport while using the interview. Some clinicians believe that structured assessment hurts rapport building. We typically explain to patients that we use these interviews because we want to ensure that we fully understand their difficulties, so that we are maximally equipped to help them. We find that most patients respect thorough assessment and that it helps rather than harms rapport building in most cases.

Additional Measures and Assessment Procedures

If you are interested in other PTSD instruments, the National Center for PTSD maintains a list of such tools and how to obtain them (www.ncptsd.va.gov/publications/assessment/). In addition to using the ADIS-IV to assess comorbidity, you may find it helpful to use the Beck Depression Inventory (BDI; Beck, Steer, & Garbin, 1988; available from www.harcourtassessment.com), which can be administered repeatedly during treatment to monitor comorbid depression. The Eating Attitudes Test (EAT; Garner, Olmsted, Bohr, & Garfinkel, 1982) is an easy, short, screening instrument that can be a helpful starting point for assessing eating disorders (information on obtaining EAT can be found at www.river-centre.org). An elevated score highlights the necessity of further eating disorder assessment. Anderson, Lundgren, Shapiro, and Paulosky (2004) have compiled additional information about the clinical assessment of eating disorders. A structured assessment tool, such as the Structured Clinical Interview for DSM-IV Axis II Personality Disorders (SCID-II; available from www.appi.org) is also valuable for early detection of Axis II disorders. In summary, we recommend completing an initial assessment using the CAPS for PTSD, the ADIS-IV for comorbid disorders, and whatever additional validated questionnaires you prefer.

Ongoing Assessment throughout Treatment

We use ongoing assessment to determine whether treatment is proceeding as expected. Ongoing assessment should focus on the two or three primary problem areas identified in your initial evaluation. We also recommend readministering the CAPS when you consider ending treatment, to ensure that your impression of improvement (based on your ongoing assessment) is supported, and to more clearly identify residual symptoms (e.g., insomnia, anger, anhedonia, numbing/detachment) that may warrant further specific intervention.

Ongoing assessment of PTSD can be tricky. CBT is oriented toward decreasing patients' avoidance, because avoidance is a poor long-term strategy for managing posttraumatic reactions. Avoidance is not totally ineffective, however. Thus, some patients experience an increase in symptoms early in treatment as they become less avoidant. Such patients often respond to treatment, and increased symptoms do not necessarily mean that treatment is off course. Assessing intermediate indicators of good and poor response can help you determine whether treatment is progressing as expected. For example, continually assessing the degree to which patients show expected reductions in anxiety during exposure sessions, as well as general reductions of avoidance behaviors, is an important gauge of progress. Evidence for this comes from in-session tracking of anxiety during exposure, of anxiety levels during home practice, and of specific avoidance behaviors (e.g., starting to use the soap that the perpetrator used would indicate decreased avoidance). Many examples of this type of assessment are provided throughout Chapters 6 and 7.

It is also useful to assess the degree of guilt, anger, shame, and so forth, triggered by trauma-related stimuli and memories. Evidence of change or lack of change can be obtained from cognitive restructuring forms, by assessing nonanxiety emotions after exposure sessions, and by observing patients' behavior. It also can be helpful to have severely depressed patients maintain daily mood ratings and/or to regularly administer a BDI to track levels of depression. The most important component of ongoing assessment is that it be specific. Having clear behavioral targets helps you to assess improvement (e.g., when a patient who was mauled by a dog visits a friend with small dogs and gradually experiences less anxiety).

USING NOMOTHETIC MODELS TO DEVELOP EVIDENCE-BASED IDIOGRAPHIC FORMULATIONS

What Is the Nomothetic Model and Why Is It Useful?

A nomothetic model (or formulation) is used to conceptualize a problem by hypothesizing a common cause of the problem across individuals. The nomothetic formulation of PTSD (described in detail in Chapter 2) views PTSD symptoms as an understandable reaction to traumatic experiences based on what is known about the development of normal fear. Symptoms are maintained in large part by avoidance and failure to process traumatic experiences fully.

To the degree that they are supported by research, the nomothetic PTSD models in Chapter 2 should improve your accuracy in understanding a given patient, above and beyond reliance on models with no empirical support. Yet nomothetic PTSD formulations are not without limitations. A nomothetic formulation is like a compass, in that it points in a general direction but does not indicate a specific path. For example, the nomothetic formulation does not identify the specific stimuli, thoughts, and behaviors that maintain PTSD symptoms for a specific patient. In addition, nomothetic formulations present a variety of possible causal factors that might or might not play a role for an individual patient (Haynes & O'Brien, 1990). Thus, although nomothetic formulations provide the confidence of scientific support and point to specific treatment strategies, individualized (i.e., idiographic) formulations are needed to tailor treatment strategies to patients' idiosyncratic posttraumatic reactions, to develop plans for monitoring treatment progress, and to amend the treatment strategies when things do not go according to plan.

Creating Evidence-Based Idiographic Formulations for Patients with PTSD

In constructing a case formulation, the overarching goal is to offer an explanation of your patient's various problems that points to a clear, evidence-based treatment plan (Persons, 1991). For complicated PTSD cases, integrating the array of information you have gathered about your patient in an organized and coherent manner can be challenging. Often you will find yourself entertaining multiple hypotheses about the causes of your patient's distress, and no single explanation will account for all aspects of the case. Adhering to the following steps in building your case formulation can simplify the process (Persons, Davidson, & Tompkins, 2001). We provide an overview of the steps, then explore them in detail.

Your first step entails organizing your assessment information into a helpful format. Next, you formulate working hypotheses, which are the cornerstone of your case formulation. Working hypotheses are the tentative explanations that you generate about your patient, based on both your observations and relevant nomothetic models. You then generate a treatment plan based on your formulation. Finally, you implement your plan with ongoing assessment, which helps you determine whether the treatment is proceeding successfully, or whether modifications to the formulation and treatment plan are needed.

After discussing each of these components in greater detail, we demonstrate the implementation of these steps using the two case examples described at the start of this chapter.

Organizing Your Assessment Information

Of the many ways to organize assessment information, we recommend including the following components (Persons et al., 2001):

1. *Identifying information.* Includes name, age, gender, ethnicity, marital status, living situation, occupation, employment status, and so forth.

2. *Problem list.* A detailed problem list includes problems the patient is facing in the following areas: psychological symptoms, interpersonal and occupational functioning, medical conditions, and financial and legal status. You will have gathered information necessary to generate a detailed problem list during your assessment. It is important to recognize that patients with PTSD sometimes do not initially view their PTSD as a "problem." Thus, your problem list may include problems not initially endorsed by the patient.

3. *Diagnoses.* List all diagnoses for which the patient meets criteria. Some patients meet partial criteria for PTSD. In such cases, list PTSD symptoms, so that you keep them in mind when generating your hypotheses. Avoidance may curb active symptoms in PTSD and in other anxiety disorders. For example, a patient who is very cognitively and behaviorally skilled at avoiding trauma stimuli may not report extensive reexperiencing symptoms; thus, he or she may not meet full criteria for PTSD. Listing PTSD symptoms can be a reminder that several viable hypotheses may explain your patient's symptoms. The case of Morgan demonstrates this point.

4. *Strengths and assets.* Given the challenging nature of CBT for PTSD, it is helpful to identify the strengths on which your patients can rely during treatment.

Developing Your Working Hypotheses

You will want to keep several factors in mind when generating your case formulation hypotheses. First, basing your working hypotheses on empirically supported nomothetic models helps you to minimize clinical judgment errors (Wilson, 1996; Persons, 2005). For instance, hypotheses for patients with PTSD that rely on the nomothetic models of PTSD described in Chapter 2 will have a strong base of empirical support behind them. When other disorders are comorbid with PTSD, we recommend that you integrate nomothetic models for the comorbid disorders that have empirical support (e.g., the nomothetic formulation of panic disorder; Barlow, 2002), BPD (Linehan, 1993a), bulimia nervosa (Fairburn, Marcus, & Wilson, 1993), and so on. The case of Sophie provides an example of this process.

You may find it helpful to list all relevant nomothetic models before generating your working hypotheses. As noted earlier, the first source for identifying relevant nomothetic formulations is your list of diagnoses. Relevant nomothetic models are not necessarily limited to the disorders for which patients meet criteria, however. For example, the biosocial model of BPD (Linehan, 1993a) often is very useful in treating patients with complicated PTSD, even when such patients do not meet sufficient criteria for a diagnosis of BPD. Thus, the list simply catalogs the models that may be useful in generating the idiographic formulation.

In developing a PTSD case formulation, we find it helpful to consider a primary hypothesis that focuses on the effects of trauma. In other words, when a patient presents with multiple problems, all of which began after a traumatic event or developed over time in concert with multiple traumatic events, we consider a case formulation that places PTSD and trauma at the focal point. The conceptualization is, in a sense, anchored or grounded in PTSD, and reactions to the traumatic event have a central role in our understanding of the various problems. This strategy helps to organize the case conceptualization. Instead of viewing a patient as presenting with two, three, four, or five separate disorders or problems, we conceptualize many problems as arising out of attempts to avoid trauma-related stimuli, thoughts, or emotions, and/or other efforts to cope with the cognitive, behavioral, and emotional sequelae of the trauma. For example, patients often present with depressed mood in addition to PTSD. Depressed mood might be conceptualized as resulting from patients' avoidance behaviors, given that they have limited their social interactions to limit anxiety. Or it might be conceptualized as resulting from patients' beliefs about the hopelessness of recovering from PTSD, or about never being able to form relationships because they view themselves as damaged.

Similarly, an eating disorder that begins shortly after a traumatic event may be conceptualized as an attempt by a woman, who views her self-worth as diminished because of the event, to enhance self-esteem via weight loss, a culturally prescribed method of self-improvement for women (Fairburn et al., 1993). Or the eating disorder might be conceptualized as an avoidance strategy, if evidence suggests that the patient's eating disorder behaviors enable her to avoid trauma cues, such as memories of the traumatic event.

Some patients' traumatic experiences postdate the onset of other disorders. Obviously, in these cases, the traumatic experience did not cause the other disorders. The earlier onset disorder, however, may have predisposed the individual to develop PTSD after the trauma. In particular, a pattern of avoidant coping established as part of another disorder may contribute to the development of PTSD. For example, Clara developed PTSD after a severe auto accident when she was 30. Clara had a 10-year history of obsessive–compulsive disorder (OCD), with prominent avoidance behaviors related to her obsession with contamination. Thus, Clara had learned to use avoidance as her primary strategy for managing anxiety. After the accident, Clara used the same strategy for her trauma-related anxiety. She avoided riding in a car and used cognitive strategies to push her trauma memories out of her mind. Similarly, Sarah, whose social phobia dated back to childhood, had an established pattern of avoiding situations that made her anxious. After she was mugged, she applied this avoidant coping strategy to deal with the assault; thus, she went out of her way to avoid the street where she was attacked, the clothing she wore that day, and men who reminded her of the assailant, and she avoided talking about it with her family.

PTSD also may contribute to the maintenance of preexisting disorders. For example, Roger suffered from depression for many years prior to surviving a train crash. After the crash, he increased his avoidance of social activities to avoid questions about the crash. This contributed to his isolation and worsened his depression. Georgia had been "shy" as a child. As an adult, she avoided situations that involved public speaking. Although the fear had limited her professional advancement, she was not bothered by this fear until age 36, when she was raped. After the rape, her social anxiety increased and generalized to situations that previously were not as anxiety provoking for her, such as starting and maintaining conversations, and using public restrooms. She also reported feeling ashamed in situations in which she thought the attention of others was focused on her—a qualitative difference from her social anxiety before the rape.

In cases such as these, we typically focus on PTSD first, if it is the principal diagnosis (i.e., the disorder causing the most distress and functional impairment) and it appears to be influencing other disorders. Successfully resolving PTSD often brings about substantial improvement in other areas of patients' lives. In addition, it can be difficult to make progress with other disorders without treating PTSD. If another disorder is the principal diagnosis, however, then it may be the initial focus of treatment. For example, in the case of Morgan (see description at start of the chapter), her traumatic events post-dated her eating disorder, which was the principal diagnosis. In her case (see below for more detail), the therapist decided to target the eating disorder first.

Keep in mind that your working hypotheses form the basis of your *tentative*, initial idiographic formulation. Use ongoing assessment to test the accuracy of your hypotheses and revise them as necessary based on these data.

Developing Your Treatment Plan and Testing Your Working Hypotheses with Ongoing Assessment

Your idiographic treatment plan should be based on nomothetic treatment protocols that have empirical support, ideally from randomized controlled trials. Researchers have rarely tested the effectiveness of implementing nomothetic treatments in an individualized (or idiographic) manner (Persons, 1991). For this reason, we advocate adhering as closely as possible to both the nomothetic formulation and treatment. In other words, for patients whose presentations are straightforward, you can apply the nomothetic formulation directly. In such cases, your most efficient strategy is to generate hypotheses that closely resemble the nomothetic formulation and to deliver treatment in a manner that closely resembles that used in clinical trials (e.g., deliver straightforward psychoeducation followed by straightforward exposure). In other cases, however, greater degrees of idiographic formulation are required from the start of treatment.

In addition to relying on nomothetic data to guide the treatment plan, we recommend that you also adopt a scientific approach to treatment of your individual patients, as described by many researchers (e.g., Hayes, Barlow, & Nelson-Gray, 1999; Persons, 2005). This entails gathering structured data regularly throughout treatment (i.e., ongoing assessment) and using this data to determine whether treatment is working. If it is not working, you critically revisit the original formulation rather than ignoring the lack of improvement or proceeding on the notion that more of the same is better.

It is helpful to divide your treatment plan into the following sections: stated goals, which are the general goals articulated by the patient; initial treatment goals, which are specific early steps that the patient can agree to tackle; and long-term goals, which the patient may or may not be able to support at the start of treatment. The distinction between initial and long-term treatment goals is often not needed with other disorders. Yet many patients with PTSD who present for treatment are unaware that they have PTSD. They also may be prepared to address only related problems. Most patients, however, are amenable to psychoeducation or an initial treatment plan that includes exploring the decision to proceed with trauma-focused treatment. Thus, initial treatment goals often target barriers to proceeding with trauma-focused treatment, including the development of basic emotion regulation skills, if patients appear to have deficits in this area. For example, Adriana presented for treatment of martial discord and was unwilling to address her prominent PTSD symptoms, even though they contributed to her marital problems. Her initial treatment goals included learning skills to manage negative affect (including anger) and PTSD psychoeducation. The therapist listed processing of Adriana's traumatic events as a long-term goal. Long-term goals are generally the ones that we tie to ongoing assessment.

We now return to the two cases introduced at the start of this chapter to demonstrate strategies for developing the case formulation and the associated treatment plan. You may find it helpful to review the cases before proceeding with the next section. In the "Working Hypotheses" section, we include the nomothetic formulation (in parentheses) that supports each idiographic hypothesis.

CASE FORMULATION: SOPHIE

Identifying Information

Name: Sophie
Age: 50
Gender: Female
Ethnicity: African American
Marital status: Married, third marriage
Education: High school graduate
Children: One daughter, age 20
Residence: Resides with husband
Financial status: Moderate financial resources
Legal status: No legal proceedings
Employment status: Full-time plus a part-time job
Leisure activities: Sophie used to enjoy embroidery and walking but has given up most leisure pursuits. She spends most of her free time alone.

Problem List

- Reexperiencing symptoms, including intrusive thoughts and memories
- Difficulty trusting people, including husband
- Reluctance to travel far from home due to feeling unsafe
- Feeling paranoid. Sophie complains of feeling on guard around others and spends a lot of time worrying about whether to trust others, and whether her computer files, medical records, phone calls, etc., are safe from others who may try to access them in order to harm her.
- "Mood swings"
- Loneliness. Sophie has "no friends" and feels detached from her husband. She believes it is dangerous to befriend other women, because they will betray her, for example, by gossiping about her or not being available when she needs them.
- Irritability and anger outbursts

Diagnoses

Axis I: PTSD, social phobia
Axis II: BPD
Axis III: None

Axis IV: None
Axis V: 60

Relevant Nomothetic Formulations

- Biosocial model for BPD from DBT (Linehan, 1993a)
- Cognitive-behavioral models of PTSD (Resick & Schnicke, 1992; Foa et al., 1989)
- Cognitive-behavioral model of social phobia (Beidel & Turner, 1998)[1]

Working Hypotheses

The therapist hypothesized that Sophie's undisclosed childhood trauma was associated with considerable shame and guilt (CBT for PTSD), which is why she would not discuss it. She also hypothesized that Sophie may have experienced invalidating reactions to prior disclosures that contributed to her reluctance to disclose (DBT for BPD). The therapist presumed that avoidance of thoughts, memories, and stimuli related to traumatic events underlay reexperiencing symptoms and hypervigilance (CBT for PTSD). The therapist also hypothesized that negative thoughts, including self-blame and negative appraisals of self-worth related to the traumatic events, underlay social anxiety (CBT for PTSD, CBT for social phobia) and contributed to avoidance (and hence processing of) trauma memories (CBT for PTSD). Based on Sophie's complaints that she felt her emotions were out of her control, the therapist hypothesized that emotion dysregulation had evolved from an invalidating childhood home environment (DBT for BPD). An invalidating family environment may have contributed to shame and self-blame in reaction to the earlier trauma. The therapist hypothesized that paranoia evolved out of an interaction between trauma-related hypervigilance and prior perceived betrayals. The therapist also hypothesized that avoidance of traveling far from home resulted from feeling generally unsafe (CBT for PTSD) given that Sophie did not report uncued panic attacks.

The therapist reviewed the formulation with Sophie, emphasizing the role of invalidating reactions from others in contributing to her distress (DBT for BPD). The therapist explained that because "bad things" had happened, including the things in childhood that Sophie was not ready to discuss, it was understandable that she felt unsafe and untrusting of others, particularly if people in her life gave her the impression that she should be over it by now (CBT for PTSD). The therapist explained that bad things that happen early in life can trigger strong emotional reactions. If you do not feel safe talking about your emotional reactions, and if people do not teach you how to cope, these emotional reactions persist and lead to a pattern of extreme ups and downs, so that you feel like you are on an emotional roller coaster. The therapist and Sophie agreed to a treatment plan that emphasized smoothing out the emotional roller coaster, while also learning more about PTSD to see whether it made sense to include PTSD treatment in her plan. The therapist presumed Sophie's social phobia was mediated by PTSD-related guilt and shame (CBT for PTSD). Thus, she had good reason to expect

---

[1]*Note.* To provide guidance as to how nomothetic formulations were used to generate working hypotheses, we include an abbreviated name of the above formulations following sections that relied on said nomothetic formulations (e.g., DBT for BPD).

that social phobia would respond to the interventions for PTSD, so treatment for social phobia (CBT for social phobia) was postponed pending reassessment after PTSD treatment.

Strengths and Assets

Despite her level of anxiety and difficulty with trust, Sophie had been able to maintain both full-time and part-time employment, and sustain her current marriage for 8 years. She had successfully extricated herself from her previous abusive marriage and obtained employment despite having no prior work history. She also had cared for her young daughter on her own for several years before remarrying. She expressed considerable motivation to improve her social and emotional functioning. She also was able to develop trust in her previous mental health provider and continued to see her for several months, demonstrating her willingness to take some risk in pursuit of her desired changes.

Treatment Plan

As a reminder, we find it helpful to think it terms of three types of goals when treating PTSD. The first set of goals consists of the aims articulated by Sophie during assessment when her therapist asked, "What do you want from treatment?" The next set comprises the initial treatment goals Sophie and her therapist generated together, based on the assessment, the working hypotheses, and what Sophie was ready to tackle. These also include skills that may help Sophie progress toward long-term goals. We list relevant treatment strategies with these goals so that you can see how treatment strategies link to goals. If you are unfamiliar with the treatment strategies for comorbid problems, you may find it helpful to refer to Chapter 9.

The final long-term goals are those that the therapist believes need to be accomplished, based on the working hypotheses. Patients vary in their readiness to agree to long-term goals at the start of treatment. Often, agreement about long-term goals is reached while addressing short-term goals. Long-term goals are those that we most often tie to ongoing assessment. Thus, we include the method for assessing progress, along with relevant treatment strategies.

Sophie's Stated Goals during Assessment

- To feel less paranoid
- To be willing to drive alone on shopping trips or on longer trips with husband
- To feel less lonely
- To feel more in control of emotions (particularly anger)

Initial Treatment Goals and Relevant Treatment Strategies

Goals	Relevant strategies
1. Sophie will understand how emotions become "out of control" and learn to better control emotions.	1. Psychoeducation: the biosocial model, the balance of emotion and reason, the purpose of emotions (from DBT;

Linehan, 1993a); learn basic skills for managing emotions (from DBT); self-validation, mindfulness, acceptance, distraction and self-soothing, planning pleasurable activities, and so forth (from DBT).

2. Sophie will understand what PTSD is and what makes it continue, so that she can decide whether to proceed with PTSD treatment.

2. PTSD psychoeducation (from CBT for PTSD; Foa & Rothbaum, 1998).

3. Sophie will trust the therapist with further disclosures regarding her trauma history.

3. Individual and group sessions focused on education, validation, and concrete skills related to current distress (from DBT and CBT for PTSD).

Long-Term Therapy Goals (Ongoing Assessment Methods) and Relevant Treatment Strategies

Goals

1. Improve social functioning (assessment: track leisure activities, number of friendships, and satisfaction with friendships)
2. Increase opportunities for social contact by increasing leisure activities (assessment: track leisure activities).

3. Reduce distress around past traumas (assessment: once identified; graph habituation to *in vivo* stimuli and memories).

4. Increase mobility (assessment: track number of minutes spent driving per week and associated anxiety).

Relevant strategies

1. Cognitive restructuring around trust-related beliefs (from CBT for PTSD).

2. Activity scheduling (behavior therapy for depression; Hoberman & Lewinsohn, 1985; Persons et al., 2001).

3. Imaginal exposure (from CBT for PTSD), *in vivo* exposure (from CBT for PTSD), cognitive restructuring of guilt and shame-related thoughts (from CBT for PTSD).

4. *In vivo* exposure to driving (from CBT for anxiety disorders; Barlow & Craske, 2000).

CASE FORMULATION: MORGAN

Identifying Information

Name: Morgan
Age: 29
Gender: Female
Ethnicity: Caucasian
Marital status: Single, in new relationship with 33-year-old male

Education: Bachelor's degree in economics
Children: None
Residence: Resides with female roommate
Financial status: Moderate financial resources
Legal status: No legal proceedings
Employment status: Full time
Leisure activities: Taking care of dog, reading, cycling

Problem List

- Overconcern with shape and weight despite being somewhat underweight
- Inability to eat normal quantities of food without vomiting
- Interpersonal difficulties with (1) roommate, because she was distressed by Morgan's vomiting in their shared bathroom and missing food after binges and (2) new boyfriend, who started pressuring Morgan to gain weight for health reasons after she fainted while mountain biking.
- Feeling "stressed" and anxious. Worrying about weight, job, interpersonal problems with roommate, getting laid off, financial future, family, and so forth.
- Depressed mood
- Unable to mountain bike, per orders from internist, because of need for weight gain and because she is relying on potassium supplements to correct her electrolyte imbalance.
- Unable to enjoy sex due to numbing during intimacy; thus, not having sex with boyfriend interferes with the relationship.
- Unable/unwilling to visit New York City, despite a desire to see friends who still lived there.
- Avoidance of all furniture and belongings from apartment in New York City (i.e., objects in storage; Morgan unwilling to unpack or use items).

Diagnoses

Axis I:	Bulimia nervosa
	Generalized anxiety disorder (GAD)
	Major depression, mild
	Rule out PTSD
Axis II:	No diagnosis
Axis III:	Recent electrolyte imbalance
Axis IV:	Interpersonal disputes with roommate and boyfriend
Axis V:	55

Relevant Nomothetic Formulations

- Cognitive-behavioral model of bulimia nervosa (Fairburn et al., 1993)
- Cognitive-behavioral model of GAD (Roemer, Orsillo, & Barlow, 2002)
- Cognitive-behavioral model of PTSD (Foa et al., 1989)
- Cognitive-behavioral model of depression (Beck, Rush, Shaw, & Emery, 1979)

Working Hypotheses

The therapist generated two hypotheses, which she subsequently shared with Morgan. The first focused on two facts: (1) that Morgan's eating disorder predated her first traumatic event, and (2) that she did not report significant reexperiencing symptoms related to the rape. These facts suggested that Morgan's bulimia nervosa initially developed independent of her PTSD. The therapist also noted that much of Morgan's description of her eating disorder closely matched the nomothetic model of bulimia nervosa (see Chapter 9 for more discussion of CBT for bulimia nervosa), and she hypothesized that Morgan believed that altering her weight and shape would improve her self-esteem (CBT for bulimia). Per the nomothetic model, her therapist presumed that overconcern with weight and shape was the driving force behind Morgan's dietary restriction, and that restriction resulted in binge eating. The therapist viewed Morgan's vomiting as a strategy that began initially to compensate for overeating, but which now also served to manage negative emotions in general. Research indicates that many patients with comorbid depression and anxiety respond to CBT for bulimia nervosa and also often experience a reduction in depression and anxiety after treatment. Thus, the therapist hypothesized that Morgan's depression and anxiety would be reduced even if treatment focused on her eating disorder. If anxiety and depression were not reduced after successful treatment for the eating disorder, then a reformulation would be required (CBT for PTSD, CBT for depression). This hypothesis, which did not postulate a central role for the rape in Morgan's current distress, was the most parsimonious and generated the simplest treatment plan.

The second hypothesis related the eating disorder to traumatic events and anxiety, even though the eating disorder appeared to have developed prior to the first trauma. This hypothesis was based on the observation that Morgan reported very high levels of avoidance related to her traumatic events (CBT for PTSD), including numbing during sex and avoidance of sex; and avoidance of talk about New York, travel to New York, and objects from her New York apartment. Thus, the therapist considered the possibility that high levels of avoidance were limiting reexperiencing symptoms that might otherwise be present and contribute to a diagnosis of PTSD. The therapist hypothesized that overconcern with weight and shape, food restriction, binge eating, and purging were established strategies for coping with threats to self-esteem and negative emotions at the time of the rape (CBT for bulimia; CBT for GAD), and that Morgan relied on these same strategies to manage emotions (e.g., anxiety, guilt, and shame) associated with her first and subsequent traumatic events (CBT for bulimia, CBT for PTSD). More specifically, Morgan's focus on weight and shape facilitated cognitive avoidance of trauma stimuli (i.e., memories and thoughts) and countered low self-esteem associated with the rape (CBT for PTSD). Morgan likely also used food restriction, binge eating, and purging to reduce anxiety evoked by trauma-related stimuli.

As part of the second hypothesis, the therapist also speculated that if Morgan was using her binge–purge behaviors as a coping strategy, then she might have difficulty tolerating the increase in anxiety associated with stopping her disordered eating behaviors. In addition, the therapist hypothesized that decreased avoidance of rape stimuli (via decreased focus on weight and shape, and discussion of rape as part of trauma treatment) would result in an increase in reexperiencing symptoms related to the rape (CBT for PTSD). This more complex hypothesis would generate a more complicated treatment plan. It also placed trauma at the center of the conceptualization; therefore, because Morgan did not meet full criteria for PTSD, it seemed a less likely scenario.

The therapist presented to Morgan the first hypothesis and an abbreviated version of the second hypothesis (focusing on anxiety vs. shame because Morgan appeared to have trouble discussing the rape). Morgan agreed to start with a treatment plan based on the first hypothesis but to revisit the second hypothesis if treatment did not progress as expected.

Strengths and Assets

Morgan was employed full-time and financially stable. Her new boyfriend appeared supportive and encouraged her to seek treatment for her eating disorder. Morgan also expressed a strong desire to change her behavior.

Treatment Plan

Morgan's Stated Goals during Assessment

- To feel less concerned about shape and weight
- To stop vomiting
- To feel more in control of eating and be able to eat a wider variety of foods
- To feel less stressed
- To resume mountain biking with boyfriend
- To improve relationship with roommate

Initial Treatment Goals and Relevant Treatment Strategies

Goals	Relevant strategies
1. Morgan will understand how her eating disorder developed and why it continued.	1. Psychoeducation the cognitive-behavioral model of bulimia nervosa (from CBT for bulimia nervosa; Fairburn et al., 1993).
2. Morgan will verbalize greater willingness to "give up" her eating disorder.	2. Decision analysis (Ahijevych & Parsley, 1999; Clark et al., 1998; Janis & Mann, 1977).
3. Morgan will understand the function of self-monitoring and show greater awareness of current eating behaviors.	3. Self-monitoring (from CBT for bulimia nervosa).

Long-Term Therapy Goals (Ongoing Assessment Methods) and Relevant Treatment Strategies

Goals	Relevant strategies
1. Decrease dietary restraint and binge eating (assessment: self-monitoring, plus graphing of number of days per week specific dietary goals were achieved).	1. Establish regular pattern of eating by assigning three meals plus planned snacks per day (directly drawn from CBT for bulimia nervosa); stimulus control strategies (from CBT for bulimia nervosa); create forbidden foods

hierarchy and introduce foods back into diet with specific behavioral assignments (from CBT for bulimia nervosa); increase overall number of calories eaten per day (from CBT for bulimia nervosa); cognitive restructuring (from CBT for bulimia nervosa).

2. Reduce vomiting (self-monitoring and graphing).

2. Delay and alternatives (from CBT for bulimia nervosa); cognitive restructuring (from CBT for bulimia nervosa).

3. Decrease overconcern with weight and shape (assessment: track via comments on self-monitoring).

3. Cognitive restructuring (from CBT for bulimia nervosa).

Note. After making significant improvement (i.e., reducing vomiting to one to three times per week, reducing binge eating, establishing regular pattern of eating), Morgan's progress stalled and she lost weight secondary to reduced binge eating and inability to increase overall caloric content of meals regularly. Morgan also reported feeling that something was missing in treatment. She and her therapist revisited the formulation and decided that the evidence now supported the second hypothesis. After deciding to proceed with treatment of posttraumatic symptoms, Morgan confessed that she and her boyfriend had begun having sex, and that she was having difficulty with this. She had been trying to stop numbing during sex and was now having reexperiencing symptoms. This new information supported the second hypothesis. Morgan's stated goals had shifted at this point in treatment.

Treatment Plan 2

Morgan's Stated Goals

- To feel less concerned about shape and weight
- To stop vomiting
- To decrease food restriction and gain weight
- To feel less anxious and worried
- To resume mountain biking with boyfriend
- To enjoy sex
- To stop working so hard to avoid trauma reminders
- To be able to go to New York without trepidation

Initial Treatment Goals and Relevant Treatment Strategies

Goals	Relevant strategies
1. Morgan will understand the nature of posttraumatic reactions, why they persist, and how they might relate to her eating disorder, so that she can decide whether PTSD treatment makes sense for her.	1. PTSD psychoeducation (CBT for PTSD); use PTSD psychoeducation to identify connections between eating disorder and PTSD (e.g., weight loss decreases secondary sex characteristics, which lowers anxiety about further sexual

assaults; generate list of eating disorder strategies that have been most helpful, and review pros and cons of starting session with PTSD strategies versus eating disorder strategies.

Long-Term Therapy Goals (Ongoing Assessment)

Goals	Relevant strategies
1. Reduce distress around past traumas (assessment: graph habituation to trauma-related stimuli and memories).	1. Imaginal and *in vivo* exposure (CBT for PTSD); cognitive restructuring of safety-related thoughts, as well as guilt and shame-related thoughts (once identified) (CBT for PTSD).
2. Increase caloric intake and weight (assessment: self-monitoring, plus graphing of number of days per week specific dietary goals were achieved; weekly weighing in session and graph).	2. Continue weekly eating assignments, review of self-monitoring, and verbal reinforcement for increasing caloric intake (from CBT for bulimia nervosa); stimulus control strategies (from CBT for bulimia nervosa); cognitive restructuring (from CBT for bulimia nervosa).
3. Eliminate vomiting (self-monitoring and graphing).	3. Delay and alternatives (CBT for bulimia nervosa); cognitive restructuring of thoughts related to food intake, vomiting, and body shape/weight (CBT for bulimia nervosa).
4. Decrease overconcern with weight and shape (assessment: track via comments on self-monitoring).	4. Cognitive restructuring (CBT for bulimia nervosa).

USING THE CASE FORMULATION TO DECIDE ON THE FOCUS OF TREATMENT: WHERE TO START?

When your patients present with multiple problems, you must decide where to begin treatment and how to order treatment strategies both within and between sessions, so that treatment does not become disorganized or overwhelming for the patient. A layering approach often works well. You introduce initial interventions strategies and rehearse them for several sessions, then reduce the amount of session time you devote to those strategies as you layer new strategies onto the earlier ones. For example, therapists may need to devote one, two, or even three entire sessions to self-monitoring at the start to present the rationale, elicit and address patient concerns, review results from monitoring, and teach the patient how to use monitoring, assess obstacles, and address obstacles. Yet once self-monitoring is in place, significantly less time is needed for review of self-monitoring, and new tasks can be added. Similarly, *in vivo* exposure may occupy a good deal of session time early in treatment, but once your patient knows what to do, you may only need to reinforce approach behaviors, highlight successes, and briefly problem-solve obstacles.

Several factors influence which problems you decide to tackle first. First, consider the presenting problem. Often, the primary presenting complaint of patients with PTSD is something other than PTSD (e.g., somatic complaints such as headaches, dizziness, gastrointestinal problems; loss of interest in sex; panic attacks; depression) or an aspect of PTSD that is not clearly related to the trauma (e.g., trouble concentrating, irritability, anhedonia, insomnia). It is often critical to address some aspect of the primary concerns, because early in treatment, when patients have little understanding of PTSD, they may have difficulty hearing that their primary concerns are due to PTSD. Such a message may instead be interpreted as suggesting that the primary complaint is "all in their head" or that patients' interpretations of their problems are invalid. By directly addressing some aspect of the presenting complaints, you validate perceptions of the sources of suffering. This serves to enhance your credibility, strengthen the therapeutic alliance, and improve adherence to the treatment plan.

Second, consider the ease of implementing the treatment plan. Generally, patients are more likely to comply with and practice simpler treatments. Also, some treatments are inherently more complex and intellectually challenging than others, so it is important to consider the patient's intellectual capabilities in planning the treatment. Many patients with PTSD experience impairments in concentration and memory that can also make cognitive treatment challenging. Third, consider the likely effect of the interventions on functioning, or, in other words, which treatment is likely to produce the biggest "bang for the buck."

In Morgan's case, the first formulation had the advantage of directly addressing the patient's stated goals, while avoiding the inherent complication and burden of simultaneous treatment of PTSD and an eating disorder. Furthermore, the empirical literature suggests that anxiety and depression will diminish with treatment of an eating disorder, so Morgan's therapist predicted that this approach would have a broad effect on functioning.

In Sophie's case, the therapist considered treatment for social phobia, because social isolation was a prominent complaint. Despite the relative simplicity of social phobia treatment (in contrast to treatment for BPD and PTSD), however, there was little reason to expect that either BPD or PTSD would respond to such treatment. Moreover, there was reason to doubt that social phobia treatment could be effective for social phobia while BPD and PTSD remained active (Zayfert, DeViva, & Hofmann, 2005); thus, the effect on functioning might be limited. As a result, the therapist opted for the more complicated treatment plan described earlier, because it targeted Sophie's stated complaints *and* advanced the agenda of fully engaging Sophie in treatment for PTSD.

In contrast, in the case of Stuart, a 32-year-old man with PTSD, social anxiety, and alcohol abuse, the therapist opted to start with social phobia. Stuart reported a long history of social phobia that led him to drop out of college and rely on drinking to cope with his anxiety. During this time, Stuart experienced an emotionally abusive relationship that became violent when he attempted to end it. He presented for therapy after 10 years of abstinence from alcohol, seeking treatment for social anxiety and depression. Assessment also revealed that he met criteria for PTSD related to the abusive relationship. Stuart's PTSD-related distress and functional impairment were rated as mild compared to the extreme rating for his social anxiety and depression. His therapist hypothesized that the PTSD developed as a result of the same avoidant coping strategies that he used to cope with anxiety in social situations. Thus, the initial treatment plan targeted social anxiety concurrent with treatment for depression. The therapist also planned to monitor the PTSD and reassess Stuart at the conclusion of the initial treatment components.

Another reason to select a disorder other than PTSD as the initial treatment target is if that disorder is one that tends to respond readily to treatment. For example, Timothy, a 40-year-old college professor, was referred for treatment of OCD whose onset occurred in childhood. He also met criteria for GAD, panic disorder, social phobia, depression, and PTSD secondary to 9/11. His therapist suggested that they begin by treating his panic disorder because of that treatment's high likelihood of success. In this case, because Timothy was demoralized by the array of problems he faced, his therapist hoped that initial successful experiences would build Timothy's trust in CBT and allow him to move forward confidently to work on his other problems.

SEQUENTIAL VERSUS SIMULTANEOUS TREATMENT

When patients present with multiple problems, you have several options as to how to proceed: (1) focus first on one problem, then move to the next problem (i.e., deliver treatment sequentially); (2) monitor one problem closely while treating the other; or (3) attempt to deliver treatment for both problems simultaneously, either by lengthening treatment sessions to allow time for multiple interventions or by alternating sessions or chunks of sessions. The first hypothesis in Morgan's case illustrates option (1) in that the therapist planned first to treat the eating disorder, then offer treatment for GAD or major depression if these disorders had not improved after the first phase of treatment.

Sophie's treatment plan illustrates a blend of simultaneous and sequential approaches. Her treatment was simultaneous in that initial sessions focused on both BPD symptoms and psychoeducation about PTSD. Eventually, the treatment would shift to a greater PTSD focus, although some components addressing BPD likely would be included throughout. Social phobia treatment would be offered to Sophie sequentially, after completion of PTSD treatment, if social phobia persisted after PTSD was resolved.

Each approach has its advantages and disadvantages. The sequential approach is simpler. As demonstrated by Morgan, however, the simpler approach does not always work, and a simultaneous approach may be needed. Alternatively, you may need to alter the order of sequential treatments. For example, Morgan and her therapist had several choices once they adopted the second hypothesis: They could stop all eating disorder treatment; they could monitor the eating disorder to make sure that Morgan did not lose the gains she had made; or they could (as they did) attempt to treat the eating disorder and PTSD at the same time, by alternating chunks of sessions. Morgan and her therapist chose the simultaneous approach, because they feared that without ongoing treatment, Morgan would lose ground. Morgan believed that being held accountable to her therapist would help her keep the eating disorder at bay. When a secondary problem cannot be ignored because of safety (e.g., dangerous eating behaviors, substance abuse), but treating the secondary problem first has failed, then a simultaneous approach is warranted.

The simultaneous approach is preferable right from the start if problems appear to interact, or if the patient appears capable of addressing both problems together. For example, Clara feared blood, because it reminded her of her auto accident and was a po-tential contaminate (i.e., OCD fear). Thus, exposure to blood meant exposing Clara to both fears. As a result, Clara's therapist decided to adopt a simultaneous approach. In the case of Sophie, the therapist judged that she was capable of learning about both PTSD and strategies to manage emotions at the same time. At times, you may also choose to combine psychoeducational material for different problems, so that a more comprehensive treatment rationale can be developed.

SESSION PLANNING: DEVELOPING AN INITIAL TEMPLATE

It is useful at the beginning of treatment to lay out an initial template regarding how the first several (approximately five) sessions will be spent. This is helpful for several reasons. First, it facilitates orderly treatment and challenges you to think through the ordering of strategies. Second, you can share portions of the initial template, so that your patients can anticipate how treatment will proceed and give informed consent. Given that patients with PTSD are highly anxious, sharing a treatment template con-veys a level of organization, competence, and thoughtfulness regarding treatment that can reduce patients' anticipatory anxiety about treatment. Finally, you can compare the actual progression of treatment to the template. Treatment that proceeds smoothly pro-vides some additional evidence supporting your formulation and treatment plan. If you encounter obstacles, however, these may be early warning signs that you missed something in your formulation.

BUILDING THE FORMULATION WITH YOUR PATIENT AND INFORMED CONSENT

Therapy proceeds more smoothly when you and your patient agree on the formulation. Research also suggests that a shared formulation may decrease risk for dropout (Epperson, Bushway, & Warman, 1983; Pekarik & Stephenson, 1988). Finally, a shared formulation sets the stage for you to outline the different possible treatment ap-proaches, so that your patient consents to treatment as a truly informed individual. Several factors are crucial in the formulation and consent processes. First, consider any problems that your patient has with the formulation and validate your patient's per-spective. Second, when you are entertaining multiple hypotheses, if at all possible, in-form your patient about all of them and enlist his or her collaboration in building the formulation. Patients who collaborate in formulating and testing hypotheses often feel more in control of treatment decisions and are not surprised by decisions to redirect treatment if the initial hypotheses are not supported. Third, provide the patient with in-formation regarding alternative treatment approaches and relevant research, so that consent is in fact informed.

Despite endorsing nearly all symptoms of PTSD and scoring high on the CAPS, Sophie did not readily appreciate the relevance of the PTSD diagnosis for her present-ing complaints. Sophie's response to learning that she met criteria for PTSD demon-strates the difficulty that some patients have coming to terms with the diagnosis, and the potential challenge of building a shared conceptualization. Typically you will not find it helpful simply to reiterate arguments as to how a PTSD conceptualization accounts for the patients' symptoms. Rather, listen for the truth in the patients' view of their own problems, validate their confusion or discomfort with the PTSD model, and offer an approach that incorporates the patients' concerns. For example, Sophie's therapist said to her, "It's understandable that you feel confused by my discussion of PTSD. You've been telling me about how you are bothered by your anger outbursts and difficulty trusting people, and it's hard to see how these could be related to the bad things that happened such a long time ago."

Sophie agreed to a plan to help her feel "less like she was on an emotional roller coaster." The initial sessions targeted her stated primary complaints (i.e., paranoia, irritability, mood swings), using "integrated DBT" (Becker & Zayfert, 2001). The initial five sessions were designed to make progress on a goal that made sense to Sophie. These sessions also served to build trust in the therapist and increase Sophie's sense of control over the therapy process. The therapist explained this to Sophie by saying:

> "Given that you're not sure if you want to proceed with therapy, and you're not sure you can trust me in particular, these first few sessions will give you a chance to see if you think I can be helpful to you. I'll be sure to check in with you at the end of each session to see how you are feeling about our work together, and to make sure we're on track with where you want to go."

While teaching Sophie skills that would be important for general emotion regulation and for increasing her ability to engage in CBT, the therapist also sought to gradually educate Sophie about PTSD to eventually persuade her to engage with more direct PTSD treatment strategies.

Telling a patient that you intend to persuade him or her of something that they do not currently believe is not consistent with the aim of building trust in the therapy relationship. Thus, this covert goal of increasing Sophie's acceptance of the PTSD conceptualization and willingness to engage in PTSD treatment presented a dilemma for the therapist who wanted to establish an openly collaborative and trusting relationship with Sophie. It is best to be as frank and direct about this as possible. Thus, the therapist said to Sophie:

> "I realize that the diagnosis of PTSD has been confusing for you. I'm guessing you have a lot of questions, and there's probably a lot about it that doesn't feel right and still isn't making sense to you. It's kind of hard to know whether PTSD treatment is right for you if you don't really even know what PTSD is or how it comes about. It might be helpful if we plan to spend some of our session time going into things in a bit more detail and also answering your questions about PTSD. That way, you can figure out whether PTSD treatment makes sense for you at some point down the line. What do you think? Would you be willing to do this?"

This opened the door to plan sessions in which the therapist presented a nomothetic formulation of PTSD, with the aim of increasing Sophie's willingness to commit to PTSD treatment.

Morgan provides a good example of the multiple hypothesis issue. Rather than prematurely committing to a case formulation, Morgan's therapist openly discussed the different hypotheses. For example, she stated:

"Having reviewed everything that you have told me, I have two different hypotheses about what is going on here. What I would like to do is present both of them to you, tell you which one I think is more likely and how the treatments would differ, then get your opinion on all of this. How does that sound to you?"

Although there are likely multiple advantages to being up front about multiple hypotheses when they are generated, there is one major advantage: You will be less likely to become overcommitted to either hypothesis. Being up front encourages both you and the patient to proceed, in a scientific manner, gathering data as treatment proceeds to determine whether the treatment based on the hypothesis is working. If the hypothesis is not working, you and your patient can then review the evidence to see whether the treatment was not correctly implemented or whether the initial formulation was not correct. In the case of Morgan, additional information pointed toward the second hypothesis by the time she and her therapist chose to change the formulation.

We recommend that you be encouraging and up-front about the research supporting the proposed treatment plan and alternative paths. One of the advantages of relying on nomothetic models and treatments with empirical support is that we can provide research-based hope. We encourage you to be honest with your patients, however, about the fact that treatment is somewhat different for each patient, and that researchers have yet to study the type of individualized treatment they will be receiving. One way to explain this is to return to the compass metaphor. In other words, research has provided us with a very good compass regarding the direction in which we need to walk, but it has not yet carved a path around every tree and stream that we will encounter.

CONCLUSION

Nomothetic formulations of PTSD are the foundation of CBT for trauma survivors. Quite often, however, trauma survivors present with a constellation of problems that necessitate an idiographic formulation that integrates nomothetic formulations for other disorders as well. Our aim in this chapter was to offer some ideas and examples of how you might construct nomothetically based idiographic formulations and treatment plans in practice. In the rest of the book, we describe in detail the elements of PTSD treatment.

FOUR

Embarking on Treatment
Clearing the Path for Success

You face a number of challenges in implementing CBT for PTSD in clinical practice. One challenge, tailoring CBT for individual clients, is the focus of most of this book. Other challenges, however, also need to be addressed. For instance, establishing a trusting relationship, key to successful treatment, can be difficult to achieve with some patients with PTSD. You also need to allay any discomfort you feel about increasing your patients' distress, even temporarily. In addition, you face an array of decisions when treating patients with complicated PTSD, such as deciding whether a patient is ready to start exposure, and whether to start with exposure or cognitive restructuring. Finally, you may find that life problems or practical concerns (e.g., insurance limitations) raise potential barriers to treatment. In this chapter we consider these disparate issues that may arise when embarking on CBT for PTSD.

BECOMING A TEAM: THE THERAPEUTIC RELATIONSHIP

A strong therapeutic relationship is critical in CBT for PTSD. We have noticed that some trainees initially are so focused on the techniques of CBT that they forget the importance of the therapeutic relationship. When implementing CBT for PTSD, you are asking your patients to quickly make large changes by facing their past in a manner that is challenging. Your patients will be reluctant to attempt the tasks employed in CBT if they do not trust you.

For example, when Steve's therapist proposed exposure, he looked her directly in the eye and stated, "I wouldn't do this if anyone else asked me. You'll be there for me, right? I feel like I am jumping off a cliff. I need to know that you are going to be jumping with me." Steve's therapist responded that (metaphorically) she would be holding his hand as he jumped. After completing his first exposure session, Steve noted that the only reason he had been willing to try exposure was because of his profound trust in his therapist. We hear this frequently.

Similarly, a strong therapeutic relationship helps you to create a setting that is conducive to learning safety during exposure. For example, Julia was very reluctant to complete exposure. Her therapist encouraged Julia to proceed by gently saying, "Tell me exactly what happened." Later, while processing her brief thought that the therapist was "mean," Julia also noted, "Although I thought you were being mean, I *knew* you wouldn't ask me to do anything that wasn't for my own good; I also knew that if I said I really needed to stop, I could, and you would be there for me." Had Julia *not* trusted her therapist, her experience could have been markedly different, and she might have felt forced.

In many cases, a solid therapeutic relationship develops naturally during the psychoeducation phase of treatment (see Chapter 5) and strengthen during cognitive restructuring and exposure, as long as you employ good clinical skills. In other cases, however, you may find that your patients have profound problems with trust.

Maintaining a Nonjudgmental Stance

You may find it difficult to like some patients with PTSD. In working with other clinicians (e.g., psychiatrists, primary care physicians, or therapists who cover for us when we are on vacation), it has become clear to us that some clinicians really seem to dislike our patients! Embracing the least judgmental conceptualization of patient behavior is an important strategy for facilitating the therapeutic relationship and developing a positive view of your patients (Linehan, 1993a). To help us maintain a nonjudgmental stance, we rely on the biosocial model of emotion regulation problems (Linehan, 1993a), which proposes that emotion regulation difficulties develop as a result of an inborn biological vulnerability to emotional sensitivity coupled with an invalidating environment. Symptoms and dysfunctional behaviors are conceptualized as evidence that patients have inadequate skills to manage their emotional reactions.

It is very easy to conceptualize the behavior of PTSD patients in a judgmental manner. For example, Amy angrily stormed out of the waiting room, sobbing when her therapist was 60 seconds late for her appointment. Other clinicians who observed this behavior concluded that Amy was being deliberately manipulative, and that they would not want to deal with such a manipulative patient. Amy's therapist used the biosocial model to maintain a nonjudgmental stance. She interpreted this behavior as indicating that Amy felt invalidated or rejected when her therapist was late, and that she lacked the necessary skills to communicate her distress appropriately. The therapist also surmised that Amy's behavior indicated that she was a poor manipulator, because skilled manipulators usually accomplish their goals without appearing manipulative. This view reduced any frustration that Amy's therapist might have experienced. Difficult or "manipulative" behaviors become less annoying when they are conceptualized as unskilled attempts to meet valid needs. Thus, it is easier to continue liking your patients even when they behave in ways that might produce negative reactions.

Maintaining a nonjudgmental stance also may help you and your therapeutic relationship in the several other ways. First, you will be less frustrated by avoidance behaviors. Second, you will find it easier to tolerate objectionable features of your patients' histories, particularly those that they themselves seem to cause. Third, research indicates that a nonjudgmental stance may facilitate a reduction in parasuicidal urges (Shearin & Linehan, 1994).

Finally, maintaining a nonjudgmental stance reduces the risk of inadvertently *appearing* judgmental, which could exacerbate shame in your patients. Thus, you provide a safer environment to explore the function of your patients' behaviors. For example, Linda was raped after leaving a party with a group of men, because she was mad at her boyfriend, who was late. Maintaining a nonjudgmental stance allowed the therapist to help Linda process the rape and her behavior without appearing critical. Linda's therapist maintained this stance by viewing Linda's behavior as an unskilled attempt to manage the intense negative affect triggered by her boyfriend's behavior (temperamental vulnerability). She also hypothesized that Linda felt invalidated by her boyfriend's behavior. When viewed using the biosocial model, Linda's behavior becomes understandable, if not functional.

Using Validation to Build Trust and Reduce Misunderstandings

Validation is another DBT strategy that can be helpful in establishing and maintaining your therapeutic relationship, particularly with patients who have difficulty trusting others (Linehan, 1993a). Many patients with PTSD have experienced invalidating environments, as described in the biosocial model. As such, they often are exquisitely attuned to potential invalidation. Moreover, as Linehan points out, they may feel misunderstood if you ask them to make changes that seem unachievable. Validation involves communicating to your patients that their behaviors are completely understandable given their circumstances. More specifically, when you validate, you observe what is happening, reflect your observation, then note that your patient's response is understandable.

Validation occurs at some level in all good therapy. In DBT, however, validation is a core intervention (Linehan, 1993a). We have found that explicit use of validation, as promoted by Linehan, often preempts misunderstandings and fosters the trust needed in CBT for PTSD. For example, after Amy stormed out of the waiting room, the therapist telephoned her and noted, "It looks like I really upset you by being late" (i.e., observation and reflection). Amy angrily confirmed this and said that she always knew her therapist really did not care about her. Her therapist continued: "I obviously really upset you, and I can really understand why you would feel that way and think that I don't care" (i.e., communicating that Amy's response is understandable). Amy's therapist did not initially challenge Amy's interpretation by saying that she *did* care. Rather, she validated Amy's perspective, until it became clear that Amy had registered the validation. At that point, Amy noted that she could think of some reasons why her therapist might have legitimate reasons for being late, and that the phone call probably meant that her therapist did care. Amy then agreed to reschedule; subsequently, when her therapist was a bit late, Amy did not flee the waiting room.

ADDRESSING YOUR OWN ISSUES

A number of therapist factors may influence treatment. For example, if you fear that trauma-focused treatment will "retraumatize" your patients, you will be unlikely to use this approach. PTSD experts also have focused on the need for ongoing supervision and support for less experienced therapists (e.g., Foa, Zoellner, Feeny, Hembree, &

Alvarez-Conrad, 2002). Moving beyond issues of expertise, others have noted that successful implementation of CBT for PTSD requires that therapists both believe in the treatment (i.e., believe that the treatment will not harm your patients and have confidence that it will work) and tolerate intense arousal during treatment (Litz, Blake, Gerardi, & Keane, 1990). Below we provide information to help you address possible concerns that you may have about CBT for PTSD.

First Do No Harm: "Will CBT 'Retraumatize' My Patients?"

If you are like many clinicians, you may have concerns that CBT for PTSD could "retraumatize" some of your patients. Obviously, you will find it difficult to administer a treatment if you believe it poses substantial risk of harm. The term "retraumatization" is used to indicate that a patient experiences dramatic worsening of symptoms and deterioration of functioning, in this case, as a result of the treatment itself (Chu, 1998). A session may be considered "re"-traumatizing if recollections of a past traumatic event are elicited in a manner that continually escalates fear and helplessness rather than promote new learning about safety. The evidence for retraumatization in CBT is difficult to interpret, because CBT does sometimes result in a *temporary* increase in symptoms, even when it is proceeding well. For example, approximately 25% of patients experience a temporary increase in intrusive symptoms (e.g., nightmares, flashbacks) after starting exposure (Foa et al., 2002). Yet, research indicates that these patients benefit from exposure at rates similar to those of patients who do not experience this exacerbation.

Nonetheless, we know of patients who appear to have experienced a more profound and lasting negative reaction to trauma-focused treatment. For example, Harriet, a single, 50-year-old woman, was completing imaginal exposure to being raped. According to Harriet, she began flashing back and repeatedly "begged" to stop, but her therapist said she "needed to keep going." Harriet appeared not to have felt that she had a choice about continuing or stopping exposure, and she did not experience a sense of safety during exposure. She noted, "He said I had to keep going, and it was just like my rape. I was out of control." Within days of this session, Harriet began experiencing nightmares and stopped eating. Shortly thereafter, she experienced a complete relapse in a previously treated eating disorder. Harriet also began abusing alcohol and was unwilling to resume PTSD treatment, even after she switched therapists. We should note that the vast majority of patients who complete exposure in both research studies and clinical settings do so without experiencing long-term negative effects. Thus, we believe that when the treatment is delivered appropriately, the risk of retraumatization from CBT for PTSD is minimal.

Lasting negative reactions to trauma-focused therapy appear to happen when certain therapeutic conditions are absent. As we noted in Chapter 2, to benefit from exposure, patients must experience both activation of their fear network and a corrective experience of safety. Patients who experience prolonged negative reactions have failed to experience and integrate corrective information (i.e., safety) with regard to their traumatic memory. This appears to be what happened with Harriet. Conditions that appear to contribute to this failure are a lack of trust in the therapist and a sense of lack of control over the exposure process. In other words, if patients feel out of control during exposure (i.e., do not believe they have the choice to continue or stop on a moment-by-moment basis) or do not trust that their therapist truly has their best interests at heart, they are less likely to experience the corrective experience of safety and may be at risk for negative reactions.

In summary, patients may be reluctant to proceed with exposure based on their fear and may need significant encouragement to engage in exposure. They are less likely to have a corrective experience, however, if they feel out of control and do not trust you. Thus, you must strike a balance between encouraging them to proceed with exposure and making sure that the conditions necessary for a corrective experience of safety (i.e., real safety, control, and trust) are present. In our experience, when these conditions are present, patients are remarkably resilient in proceeding with exposure.

Confidence: A Vital Component of CBT for PTSD

Clinicians are trained to alleviate suffering, yet CBT for PTSD requires that you encourage patients to engage in a task that is inherently distressing. Unfortunately, patients tend to detect ambivalence and a lack of confidence, which may result in you and your patients colluding in avoiding difficult tasks. To implement CBT for PTSD you *must* be willing to push patients gently to face their traumatic events. You also need to tolerate the possibility that patients may sometimes *briefly* feel that you are being "mean."

For example, during imaginal exposure, the therapist encouraged Julia to describe her rape in detail as opposed to saying "Then he took off my panties and raped me." Crying, Julia stated, "I don't think I want to." The therapist validated this urge, saying "That's understandable," then gently asking, "Can you tell me exactly what happened?" Julia later noted that, at the time, she thought her therapist was being mean. She also thought, "I can't believe she is going to make me do this." Yet after exposure, Julia felt as if she had lost a "50-pound load" and was grateful that her therapist had "pushed me to do what I needed to do." Julia also appreciated learning that her therapist could know "every horrible detail" and still "look at me the same way and care about me." If the therapist had lacked confidence, Julia might have stopped and would not have benefited. She also might have lost trust and confidence in her therapist. In summary, CBT for PTSD requires that you firmly believe that short-term, aversive tasks result in long-term improvement in functioning, and that the long-term relief is worth the short-term pain.

Developing Confidence

You can develop confidence by seeking supervision from an experienced CBT therapist, attending continuing education workshops, and/or reviewing the literature. If you were trained originally in other approaches, you may not be accustomed to relying on the scientific literature for confidence. The research supporting CBT for PTSD, however, can be helpful. The first time one of us used exposure (C.B.B.), she had to tell herself over and over during the session, "The research says this works, the research says this works." Even after our years of experience, the research still helps us guide patients through the treatment.

Another powerful means of developing confidence is to experience successful outcomes when you use CBT with either yourself or your patients. Thus, consider trying out exposure and cognitive restructuring in your own life. Personal experience with exposure is particularly compelling and useful for developing confidence. For example, you can address common fears (e.g., fears of animals, heights, closed spaces, or public speaking) by implementing exposure on your own (following the procedures in Chapter 6) or with an experienced behavior therapist (you can locate one via the Association for Behavioral and Cognitive Therapies, www.abct.org). You also can discover the effects of exposure in situations that generate only moderate anxiety. For example, repeatedly riding the same roller coaster can demonstrate how physical sensations and anxiety decrease in response to repeated exposure. Some subways have very steep escalators, and many people feel anxious at first when they ride them. Riding these repeatedly also will demonstrate the effects of exposure firsthand.

Finally, you can increase your confidence by implementing exposure for a simpler anxiety disorder. Exposure therapy for panic disorder, specific phobia, and some cases of obsessive–compulsive disorder (OCD) involves concrete tasks that promote rapid anxiety reduction. These forms of exposure also are often more straightforward than those for PTSD, because the treated fears are clearly irrational. Thus, if you have never implemented exposure clinically, you may find that beginning with exposure for other disorders is easier and more comfortable.

Ability to Tolerate Arousal

CBT for PTSD also requires that you tolerate anxiety and other negative emotions. Obviously, the more confident you feel, the less anxiety you experience. Nonetheless, no treatment is 100% successful, which means that some of your patients may not benefit. Thus, at times, when you find yourself encouraging a patient to engage in exposure, you may feel anxious and wonder, "Is this going to work for this person?"

For example, you may feel anxious if you decide to use exposure with a patient who is not an ideal candidate, but for whom there are no other good treatment options. For instance, as a child, Steve had been sexually assaulted by his babysitter. After extensive psychodynamic therapy and many trials of medication, he was referred for CBT as a last resort. Steve was highly suicidal, very hostile, and kept two loaded revolvers under his pillow. Steve refused to give up his revolvers permanently, and his suicidality and depression failed to respond to new medications or CBT for depression. Steve's therapist and his psychiatrist decided that because nothing else had worked, there seemed to be little reason to not try exposure, as long as safety precautions were taken. For example, Steve agreed to give the revolvers to a friend for 1 week, though he was unwilling to give them up longer. His psychiatrist also made sure she was available to admit Steve to the hospital if his suicidality escalated. During the first exposure session, Steve's experienced therapist felt significant anxiety and urges to avoid using exposure.

Steve benefited tremendously from his first exposure session, and subsequent sessions were much less anxiety provoking for the therapist. This example, however, highlights the reality that exposure may require you to confront your own anxiety. Exposure also may require you to tolerate other negative emotions that can be triggered by particularly horrific events. For example, in listening to Kelly describe an exceedingly brutal gang rape in detail, her therapist experienced horror and profound sadness. The therapist later processed his own experience of listening to Kelly's experience in confidential consultation with another trauma therapist.

"I FEEL CONFIDENT: WHICH TECHNIQUES SHOULD I USE?"

To a large degree, your decision to employ certain CBT techniques will be guided by your case formulation. At times, however, you may be unsure about whether to start with cognitive restructuring or exposure, or whether your patient is a good candidate for either intervention. This section addresses these treatment issues.

"Is My Patient Ready for Exposure?"

We believe that exposure is vastly underutilized and that its deployment is often postponed much longer than is ideal. Patients with PTSD regularly relive their traumatic experiences in an uncontrollable manner, and exposure offers them a very good chance at recovery, often surprisingly quickly. At the same time, patients with PTSD often present with an array of complicating factors that understandably raise concerns. At present, clear empirical guidelines are not available regarding which patients at what point in therapy should start exposure for PTSD, and no consensus has emerged regarding clinical guidelines (Frueh, Mirabella, & Turner, 1995; Litz et al., 1990). Thus, decisions regarding exposure require that you balance competing concerns.

When PTSD is the principal diagnosis, begin by assuming that exposure is the most efficient and rapid avenue to symptom relief, and that it should be implemented as quickly as possible. Determination of "as quickly as possible" involves consideration of several other factors beyond the primacy of PTSD, including safety, willingness, and ability. You will begin to assess these factors at the start of treatment and continue to evaluate them throughout treatment. For example, after initially determining that a patient seems to be a good candidate for exposure, you may reassess that patient's ability to complete exposure if things do not go according to plan. Also, you typically can assess willingness only after you have presented your case for exposure (see Chapters 5, 6, and 7).

Safety

Suicidality, aggression/homicidality, substance abuse, food restriction, self-injury, and impulsive or reckless behaviors (e.g., reckless driving) are examples of behaviors that can pose a danger to your patients or others. Whenever a patient with PTSD reports a history of such behaviors, formulate a plan for managing these behaviors. The plan might include referral for other treatment or a temporary focus on establishing safety. For example, Bill reported that he was using cocaine nightly, and assessment revealed that he met criteria for substance dependence. Given the risks involved with cocaine dependence and the possibility that the cocaine use might prevent Bill from benefiting from PTSD treatment, the therapist referred Bill for detoxification and substance abuse treatment before proceeding with CBT for PTSD. Amalia reported frequent anger outbursts during which she threw dangerous objects such as knives, scissors, or pans at others; her therapist decided that this presented an unacceptable level of risk and postponed trauma-focused therapy in favor of teaching Amalia anger management skills. Alternatively, the plan might involve monitoring the dangerous behavior during treatment or creating a plan to increase safety (e.g., having Steve give his guns to his friend). In such cases, exposure might proceed relatively quickly. Li Ming was noticeably underweight and admitted to previous extreme low weight (40 pounds below normal adult weight). Her therapist agreed to proceed with PTSD treatment after Li Ming agreed to monitor food intake and body weight. Likewise, Becky had a history of suicide attempts but had not been suicidal in quite some time. Given her history of prior suicide attempts and of increasing suicidality during periods of high stress, Becky and her therapist decided to proceed with exposure while implementing daily monitoring of suicidal urges during treatment.

In some cases, the threats to patients may be from others. Assessing the validity and imminence of such threats can be difficult, because patients with PTSD, given the nature of the disorder, are biased toward perceiving threat. For example, Kendra reported remaining watchful and on guard for her ex-husband, who had physically abused her until their divorce. She stated that she saw him around town and felt threatened by him. Careful questioning revealed that Kendra had never actually seen him, but she had seen vehicles that looked like his. In fact, Kendra was not certain of his actual whereabouts or whether he was a threat. Similarly, Pamela reported that her ex-husband, the perpetrator of 25 years of physical abuse, continued to drive by her house and make his presence known to her. Although she was certain of his identity, she also noted that he had not violated the distance limits set by their divorce decree, had not made a threat in 3 years, and in fact was now married to another woman. In both cases, the women's therapists opted to proceed with treatment while continuing to assess threats periodically.

Conversely, however, some patients with PTSD underestimate or disregard threat. For example, Gregory continued to visit his mother weekly despite his stepfather's periodic assaults that left him bruised and bleeding. His therapist focused on helping Gregory problem-solve options for maintaining a relationship with his mother, without tolerating being battered by his stepfather.

When deciding how to proceed, consider the recency of the behavior, the level of threat, and the conditions under which the behavior tends to increase. CBT for PTSD often will need to be postponed until the risk posed by very dangerous behaviors is no longer imminent. However, "often" does not mean "always." For example, significant suicidality typically is considered a contraindication for exposure. But, as noted earlier in Steve's case, the therapist successfully implemented exposure after arranging several safety precautions. Similarly, Lucy reported that she regularly scratched herself to the point of drawing blood. Her therapist determined that this behavior did not pose imminent risk of serious harm, and was related to her PTSD. Thus, treating the PTSD would likely reduce the self-injurious behavior. The therapist decided to proceed with CBT for PTSD while monitoring the scratching behavior, and to address the scratching behavior in the course of treatment.

Willingness

Patients with PTSD seek treatment for many reasons; often, PTSD is not among them. For many individuals, a conceptualization that links their presenting complaint to the trauma is unexpected and discomforting. Such patients may not be willing to embark on trauma-focused treatment, particularly if they feel that they have dealt with the event successfully, or if they fear that exposure might disrupt the tenuous level of functional stability they have achieved. It may take some time for such patients to be willing to proceed with exposure.

Some patients may become unwilling to engage in exposure if they experience an increase in symptoms with exposure. They also may dropout if they believe that you will disapprove of their decision, or that there are no other treatment options. For example, after her first exposure session, Emma stated, "I can't continue this—I can't go back to how I was 10 years ago. My husband and I discussed it, and I realize I can't risk it." For such patients, it is important first to validate fears about disrupting functioning. Next, remind patients that an increase in symptoms in the beginning of treatment does not predict outcome. Finally, communicate to patients that they have control over treatment decision making. Some patients find it helpful to weigh the pros and cons of exposure treatment (see "Decision Analysis" in Chapter 9). During this process, strike a balance between reminding patients that their chances of benefiting are good, and acknowledging that you cannot predict with certainty what will happen. The only way to find out is to try. In our experience, when validation is balanced with honest education about treatment options, patients feel supported and in control of their treatment decisions. In response, they often are willing to proceed with treatment, and do not feel coerced.

Patients who continue to hope that they can fix their PTSD without having to think about the traumatic event may be unwilling to think about what happened, or may engage in well-rehearsed dissociative responses that, although apparently automatic, are nonetheless a form of unwillingness. For example, when prompted to begin imaginal exposure to her abuse memory, Isabella typically began shaking her leg, staring unblinkingly, and slowing her speech to the point of being almost nonresponsive. When discussing her reactions to the exposure task, she described herself as deciding to "blank out." For such patients, willingness to contemplate the event may involve not only reaching a decision to engage willingly in exposure but also effortful practice at experiencing the memories, emotions, thoughts, and sensations that accompany the memories (i.e., patient ability; see below).

It is easy to miss dissociative behaviors, because patients may be skilled at disguising them. For example, patients may appear to be fully engaged in a discussion, yet have no recollection of it the next day, which indicates that they were probably dissociating at the time of the discussion. You may not be able to detect dissociation in such patients until you get to know them well enough to recognize subtle changes in affect, lack of responsiveness to humor, or flattened facial expression that may signal its occurrence. Even when you detect such dissociation, however, you may find that once it has begun, there is little you can do to stop it. Efforts to prevent dissociation by teaching your patient to maintain present awareness often are more successful than interrupting a dissociative episode once it has begun.

Other behaviors also may indicate a lack of willingness to engage in exposure. For example, unwilling patients may drop out of treatment or attempt to persuade you that therapy will not work. Patients with PTSD often have difficulty believing that anxiety will decrease as a result of treatment—no matter how logical the rationale. Many patients believe that approaching trauma memories and stimuli will make matters worse. Thus, they may try to convince you that discontinuing their avoidance is ludicrous and dangerous. This behavior suggests that patients have not fully accepted the rationale.

In some instances, shame may underlie unwillingness. Patients who believe that their trauma is very shameful fear losing the relationship with you as it becomes more important to them. In such cases, as the therapeutic alliance strengthens, your patients paradoxically appear less, rather than more, willing to engage in trauma-focused interventions.

Addressing willingness involves two steps. First, you need to assess willingness, which may be a matter of simply asking patients, "Are you willing to do this?" In other words, given the available information, and their personal goals, are they (1) persuaded that exposure will work for them to achieve their goals and (2) willing to experience intense emotions for the promise of eventual symptom relief. As highlighted earlier, however, unwillingness also may require additional assessment (e.g., to determine that shame is driving the unwillingness).

If you determine that a patient is unwilling to try exposure, begin by revisiting the rationale for exposure. Your patient may have misunderstood the rationale, failed to retain it, or may have unanswered questions. Second, you may want to explore patients' concerns about lack of control over the exposure process or fear that you will "force" them to complete exposure. Third, if you suspect that shame may underlie unwillingness, you may find it useful to introduce cognitive restructuring first (see Chapter 8). This enables you to address thoughts underlying shame and thoughts about the consequences of disclosure that may inhibit patients' willingness to do exposure. In addition, you may explore the pros and cons of engaging in exposure (see "Decision Analysis" in Chapter 9).

Increasing a patient's control over exposure is another useful strategy to increase willingness. As with any therapy task, exposure must be conducted voluntarily, and you need to alleviate any of your patient's concerns that "you will force me to think about it." Voluntary participation in exposure is both ethical and practical, because control over exposure may be important for its success. For instance, one perspective regarding why exposure works (Mineka & Thomas, 1999) holds that anxiety reduction during exposure largely is due to increased perceptions of control. Also, as discussed in Chapter 2, theories of PTSD implicate loss of control over threat in the etiology of PTSD. Studies have not examined the role of patient control among individuals with PTSD. Several studies, however, have demonstrated its value in treatment of specific phobias and OCD. For example, two studies found that self-controlled exposure was superior to therapist-controlled exposure for specific phobias (Hepner & Cauthen, 1975) and OCD (Emmelkamp & Kraanen, 1977).

> Exposure therapy can of course be given only to sufferers who are willing to carry it out.
>
> —MARKS (1987, p. 458)

The prominent role of perceived loss of control in PTSD highlights the importance of increasing patients' sense of control over their lives. It follows that a therapy intervention will be counterproductive if patients do not believe that they have control of it. Indeed, as noted earlier, feeling out of control of exposure may be a risk factor for a negative reaction. Therefore, we suggest offering patients as much opportunity to control the therapy process as possible. For example, we explicitly remind patients that exposure is completely voluntary. When Julie reported anxiety about starting exposure, her therapist stated, "Don't forget, you have control over this. I can't and won't make you do exposure. This is your choice and under your control." Julie responded, "You're right. I think I can do this, though. I think I need to do this."

Patient Ability

At times, patients are willing to try exposure but seem to lack the skills needed to successfully complete it. Patients who lack the skills to experience and attend to anxiety, to the exclusion of other emotions, rarely do well with exposure. Yet they may be able to continue with exposure successfully after developing mindfulness skills, as provided in DBT (Linehan, 1993a). Mindfulness involves attending to present experiences, including emotion states. Mindfulness skills can therefore facilitate the engagement with anxiety necessary for successful exposure. We discuss the skills involved in exposure in greater depth in Chapters 6 and 7.

"Should We Start with Exposure or Cognitive Restructuring?"

Once you have decided to use exposure, you need to decide whether to start with exposure or cognitive restructuring. Typically, we start with exposure, unless there is good reason to do otherwise. The most common reason to start with cognitive restructuring is if your assessment indicates that your patient is experiencing strong feelings of guilt and/or shame in relation to the traumatic event. These feelings might impede willingness to engage in exposure, or they might interfere with habituation during exposure and result in diminished benefit for your patient (discussed in greater detail later in Chapter 8).

If you plan to include exposure and cognitive restructuring simultaneously throughout treatment, it also may make sense to initiate cognitive restructuring first, because thoughts that emerge during exposure sometimes are not addressed by exposure alone. In such cases, you use cognitive restructuring to address these thoughts immediately following an exposure, if your patient has already learned the skill.

For example, Carlos, a survivor of childhood sexual abuse, expressed a great deal of shame about the abuse during the evaluation and scored high the Trauma-Related Guilt Inventory (Kubany et al., 1996). Anticipating a prominent role for cognitive restructuring in his treatment, the therapist taught Carlos cognitive restructuring immediately following psychoeducation. Initially, Carlos challenged fearful thoughts such as "It's not safe to be home alone," and hopeless thoughts such as "I'm never going to feel good." Subsequently, Carlos's therapist noted that thoughts related to shame and guilt were expressed during imaginal exposure. For example, Carlos said, 'I let it happen, so I was a collaborator" and "It means I'm gay—I'm less of a man." Following a 60-minute exposure, the therapist was able to segue immediately into cognitive restructuring, and Carlos made significant progress challenging the first thought in the remaining 15 minutes in the session. Thus, when you are fairly certain that you need to use cognitive restructuring, it often makes sense to teach the skill in advance, so that it may be deployed when needed.

Another reason you might introduce cognitive restructuring prior to exposure relates to comorbidity (particularly depression) and/or safety concerns. For example, if your patient exhibits very severe depression accompanied by suicidal ideation and low functioning but does not require hospitalization, you may opt to spend a discrete period focusing on depression, and building momentum and trust before focusing more directly on PTSD. Cognitive restructuring is an empirically supported intervention for depression, so it makes sense to use it in this instance. This might include other cognitive-behavioral interventions for depression, such as activity scheduling (see Persons et al., 2001) or problem solving (see Chapter 9).

Typically, this phase of treatment is very brief (two to four sessions) and focuses on increasing functional activity and elevating hope about the potential of CBT for PTSD to reduce suffering. Consider moving forward to exposure as soon as you detect increasing hope and a modest improvement in functioning, rather than waiting for depression to resolve fully. This is unlikely without focused PTSD treatment. If improvement is not achieved quickly, a higher level of intervention, such as a partial hospital program, may be necessary. Also, if your patient's depression has clear links to life issues beyond PTSD, such as a failing marriage, chronic pain, or family problems, or if depression is the principal diagnosis (see Chapter 3), then it may be necessary to focus your initial treatment plan on improving mood. After a full course of treatment for depression, reevaluate PTSD and determine whether CBT for PTSD is still indicated.

Cognitive restructuring may also be helpful in enacting behavior changes that might increase physical safety or reduce anger. For example, Gloria's trauma symptoms were related to the loss of her husband on 9/11 and childhood physical abuse by her stepmother. Yet the therapist was reluctant to start with exposure, because Gloria was engaging in cutting that followed her frequent contact with her elderly, emotionally abusive father. The therapist used cognitive restructuring to address Gloria's thoughts that she was obligated to take care of her father in old age. As a result, Gloria decreased contact with her father, and her urges to cut also rapidly declined. Similarly, Nihla, who was sexually abused by her cousin, continued to have regular contact with him at family functions and via telephone, even though he was often subtly sexually suggestive during these encounters. These contacts fueled Nihla's anger, so her therapist began by addressing Nihla's thoughts that she was obligated to maintain a relationship with her cousin. Subsequent interventions also targeted anger.

Finally, the decision to introduce cognitive restructuring first also relates to practical issues of timing. If you are beginning treatment with a new patient right before you leave for vacation, then this might not be a good time to start exposure. Thus, you might decide to introduce cognitive restructuring during the few weeks before you leave. This ensures that you will be available to monitor your patient during the first weeks of exposure, and it also maintains active therapy tasks during the interim. Although postponing the start of therapy until after your return is also an option, the gap may increase risk of dropout.

There are also instances in which cognitive restructuring may be unwise. For example, patients with obvious cognitive limitations often have great difficulty engaging productively in formal cognitive restructuring. You may also encounter this in patients with no apparent cognitive deficits at the outset. If you have clear information that your patient has cognitive limitations (e.g., a history of traumatic brain injury, developmental disability, or dementia), consider moving directly to exposure, even when other indications for cognitive restructuring are present.

"Should We Start with *In Vivo* or Imaginal Exposure?"

There are good reasons to start with *in vivo* exposure in many cases. It often is easier for patients to maintain their focus of attention on the concrete, observable stimuli of *in vivo* exposure compared to the abstract exposure stimuli (i.e., memories in their mind) of imaginal exposure. Memories also are typically more complex than *in vivo* exposure stimuli. As such, an *in vivo* exposure stimulus can be easier to attend to for an extended period than a memory, and *in vivo* exposure can result in rapid fear reduction, often in 30 minutes or less. Attaining rapid reduction in fear is more immediately reinforcing to the many patients who are leery of beginning exposure.

Starting with *in vivo* exposure has the added advantage of providing you with important information before embarking on imaginal exposure. From the first *in vivo* exposure homework assignment, you learn to what extent your patients are willing and able to do exposure exercises independently, whether they understand and comply with the task and record keeping instructions, and how rapidly their anxiety diminishes. You should use this important information to guide planning of treatment activities. Disregarding such observations could jeopardize the therapeutic alliance and/or patients' commitment to treatment activities and potentially result in diminishing treatment adherence and/or dropout. For example, if a patient does not carry out the *in vivo* exposure assignment, then this may forebode poor adherence when imaginal exposure homework is added to the assignment.

MANAGING PRACTICAL CONCERNS AND SYSTEMIC BARRIERS

Session Length and Frequency

Unfortunately, mental health delivery systems are sometimes not well adapted to CBT for PTSD. Nonetheless, whenever possible, we advocate implementing CBT in a manner that stays as true to the research as possible. Thus, we recommend that you use 90-minute sessions, if possible (i.e., you can obtain reimbursement), because CBT for PTSD often is delivered in 90- or 120-minute sessions in research trials (Bryant et al., 2003; Foa et al., 1991, 1999; Paunovic & Ost, 2001; Resick et al., 2002).

Similarly, consider using twice weekly sessions, if indicated and feasible. A number of researchers administer CBT for PTSD over a shorter time period by using twice weekly sessions (Foa et al., 1991, 1999). Although it is unclear whether twice weekly sessions improve outcome in PTSD treatment, CBT researchers in other areas (e.g., eating disorders and depression) advocate twice weekly sessions at the start of treatment to encourage early momentum (Fairburn, Bohn, & Hutt, 2004). Moreover, even when your plan is for weekly sessions, some PTSD patients may benefit from biweekly sessions during the difficult phases of treatment. For example, if a patient is struggling with exposure, then you may decide to move to a biweekly schedule. Similarly, with a patient facing a crisis, you may be able to continue with exposure by meeting biweekly, one time per week for exposure and once to manage the crisis.

If you are in private practice and rely on third-party reimbursement, however, you may find such recommendations problematic. Many third-party payers refuse payment or construct time-consuming approval procedures for longer or more frequent sessions.

Thus, right from the start, you may face barriers that prevent you from implementing evidence-based CBT methods.

We advocate expending the effort needed to get past these hurdles, because CBT for PTSD can dramatically reduce your patients' suffering. In other words, do not give up. Systems barriers usually can be managed with some creativity. For example, exposure sessions often can be reduced to 50 minutes after your patient has experienced a reduction in anxiety during the first session or two. Also, some benefit plans permit either longer or more frequent sessions, though they may not permit both. Thus, some patients can be scheduled twice per week for 50 minutes during early exposure sessions.

Fortunately, insurance companies are becoming familiar with empirically supported treatment guidelines. In such instances, showing that you are familiar with the research literature and speaking intelligently about CBT helps establish your clinical competency, which facilitates authorization. If faced with care managers who are not familiar with CBT for PTSD, you may find it helpful to initiate a discussion of the research supporting CBT. This might include faxing the care manager a list of references supporting the efficacy of CBT for PTSD (see Chapter 1), offering also to fax copies of some of the original research reports, and inviting the care manager to share research on alternative treatments that the insurance company would like you to use. Do not be afraid to use the research literature to advocate for your patients. The literature supporting CBT for PTSD is substantial, and good outcome reduces long-term costs. Also, most reviewers will accept your point rather than have their fax machine tied up with page after page of original research reports.

In addition to other limitations, many plans restrict the number of sessions per year, a potential problem for any form of therapy. If you fear that premature termination will leave your patient in a state of elevated distress, however, you may be reluctant to start trauma-focused therapy. This is understandable, and you will undoubtedly see some cases in which it does not make sense to start exposure when therapy is limited (e.g., in some patients with severe suicidal ideation). Yet a surprising array of patients can benefit by moving forward with CBT, which was designed to be short-term. Many patients experience considerable benefit from just a few sessions of exposure and/or cognitive restructuring. When all else fails, you can delay treatment to the later quarter of the year, which reduces the effect of yearly benefit limitations. Finally, some governments have enacted mental health parity laws that prohibit limitations of health care benefits for specific mental disorders, such as PTSD. Under such laws, session limitations often are not permitted. You should familiarize yourself with the mental health parity laws in the jurisdiction in which you practice. There may be times when you need to remind the care manager tactfully about the law.

Inadequate Support

One systems issue with which you may struggle is inadequate support for treating challenging patients. Many patients with PTSD experience a significant number of crises during treatment, including suicidality, interpersonal disputes, and financial and legal problems. Moreover, borderline symptoms are not uncommon, even among patients with PTSD who do not meet full criteria for borderline personality disorder

(BPD). For example, patients with PTSD may engage in stressful behaviors (e.g., self-injurious behavior) and reinforce you for conducting ineffective therapy (e.g., by reinforcing you for avoiding trauma-focused treatment; Linehan, 1993a, p. 425). In summary, treating a large, or even moderate, number of these patients can be challenging.

Trauma-focused therapy also requires you to listen to horrible events in graphic detail, over and over again. Although you adjust to this, listening to a different type of event, a particularly horrific event, or one that reminds you of personal experiences, may periodically leave you feeling somewhat overwhelmed, even if you are very experienced.

In outlining treatment for BPD, Linehan (1993a) emphasizes the need for ongoing supervision and consultation. As noted earlier, therapists who treat PTSD and those who treat BPD encounter similar stressors. Thus, Linehan's advice seems relevant for PTSD therapists. Peer consultation can help to boost morale, provide alternative perspectives when therapy seems stuck, and provide a safe, confidential setting for processing your own reactions. If you are in solo private practice, consider setting up a consultation group with other therapists who regularly treat PTSD, ideally using CBT or other trauma-focused therapies. If you are implementing CBT, you will likely find it less helpful to participate in a consultation group with therapists who are reluctant to address their patients' trauma histories directly.

CONCLUSION

When you embark on CBT with a patient with complicated PTSD, you need to consider a wide range of disparate issues. We have attempted to provide guidance in addressing some of these challenges. Ultimately, your effectiveness in treating PTSD depends on your ability to balance the structure and tasks of CBT, and respond to the individual needs of your patient.

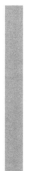

FIVE

Psychoeducation

Kate is a 50-year-old woman with a history of multiple traumatic events. As a child she witnessed her brother being beaten by her father. As an adult, Kate was physically abused by her first husband, who threatened to shoot her on numerous occasions. Three years after she divorced him, Kate began dating Mark, whom she married 3 years later. While on their honeymoon, Mark began to abuse Kate physically and sexually. Feeling defeated, Kate concluded that being abused was her "lot in life." She remained married to Mark for 10 years, often enduring daily physical and/or sexual abuse. Finally, with the help of the battered women's shelter, Kate left Mark and filed for divorce. At intake, Kate displayed a pronounced startle response and reported extreme anxiety about the assessment. She stated that a previous therapist had told her that she needed treatment for PTSD, but that it had taken her over 6 months to summon the courage to seek specialized treatment. Kate had limited contact with her adult children, who had withdrawn from her during her second marriage. She also had virtually no social life and felt depressed much of the time. She experienced panic attacks on a regular basis. A typical day consisted of going to work, where she struggled to concentrate and manage flashbacks and intrusive memories, then returning home. She spent most evenings hugging her small dog and listening for noises outside of her apartment, because she was afraid that Mark was stalking her. Kate's divorce was still pending, and she had few financial resources or personal items, because she had left behind almost all of her belongings when she separated from Mark. Moreover, she was too fearful of him to fight for her possessions or money. At the same time, having left her first husband without much more than the clothes on her back, she felt depressed about having to "start over once again" and berated herself for being "chicken and a loser." Kate also believed that she was going "crazy," and that her PTSD symptoms justified this interpretation of herself.

RATIONALE AND BACKGROUND

Psychoeducation serves several important functions in CBT. To start, by sharing information about PTSD, you begin to shape patients' expectations about the therapy process, making treatment more predictable and less anxiety provoking. In addition, patients often have expectations about therapy that may or may not accurately match up with CBT. For example, patients may expect therapy to focus on developing insights rather than on developing new skills. They also may expect to feel soothed and relaxed during therapy sessions, and not expect therapy to involve any discomfort.

Demonstrating to trauma survivors that you understand what they are experiencing also builds patients' trust in you and the treatment, which is essential to treatment success. Finally, by providing a clear and coherent treatment rationale, you help patients to become educated collaborators in their own treatment and reduce the hierarchical differential between you and your patients. Thus, you prepare patients to act collaboratively and to be more active participants in the change process.

In addition, psychoeducation imparts important information that lays the groundwork for reprocessing traumatic memories. The information presented in psychoeducation helps patients understand that their reactions to traumatic event(s) are normal, and that there are logical explanations for why their symptoms persist. Patients find this reassuring. They also are reassured to learn that there are logical, although sometimes counterintuitive, strategies for altering their symptoms. In fact, normalizing reactions to trauma is a cognitive intervention that challenges distressing thoughts about the meaning of PTSD symptoms and the possibility for change (e.g., "My reactions mean I am going crazy" or "This is hopeless; I will never get better"). Quite often patients immediately use new information to shift their interpretations, resulting in an immediate decrease in suffering. For example, after learning that her vigilance was part of a natural reaction to having survived a life-threatening situation, Kate remarked, "So, I'm not going crazy!" The information presented in psychoeducation also facilitates formal cognitive restructuring later in treatment.

Our approach to psychoeducation uses metaphor and Socratic questioning to convey material from various sources on anxiety treatment (Foa & Rothbaum, 1998; Rothbaum & Foa, 1999; Barlow & Craske, 2000). Psychoeducation covers two main areas: a brief orientation to CBT (i.e., an overview of the treatment components) and a discussion of common reactions among trauma survivors. Typically, you present a brief overview of CBT before discussing common reactions. It is appropriate to present common reactions first, however, to patients who have not decided to do PTSD treatment. Psychoeducation helps you build a persuasive case, or rationale, for exposure and cognitive restructuring, which helps to quell the understandable anxiety that patients experience. In this chapter we provide detailed information about implementing the main components of psychoeducation. You build upon this by providing a more explicit rationale for exposure and cognitive restructuring as each is introduced. This book includes additional specific suggestions for enhancing the rationale for exposure (Chapters 6 and 7) and for cognitive restructuring (Chapter 8).

ORIENTATION TO CBT

Introducing patients to CBT does not need to take a long time. Often a simple description, such as the one below, suffices. In this example, the therapist briefly describes both exposure and cognitive restructuring. Based on your case formulation, you may decide to proceed with one of these interventions initially, in which case, it may only be necessary to discuss that intervention at the outset.

Case Example: Kate

Note. Additional commentary on what the therapist is trying to achieve at each point is indicated by bracketed, italicized material.

THERAPIST: Kate, let's talk a bit about what you can expect in treatment.

KATE: OK.

THERAPIST: The goal of treatment is for you to learn new skills to cope with fear, anxiety, and other forms of distress related to your traumatic experiences, so that you can live more easily and more happily.

KATE: (*Nods.*)

THERAPIST: You can expect a few things throughout treatment. First, I always like to emphasize that we are going to approach this problem as a team. We both bring a certain amount of expertise to this problem, and we will solve it most effectively by working together as a team. I know something about PTSD and strategies and skills for reducing symptoms. You know you. No one else has the same level of expertise when it come to who you are and your own reactions. So, basically, we are in this together, and it is going to take active work on both of our parts to change things for you.

KATE: OK, that makes sense.

THERAPIST: Second, treatment extends beyond the time you will spend with me in this office. Homework is an essential part of this treatment. Some homework tasks involve activities to be done throughout the day, such as monitoring your responses to upsetting situations. Others will require you to set aside time to carry out a task or practice a skill. Daily practice of the skills is necessary to benefit from treatment. Our goal is to help you feel better as quickly as possible, and using time outside of session really helps move us forward toward our goal. Thinking back on what we just went over, does this make sense to you? Do you have any questions?

KATE: That makes sense. I don't think I have any questions.

THERAPIST: OK, now let's talk about some of the specific skills and strategies we will focus on during treatment. Our first task will be to teach you about the ways that most people respond to traumatic experiences. In particular, you will learn that PTSD symptoms are learned reactions that can be unlearned. The remainder of the treatment program involves teaching you ways to change these learned responses. This will probably make more sense once we get started, but do you have any questions so far?

KATE: (*Shakes head.*)

THERAPIST: Treatment also typically involves learning to identify and then challenge, or change, thoughts that contribute to distress. We often refer to this skill as "cognitive restructuring." You will learn to pay attention to what you are thinking in order to become more aware of thoughts that lead to distress. Then you will learn to recognize patterns in your thinking that contribute to distressing feelings. You also will learn ways to challenge your thought patterns and "talk back" to them in a way that can reduce your distress. Now, you may have been told by others to think "positively," and what I just described may sound a bit like that. So, if that is the case, let me reassure you that we are not going to adopt a "Pollyannaish" approach here. Instead, cognitive restructuring helps you systematically change the way you think in a very meaningful way. Cognitive restructuring acts with other strategies to help you rework the traumatic experience in your mind, so that you will be less distressed by it. This will make more sense once we start, but do you have any questions so far?

KATE: No, I think I am following.

THERAPIST: In addition, we will use a strategy called "exposure" that has been found to be very helpful in reducing fear and avoidance related to traumatic experiences. Two kinds of exposure are typically included in treatment for PTSD. Before I explain these, though, if you don't mind, I am going to stop for a minute and ask you a question. I think you will see why in just a second or two. Do you have any pets?

KATE: Yes, I have a little lap dog. I don't know what I would do without him.

THERAPIST: Wonderful. So let's imagine that I am afraid of dogs, but I really need to get over this fear because I am going to stay with a friend next month who has a dog. How would you help me get over my fear?

KATE: I don't know. I guess I would tell you to spend time with a dog—a little, friendly dog on a leash, to start. If you spend time with a little, friendly dog like my Charlie, you will see that dogs are not so scary. Then you could move to a bigger dog. But only when you are ready.

[*Commentary: The therapist lets Kate describe exposure instead of telling her about it. This strategy increases patient engagement and makes the process more collaborative.*]

THERAPIST: Great! We actually have a name for just what you described. We call that *in vivo* exposure, which basically means "live exposure." *In vivo* exposure involves carefully structured exposure to real-life situations that you have been avoiding in order to reduce fears related to traumatic events. So, just like you would help me approach a little dog, then a bigger dog, I will help you approach situations that you have avoided because they remind you of the trauma, but which you know will not hurt you.

We also will use a second type of exposure called imaginal exposure. Now, have you ever watched a movie with a complicated, twisty plot? For example, maybe a movie where you couldn't quite make sense out of what had happened during the movie. You may have found yourself thinking about the movie for quite period of time after the movie ended, and you may even have dreamed about the movie.

KATE: I can remember a few movies like that.

THERAPIST: Good. Let's think about what might be going on after you see a movie like that. It's almost as if your brain needs to make sense of what you see during the movie, to the point that it can't let go until all the pieces fit together. So we might say your brain needs to process the movie, to put all the pieces together and make sense of the experience.

KATE: (*Nods.*) That makes sense. It's like I can't stop thinking about it until it all fits together.

THERAPIST: Exactly. And, in many ways, traumatic experiences are a bit like a really complicated movie. Our brains need to make sense, or process, traumatic memories. Only it is hard to process these memories, because, for the most part, we want to avoid these memories. What happens when you suddenly have memories of your traumatic experiences? What do you do?

KATE: I try to shove them out of my mind.

THERAPIST: And that makes complete sense! It makes sense that you don't want to think about your memories. What do you think would happen, though, after a complicated movie if you kept shoving the movie out of your mind?

KATE: I don't know. I guess my mind couldn't make sense of it, if I kept pushing it away.

THERAPIST: Exactly, we have to give our minds some time to process the movie, and the same is true of traumatic experiences. And when we shove the memories away, our brain doesn't get a chance to do what it needs to do. That is the rationale behind imaginal exposure. Imaginal exposure involves recalling your traumatic memories repeatedly for an extended period of time. The goal of this treatment is to help you process the memories connected with the trauma and reduce your anxiety about the memories. Staying with these memories rather than avoiding them may be very distressing at first. That is a normal reaction to those abnormal and hurtful events. But over time, this therapy will help decrease the anxiety and fear associated with the memories. It will help you unlearn the anxiety response that you developed as a result of traumatic experiences.

The basic points you communicate to your patient are quite simple. A few points, however, are worth mentioning. First, one of the most critical aspects of psychoeducation is that it make sense to patients in terms of their own ways of understanding the world. Your job is to truly teach the information to your patients and to confirm that they understand. One observation that we have made in supervising new CBT therapists is that the need to communicate content in CBT appears to distract some therapists from practicing their "nonspecific" therapy skills. For example, when supervising one psychiatric resident, we discovered that she had quickly, yet superficially, reviewed the information with her patient and told her patient to take the readings home to make sure she "got it." The resident later stated, "That was really easy, quick, and boring." Not surprisingly, the patient came back to the next session saying she had misplaced the papers and really didn't understand what was happening. Thus, we encourage you to use your therapeutic skills and find your own style of presentation. General therapy skills are essential to effective CBT.

It also is important to make the material meaningful for your patients. As demonstrated earlier, the use of metaphors may help bring the information to life. Similarly, to the degree that it works for you and your patients, use humor. Although this advice is basic, we include it because *how* you deliver psychoeducation is as critical as *what* you communicate. The therapeutic relationship is just as vital to CBT as other forms of therapy, and a dry "Here are the rules—this is what we are going to do" approach may not facilitate that relationship. You lay the foundation of your relationship during psychoeducation. Later treatment components rely heavily on that foundation, so it must be as solid and stable as possible. Finally, it is important to remember to maintain a dialogue with your patient. Few people enjoy being lectured, yet the quantity of information presented in psychoeducation increases your risk of lecturing. Below are some common therapeutic tools that can help you maintain a dialogue.

- Use language that your patients use to describe problems and reactions. Avoid speaking down to your patients or using language so sophisticated that it will intimidate them. Using their words helps to create a common language.

> "You told me when we first met that for most of your life you have kept these memories and feelings 'boxed away.' It makes sense that you didn't want to think about what happened, because you always felt 'yucky' when you were reminded of that time in your life."

- Check in frequently to make sure that your patients understand. Pulling a patient "out of your pocket" (i.e., "Some patients tell me . . . ") also can make it safe for patients to admit that they do not understand.

> "Some people find it confusing when I talk about becoming aware of thoughts that contribute to distress. Does this make sense to you or is this confusing?"

- Listen to and validate concerns.

> "It makes sense that you don't want to 'go there.' You've been keeping it boxed up for so long. It's natural to fear that the dam could break—that if you let yourself think about it you will be completely consumed by your distress."

- Be empathic and supportive, reassuring yet honest. This treatment will be challenging at times, so you do not want to hide that fact.

> "As you told me, you decided to get my help because you realized that the way you were coping wasn't really working—that you felt like your life was getting 'smaller and smaller.' You came here even though it was very hard for you to decide to do this. It takes a lot of courage to face your fears. Even though there is hard work ahead of us, you have shown that you have courage and the desire to have a better life."

TEACHING COMMON REACTIONS
TO TRAUMATIC EXPERIENCES

Patients with PTSD often find it difficult to discuss their traumatic experiences, particularly during the early phases of treatment. Discussing such experiences is a critical part of CBT for PTSD. Remember, however, that the goal of psychoeducation is not to expose patients to traumatic memories and stimuli. Rather, during psychoeducation you provide information with the aim of increasing patients' awareness and understanding of their experiences.

Unfortunately, targeting the latter goal (imparting information) sometimes inadvertently includes exposure, and changes in cognitive processes can impair *some* patients' ability to learn. For example, when material discussed during psychoeducation elicits memories, the associated arousal may produce a shift in attention and focus, which results in impaired ability to concentrate on psychoeducation. This may then interfere with both the storage and later recall of psychoeducation material. Impairment in concentration may be particularly problematic for patients with PTSD who are highly aroused and thus prone to becoming cognitively overwhelmed (i.e., they "shut down" or "tune out"). Patients who are prone to dissociation also may dissociate during psychoeducation. Thus, you may sometimes find that a patient has retained little information from the first session despite appearing to understand the information during the initial presentation.

Because it is difficult to predict in advance who will have difficulty maintaining focus, you may find it helpful to approach psychoeducation as an educational process rather than a one-time lecture. Learning information often proceeds best if conducted progressively—first introducing concepts in broad strokes, with further elaboration and repetition at later sessions. Multiple modalities also can provide helpful repetition. For example, we often present information verbally, draw pictures on a board or pad, provide handouts that review key ideas, and even provide audiotapes of psychoeducation discussions for home review. The latter often is particularly helpful for patients who dissociate or "shut down" during psychoeducation.

Providing opportunities to learn through active processing and discovery rather than through passive absorption also may keep things interesting and help patients learn. When information is presented in rote and technical terms, the relevance to "real life" is not only lost for many people but it can also become more difficult to attend to the information. In our experience, the use of metaphor facilitates discussion of post-trauma reactions by providing distance from trauma survivors' own experiences and increasing engagement with the material. Distance seems to help many survivors maintain their focus, and the metaphor can provide a language for easily labeling experiences throughout treatment. In addition, metaphors naturally infuse humor into the psychoeducational process. Thus, if metaphors work for you and your patients, use them and have a bit of fun.

The prominence of the fight–flight response in anxiety specialists' understanding of anxiety and fear reactions predisposes us toward using metaphors involving dangerous animals (lions, tigers, bears, etc.). Thus, rather than starting with a general discussion of fear as an understandable reaction to survivors' traumatic experiences, we take our patients on an imaginary safari. If a safari does not fit your clinical style, pick and develop your own analogy (fire in the building; crazy, large dog in the backyard, etc.) or use a more direct presentation. Many of our patients enjoy the trip to Africa, however, and it reduces their anxiety about discussing their own symptoms and experiences. A sample dialogue is presented below. Handout 5.1 is an example of a Common Reactions to Traumatic Experiences handout. We encourage you to copy or adapt the handout for your own purposes.

In summary, your goal in this phase of psychoeducation is to (1) teach your patients that the frightening and overwhelming fear sensations they experience are part of a normal human function (i.e., the flight–fight–freeze response); (2) teach them about typical human reactions to traumatic experiences, including physical, behavioral, and cognitive components; (3) help them identify their own specific reactions and break these into categories listed on the handout, so that they can step back from their symptoms; (4) help them build their own rationale (based on the information presented) regarding why treatment involves approaching fear-producing but safe stimuli and memories; and (5) show them that you understand what they are going through and are not overwhelmed by their symptoms. As noted earlier, many patients find psychoeducation very reassuring. It demonstrates that their symptoms are understood and provides some evidence that treatment can make a difference.

Case Example: Kate

The section below demonstrates teaching the fight–flight–freeze response in a Socratic and validating way, and shows how psychoeducation teaches Kate to examine the function of her reactions (i.e., to think like a behaviorist).

THERAPIST: What we are going to talk about now is why you react to things the way you do, and why so many distressing feelings continue to bother you. By the end of this process, I think you will find that you have a better understanding of what has been going on and the reasons you feel the way you do. Our strategies for treatment also should make more sense. Now, some people find it tough to concentrate when they think about their own personal situation. So I would like to suggest that we go about this in a slightly different way. If it is OK with you and you are willing to bear with me for a bit, I would like to take us on an imaginary trip to Africa. Are you willing to give this a try?

KATE: OK, I guess so.

THERAPIST: Great. OK, we are now in Africa. Let's just assume that the purpose of our trip is a safari and that we have set up our tent and are getting ready to eat dinner. I don't know if you've camped out much, but you can probably guess that one of the first things we need when we set up camp is to get some water. Because you are a good sport, you volunteer to go down to the watering hole. Now, as you are filling our water jugs, you look up and realize that a lion has come to the watering hole. (Lions need water, too!) He is huge and growling. He is this yellow-brown color. What color would you call a lion?

KATE: Rusty gold?

THERAPIST: Sounds good. He is rusty gold with a big furry mane, but what really catches your attention are his big sharp teeth and claws. Now, how do you feel?

[*Commentary: The therapist is establishing early that this will be an interactive discussion rather than a lecture. She reinforces the patient's participation and validates the patient's imagery.*]

KATE: Scared, it's a lion!

THERAPIST: I'd be terrified! So how do you react? What do you need to do to survive?

KATE: I would run.

THERAPIST: So would I! What would you feel in your body as you were preparing to run from the lion?

KATE: Adrenaline?

THERAPIST: You are correct. Adrenaline is one of the chemicals in your body that influences your reactions at that moment. How can you tell that adrenaline has been released? What do you notice in your body?

[*Commentary: The therapist makes every effort to keep the discussion upbeat and uses any information the patient provides to lead her to the information that is central to the discussion.*]

KATE: Well, my heart is pounding.

THERAPIST: I bet it is! Why do you think your heart is pounding? How does this help you to escape from the lion?

[*Commentary: The therapist encourages the patient to link the response to function.*]

KATE: Umm, it pumps blood.

THERAPIST: Yes, it does. Why is that helpful?

KATE: Umm, I'm not really sure.

THERAPIST: Well, if your legs are going to run, what do your muscles need?

KATE: Energy?

THERAPIST: Right. Energy comes from food that is digested and sent throughout your body in the form of sugar, or glucose. When your heart pumps harder, blood circulation increases, bringing more fuel to your muscles so you can run fast. What else do your muscles need to burn that fuel?

KATE: Hmm, maybe oxygen?

THERAPIST: Yes! You need more oxygen to burn that fuel so you can run fast. The blood also brings oxygen, but how do you get it?

KATE: Well, I expect I might be breathing hard.

THERAPIST: Exactly! So right off, your breathing quickens and your heart pounds faster to bring more blood carrying fuel and oxygen to your muscles. What else do you notice?

KATE: I'm trembling and hot and sweaty.

THERAPIST: OK. So why do you think you'd be trembling?

KATE: Well, my muscles are raring to go!

THERAPIST: Right, the tension in your muscles helps you spring into action when the time is right. And sweating?

KATE: Well, I'm not sure. Would it be to keep me cool while I'm running?

THERAPIST: That makes sense.

KATE: Oh, I get it. It's like the fight–flight thing?

THERAPIST: Right. All of the physical fear sensations that you experience are a result of your body preparing you to run and fight. Although they may be uncomfortable at times, they are a survival reaction designed to help you in a life-threatening situation. The fight–flight response protects us from harm or even death when we face danger. We all have a fight–flight response—we need it to survive—and it is normal, in fact healthy, to react this way when we are faced with danger. It sounds like you've come across this term before, so you know what I mean.

[*Commentary: The therapist continues to validate patient's responses and elaborates upon them.*]

KATE: Yeah.

THERAPIST: Do you notice anything else when you are faced with the lion and your fight–flight response is activated?

KATE: Well, I tend to feel kind of queasy and lightheaded. How can that be helpful?

THERAPIST: Well, the thing to keep in mind is that when survival is at stake, your body is going to put all its resources toward helping you get away and divert resources from nonurgent matters like digesting and storing food for future energy, thinking, problem solving, or planning for the future. When you are about to be lunch, it's not a good time to digest lunch! When your digestive system grinds to a halt, it can make you queasy. And when you have to potentially fight or run away from a lion, you must have oxygen—so you breathe quickly to take in more oxygen. But when you breathe faster, you also expel more carbon dioxide. This sends a signal to the blood vessels in your brain to constrict, resulting in less oxygen actually getting to your brain cells. This is not dangerous, but it can make you feel dizzy. But all of the changes you experience are very effective for helping you survive your encounter with the lion. Your reactions also include changes in your thinking. Whereas before you were focused on getting water, now your only thought is "I've got to get out of here!" or "I'm gonna die!" Staying focused on the threat is important. If you kept thinking about getting water, you'd never survive your trip to the watering hole.

KATE: I see, it does make sense.

THERAPIST: It can be helpful to look at your fear reaction as three parts—your physical sensations, your fearful thoughts, and your fear behaviors (running, fighting back, or, as we'll talk about later, freezing). Each of these propels the other. Your pounding heart is a signal to you that something is up, which leads you to think "Danger is near!" That thought incites an urge to run. No matter where you start in this loop, it spirals into fear, with each fear component driving the next. Are there any other sensations you experience when your fear is triggered that we haven't covered yet?

KATE: Well, sometimes I get a tingling in my fingers.

THERAPIST: Yes, a lot of people say they feel that. Your body is doing an amazing thing. The small blood vessels of your hands and feet are constricting (getting narrow), which decreases the blood available there. Why do you think that would be helpful?

KATE: I'm not really sure.

THERAPIST: Well, your hands and feet are the parts of your body most likely to get cut, so your body makes sure that you will only lose a little blood if the lion manages to scratch you as you escape up the tree. The side effect of this is the tingling you feel! As I pointed out earlier, you can think about fear having three components. We just discussed the physical sensation component, so let's spend a few minutes looking at the other two components, fearful thoughts and behaviors. What are some of the thoughts that go through your head as you see the lion?

KATE: "I'm going to die—I gotta get out of here!"

THERAPIST: These thoughts are part of the fear cycle and reinforce the notion that you are in danger. You can understand the importance of fear thoughts if you think about getting rid of them. Imagine if you saw the lion and thought, "It's just a big cat, let's go pet it." What would happen if you thought that?

KATE: I might pet it, and it would eat me.

THERAPIST: Exactly! Instead of protecting yourself, you might end up as dinner for the lion! Your fear thoughts show that you understand what the lion could do to you.

KATE: That seems pretty important.

THERAPIST: Finally, there are fear behaviors. As the name "fight–flight" suggests, two of the most common fear behaviors are running and fighting. Typically we run before fighting, if both are possible. But sometimes running isn't possible. Imagine that you couldn't run from the lion because large boulders were trapping you. What would you do?

KATE: I'm not sure. I guess I would fight.

THERAPIST: Right. Chances are you would fight, particularly if you had something to fight with, such as a large stick. But what if you didn't have a weapon? What might you do then? As you may have guessed, there is a third behavior that you might turn to if you had no other options—freezing. You may find it helpful to think of the fight–flight response as the flight–fight–freeze response, because when you are unable to run or fight, you will freeze. What might happen if you freeze at the watering hole? If you are lucky, the lion won't see you. Movement attracts attention and by freezing, you might just go unnoticed.

KATE: I see.

THERAPIST: OK, so it's making sense to you that your fight–flight–freeze response would kick in when you are faced with the lion. But I bet what you really would like to know is "Why doesn't it stop?"

KATE: Definitely.

THERAPIST: Now, back to that lion. Fortunately, you got away from the lion. But over the next few days, you notice that things are different than when you first arrived in Africa. You don't want to go back to the watering hole. When you finally do go back, you feel fearful and anxious. You're on guard, with your "antennas up," watching for the lion's return. Your last encounter with the lion keeps replaying in your head—the image of the lion's teeth and claws, and the sound of its roar are etched in your memory. You see something gold colored to your right (it's a gold deer-like animal) but, rather than stopping to check it out to see if its dangerous, you bolt back to camp, thinking "Better safe than sorry!" When you return home from Africa, you notice that you feel nervous every evening around dusk, the same time that you met the lion at the watering hole. You even have a panic attack when an orange tabby cat walks in front of you; just the sight of an orange fuzzy creature triggers your fear. These situations and objects have become *triggers* or *cues* that remind you of the lion activate your fear. Let's think about why this might happen. Why do you think we experience fear when we are reminded of traumatic experiences? Why would it be a good thing to be fearful at the watering hole or at dusk?

KATE: Well, I don't want to be chased by the lion again.

THERAPIST: Of course! And, as you have correctly learned, the watering hole is a common place for lions to hang out. And lions may be more active at dusk in Africa. In these situations, it is to your advantage to be "on guard," because you are likely to encounter another lion. This is why triggers and cues remind you of the lion attack and put you on guard. Your body and mind are trying to prevent the dangerous situation from happening again. But what about when you return home? Are you more likely to encounter lions at dusk in your town?

KATE: No, there are no lions in my town.

THERAPIST: Is the tabby cat as dangerous as the lion?

KATE: (*Shakes head.*)

THERAPIST: Yet even though you were not likely to encounter a lion in these situations, you still felt fear. Dusk may have signaled the presence of lions in Africa, but it has no relationship to whether you encounter a lion in a region where none live. And when you're in Africa by the watering hole, something orange and furry could be a lion, but its not likely to be one at home. When you experience a traumatic event, many cues are present that you will learn to associate with the danger. These cues are your early warning signals of danger. They can include a wide variety of things, such as smells, noises, particular times of day, people, and colors. Your reactions to these cues can become a problem, and disturbing for you, when they continue to occur even after the danger is over. Unfortunately, many of these triggers are serving as false alarms. Rather than keeping you safe, they prevent you from enjoying life. Often they activate your anxiety without you even recognizing the trigger. Your fear may seem to come from "out of blue."

KATE: Hmm. That really makes sense. You know, sometimes my anxiety does come from out of the blue. Are you saying there are triggers and I just don't know it?

THERAPIST: Exactly. So, let's now turn to your reactions and start to identify your triggers and your fearful reactions. If we look at this handout, you will see that there are places for you to write down some of your triggers. Let's start here in session, then you can finish on your own. You'll also see that much of what we have discussed today is included. I encourage you to read the handout, possibly even several times to make sure that you understand everything. We have covered a lot of material today.

KATE: We sure have.

THERAPIST: That is why this handout includes everything, so that you can look at it repeatedly. So let's look at this first section. Can you think of places and/or things that trigger your anxiety?

KATE: Well, I had to go back to my old apartment one time to get some papers that I left behind. I knew that Mark was out of town, and I had made arrangements for the manager to let me in. Even so, I was shaking and so scared when I was in the apartment. I also got scared the other day in a store, when I saw a fishing hat like the one Mark used to wear.

THERAPIST: Those are great examples. So why don't you write down "apartment" and the "hat" over here and then make note of your fear reactions—like "shaking" on the other side. Did you have other fear reactions?

[*Commentary: The therapist reinforces Kate's correct answer and makes sure that she understands how to fill out each section before moving on to the next section of the handout. Typically, it is helpful to have patients start filling out a few items of each section in session, so that you ensure that your patients truly understand what they are supposed to do with the handout.*]

The amount of time needed for psychoeducation varies from patient to patient. Generally, we complete the main elements of psychoeducation in two to three sessions. Our preference is to move through psychoeducation as quickly as possible, so as not to collude with patients in delaying exposure. We always remain alert, however, for signs that a patient is becoming overwhelmed or not retaining the information. Signs to consider include statements that indicate the patient does not really understand the concepts, dissociation during session, and/or failure to complete the common reactions handout between sessions. When we encounter such signs, we slow down the presentation and increase repetition. As noted earlier, having patients listen to tape-recorded sessions may be particularly useful for overwhelmed or dissociating patients. We also may have the patient complete the handout in session with therapist assistance. This behaviorally demonstrates to your patients that you understand they had difficulty on their own and are willing to support them in completing the assignment. It also demonstrates that you will not be deterred by avoidance.

We do not assume that any of these problems necessarily indicate that the patient will not be able to complete trauma-focused treatment. Patients who dissociate or become overwhelmed typically do so because they are anxious. Thus, we attempt to use psychoeducation to demonstrate that careful approach of anxiety-provoking stimuli or situations (in this case, psychoeducation) will result in decreased anxiety.

CONCLUSION

Psychoeducation forms the foundation of treatment. In some cases, based on your case formulation, you may choose to conduct CBT for PTSD without cognitive restructuring. In other cases, you may find few opportunities to use *in vivo* exposure. In virtually all cases, however, you rely on psychoeducation to set the stage for what comes next. The goal of psychoeducation is to normalize symptoms and motivate patients for the next stage of therapy. The examples and handout offered in this chapter are a starting point. You are most likely to achieve these goals if you tailor your approach to the various learning styles and specific experiences of your patients.

INTRODUCTION

The traumatic events that you survived have had a lasting effect on your life. It's natural to have many distressing emotions about the trauma you experienced. At times, your feelings may seem to spiral out of control. Sometimes, you may even become so overwhelmed that you "switch off" your feelings or "numb out." One of the goals of treatment is to help you understand your reactions, so that you can stop the spiral and gain control over your emotions.

Let's talk about why you react to things the way you do, and why so many distressing feelings continue to bother you, even after the trauma is behind you. You may find that thinking about your own personal situation makes it hard to concentrate. Many people find it easier to learn about reactions to trauma by thinking about a situation other than their own. So we are going to take a trip to Africa . . .

Welcome to Africa. What are we are doing here in Africa? We are on safari. It is our first night out in the wild. We just set up our tent and have everything ready to go for dinner tonight. All we need is some water, so you volunteer to go down to the watering hole. As you are filling our water jugs, you look up and see a figure approaching. Having seen many episodes of *Wild Kingdom*, you quickly recognize it as a lion. He is very large, with a bushy orange mane, and is looking right at you and growling. You see his big teeth and sharp claws. He is so close that you can even smell him.

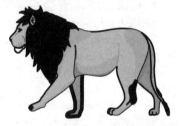

How do you react? Do you feel fear? A racing heart? An urge to run? Do you have the thought "I'm going to die!" Such reactions are part of the natural response to a dangerous situation, known as the "fight–flight" response. The fight–flight response protects us from harm or even death when faced with peril. A key point is that we all have a fight–flight response (we need it to survive!) and it is normal, in fact *healthy*, to react this way when we are faced with danger.

These reactions can become problematic and disturbing, however, when they continue to occur even after the danger is over. Before we explain why they continue, it is important that you recognize your own reactions for what they are, and that you understand why they happen. This handout will help you to identify your reactions to trauma and to understand why these reactions occur. We will often return to Africa in order to help you make sense of your daily experiences here at home. This handout will help you to identify reactions that are central to PTSD. These include fear and anxiety arousal, avoidance, and reexperiencing the trauma. You will also identify things that trigger your PTSD symptoms.

(continued)

FEAR AND ANXIETY

Let's go back to that watering hole in Africa. (Are you there yet? If not, take a moment to really *imagine* yourself at the watering hole.) How do you feel when you see that growling lion slinking toward you? Chances are you feel some fear. Fear goes by many names—the words that pop into your mind might be "panicky," "afraid," "scared," or "terrified." It's natural to feel anxious and afraid when you are faced with a potentially life-threatening danger. Anxiety and fear can feel overwhelming, so to understand what's happening, it's helpful to look at their components. Let's first look at the big picture; then we'll look at each component in detail. When you feel fear, you likely experience **sensations in your body** (e.g., shaking, sweating, breathing fast, or "palpitations")

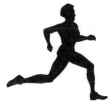

You may also have fearful thoughts . . .

I'm gonna die!

And an urge to flee . . . (This is a **fear behavior**)

So, you see, your fear reaction can be broken down into these three parts—your physical sensations, your fearful thoughts, and your fear behaviors (running, fighting back, or, as we'll talk about later, freezing). Each of these fuels the others. Your pounding heart signals to you that something is up, which leads you to *think* that there must be danger, and so, you may give in to your urge to run. No matter where you start in this loop, it spirals into fear, with each fear component further triggering the next.

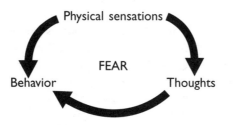

Let's look at the physical sensations associated with fear. What sensations do you feel when you see that lion coming toward you at the watering hole? Can you feel your heart pounding? Are you breathing hard and fast? How about trembling or shaking? These reactions are part of the fight–flight response, which is your body's way of preparing to handle a dangerous situation. The fight–flight response is your survival reaction, and it is going to help you get away from the lion. Now, let's imagine for a moment that there is a large tree near the watering hole, and you think you can climb it. You decide to make a run for the tree, since you happen to know from *Wild Kingdom* that lions don't usually climb trees.

Fortunately, your body is already prepared for the sprint and climb. The moment you recognized the lion, adrenaline was released to signal to your body to prepare to run or fight. So, in the few precious seconds it took you to decide to run to the tree, various parts of your body were getting ready to do their jobs. For example, your heart started beating harder and faster, and your breathing rate increased. Your heart increased the blood flow throughout your body, so that your muscles have enough oxygen to hightail it away from the lion or to beat the lion with a big stick. Breathing faster

(continued)

helps, because the large amount of air you gulp in ensures that your blood has plenty of oxygen in it. If your muscles didn't have enough oxygen, they might cramp, and that would slow you down—something that you do not want to happen when you are escaping a lion!

Your body is also doing many other amazing things. For example, the blood vessels in your hands and feet are constricting, which decreases the blood available there. Your hands and feet are the parts of your body most likely to get cut, so your body makes sure that you will only lose a little blood if the lion manages to scratch you as you escape up the tree. You may not have noticed, but while you were crouched by the watering hole, your muscles became so tense that you started to shake. This is so that you can react quickly if the lion starts charging you. The tension in your muscles helps you spring into action when the time is right. And you may have noticed that you are sweating a lot. This will help cool you down, so you don't overheat as you escape. All of the physical fear sensations that you experience are a result of your body preparing you to run and to fight. Although they may be uncomfortable at times, they are a survival reaction designed to help you in a life-threatening situation.

As pointed out earlier, you can think of fear as having three components. We just discussed the physical sensation component, so let's look at the other components, fear thoughts and fear behaviors. What are some of the thoughts that go through your head as you see the lion? "I'm going to die?" "It's going to get me??" These thoughts are part of the fear cycle and reinforce the notion that you are in danger. You can understand the importance of fear thoughts if you think about getting rid of them. Imagine if you saw the lion and thought, "It's just a big cat, let's go pet it." Instead of protecting yourself, you might end up as dinner for the lion! Your fear thoughts show that you understand what the lion could do to you.

Finally, there are fear behaviors. As the name "fight–flight" indicates, two of the most common fear behaviors are running and fighting. Typically we run before fighting, if both are possible. But sometimes running is not possible. Imagine that you couldn't run from the lion because large boulders trapped you. What would you do? Chances are you would fight, particularly if you had a weapon. But what if you didn't have a weapon? What might you do then? As you may have guessed, there is a third behavior that you might turn to if you had no other options. This is called the freezing response. You may find it helpful to rename the fight–flight response and call it the "flight–fight–freeze" response, because when you are unable to run and unable to fight, you will often freeze. What might happen if you freeze at the watering hole? If you are lucky, the lion won't see you. Movement attracts attention, and by freezing you might just go unnoticed. This is why we sometimes freeze in dangerous or fearful situations.

Now back to that lion. Fortunately, you are a good climber, and you climbed up the tree. You were able to get away even though the lion charged you. But over the next few days, you notice that things are different than when you first arrived in Africa. You don't want to go back to the watering hole. When you finally do go back, you feel fearful and anxious, and you stay on guard.

When you return home, you notice that the smell of animals at the local petting zoo make you feel very anxious, even though you know the petting zoo does not have a lion. And you feel nervous every evening around dusk, the same time that you met the lion at the watering hole. You even had a panic attack when an orange tabby cat walked in front of you back at home; just the sight of an orange fuzzy creature triggered your fear. These situations and objects have become **triggers** or **cues** that remind you of the lion activate your fear. Let's think about why this might happen.

Why do you think we experience fear when we are reminded of traumatic experiences? Why would it be a good thing to be fearful at the watering hole or at dusk? As you may have guessed, the watering hole might be a common place for lions to hang out. And lions may be more active at dusk, if

(continued)

you are in Africa. In these situations, it may actually be to your advantage to be anxious and "on guard," because you are likely to reencounter a lion in these situations. This is why triggers and cues make you anxious. Your body and mind are trying to prevent the dangerous situation from happening again.

But what about that trip to the zoo, dusk at home, or the tabby cat? In these situations you were not likely to encounter a lion at all, and you still felt fear. The smell of a lion might be a helpful cue if you were out on safari again, but at the zoo it was an unhelpful cue. And having a panic attack every time you encounter an orange cat is certainly a problem. When you experience a traumatic event, you typically develop many fear triggers. Unfortunately, many of these triggers do not keep you safe; instead, they prevent you from enjoying life. For example, you probably did not enjoy visiting the zoo and might stop going even though you used to love the zoo. These triggers may activate your anxiety without you even recognizing the trigger. In these situations, your fear may seem to come from "out of blue." Triggers can include smells, noises, certain times of day, people, colors, relationship situations (e.g., an argument), or places. Triggers can also include certain thoughts or images inside your head, or even certain emotions.

In the section below, write down any triggers that you can think of. Because it is sometimes difficult to identify triggers, you may find it helpful to think of your fearful reactions, then to think about situations that produce those reactions. Often we feel the urge to avoid situations or triggers that make us anxious. So you may also find it helpful to think of places, people, or other trauma reminders that you try to avoid.

Things that trigger my fear	My fear reactions
Places and things:	*Body sensations:*
People and activities:	*Urges:*
Sounds, smells, sensations:	*Thoughts:*

(continued)

AVOIDANCE

Active Avoidance

Imagine for a moment that you are invited to go back to Africa on safari after you narrowly escape the lion. Would you go? You might find yourself feeling very reluctant to return to Africa after nearly being attacked by lion. After all, you learned that being on safari in Africa is not always safe. Avoidance is very common after a traumatic experience. Sometimes avoidance is a good thing. For example, it is healthy to avoid getting too close to a lion. Yet at other times, you may have the urge to avoid a wide range of situations that are not truly dangerous, even though they feel scary. For example, tabby cats and petting zoos are generally considered fairly safe, yet you might find yourself avoiding them after your lion experience. The urge to avoid is a natural reaction to situations that feel dangerous.

You may be avoiding people, places, or things that remind you of your trauma. You may also be avoiding thoughts and feelings about the trauma. Sometimes thoughts and feelings seem overwhelming and dangerous. You may have the urge to avoid thinking about things that remind you of your trauma. It is useful to identify all of the situations, thoughts, and feelings that you try to avoid. Since you may use a variety of strategies to avoid, it is also helpful to ask yourself, "How do I avoid?" In the space below, describe the places, things, feelings, and thoughts you avoid:

What I avoid	How I avoid
Places, people, activities, and things	
Thoughts, feelings, memories, conversations	

Passive Avoidance ("Numbing")

Sometimes the desire to avoid memories, thoughts, and feelings related to the trauma may be so intense that you start to feel numb. You might also find that you forget certain aspects of your traumatic experience. Numbing comes in many forms and often includes feeling empty or detached from people around you. Sometimes you may find that you do not feel pleasure, even during activities that you used to enjoy. Describe these experiences in the space provided on the next page:

(continued)

Pleasurable activities that no longer interest me	Feelings of emotional detachment or numbness

REEXPERIENCING THE TRAUMA

It is very common to reexperience a trauma after surviving a traumatic experience. In the days and weeks after your encounter with the lion, you might find yourself thinking about the lion over and over. You have nightmares about the lion and can't seem to get him out of your head. Pictures of the lion suddenly pop into your mind, and sometimes you have vivid flashbacks, such that it seems like the lion attack is happening all over again even though you are at home. These experiences are typically intrusive and may seem completely out of your control. Memories, flashbacks, and distress often are triggered by external events, though they also may appear to come out of nowhere. Describe some of the reexperiencing symptoms that have troubled you in the space below:

Images or flashbacks	Dreams
Emotions	**Thoughts**

SIX

Introducing Exposure Therapy

Exposure is seemingly straightforward (i.e., you expose your patient to feared stimuli for an extended period of time). Yet understanding how exposure works and what your patient is supposed to learn from exposure is vital to maximizing effectiveness and avoiding errors. This chapter is designed to help you make sense of exposure. In particular, we explain what patients learn during exposure (both *in vivo* and imaginal), then discuss the "nuts and bolts" of conducting *in vivo* exposure with patients with PTSD. In addition, we explore common pitfalls, and strategies for handling problems with *in vivo* exposure. We provide additional details for conducting imaginal exposure in Chapter 7.

MAKING SENSE OF THE EXPOSURE PROCESS

The Case of Jill: Attack by a Bull Mastiff

Three years ago, when Jill decided to take an evening walk in her neighborhood, she saw her neighbors' bull mastiff Barney lounging on their front lawn. Jill looked at Barney and Barney growled. Suddenly, he lunged at her. Jill began running. Barney chased her, knocked her to the ground, and bit her repeatedly on her body and face, severely injuring her. Jill wrestled with Barney until a neighbor finally confined him to a yard and called the police. Jill was stunned to realize what had happened, because Barney had always been friendly and she had never thought of him as dangerous. As she was loaded into the ambulance, Jill overheard a police officer say, "She should have known better than to run from a dog."

When Jill comes to see you, after being referred for depression, she reports that she hasn't left her house for weeks, because she is terrified that she will encounter a dog. She no longer watches television, because she fears seeing dogs. She has become overprotective of her kids, forbidding them to visit friends who have dogs. As hard as she tries to put the memories of it behind her, she finds herself reminded of the attack several times a day. Even showering and putting on makeup are difficult, because seeing her extensive scars brings back memories of Barney's teeth sinking into her flesh. Jill confides that she fears "I am losing my mind," because she cannot control the memories. At night she is particularly on edge; as soon as the sun sets, she finds herself locking doors and listening for dogs barking. Sleep is difficult, because she is afraid of letting her guard down. So she piles on heavy blankets and leaves lights on in the bedroom to feel safer. When she does sleep, she dreams of being chased by animals. In your first meeting, she states that she "used to like most animals," but since the attack she believes "most dogs are dangerous" and when you probe further, she concedes, "Well, if any of them are safe, I can't tell the difference." Moreover, Jill admits that her self-confidence has deteriorated: "I used to think I could handle anything. Now I know that I am weak—I just can't cope with bad things."

What Jill Needs to Accomplish during Exposure

The primary goal of exposure for PTSD is to reduce the fear associated with thinking about the trauma and trauma-related stimuli that are not truly dangerous. Jill needs to learn that although being attacked by a dog is dangerous, the *memory* of being attacked by a dog is not. Jill also must learn that most dogs will not harm her, and that her fear will eventually decrease when she confronts anxiety-provoking but safe situations and memories, even though it feels like the fear will increase forever.

In addition to reducing fear, exposure should increase your patients' perceived control over their fear. This facilitates generalization of fear reduction across situations and time. For example, by (1) learning that she can tolerate fear, (2) learning to be less fearful of dogs during *in vivo* exposure, and (3) learning to be less fearful of the attack memory during imaginal exposure, Jill's perception of control over her anxiety reactions should increase. As we discuss later, enhancing the perception of control over anxiety may be the fundamental "shift" that treatment of PTSD (and likely other anxiety disorders) aims to achieve.

Exposure, particularly imaginal exposure, also facilitates processing of the traumatic memory. As noted in Chapter 2, patients need to "make sense" of their experience, which typically involves integrating all relevant information into a coherent narrative of the event. Imaginal exposure can affect a range of negative emotions that may accompany PTSD. For example, in Jill's case, reprocessing helps to reduce the feelings of guilt and powerlessness that pervade her everyday thinking.

Learning during In Vivo *Exposure*

Following the attack, Jill rigidly adheres to her new concept of "dogs," which unambiguously associates dogs with danger. Thus, in addition to fearing dangerous dogs like Barney, Jill also avoids dogs that are unlikely to bite her, such as her friend's friendly mutt. This "better safe than sorry" approach to dogs makes sense given her experience. However, it is inaccurate and leads Jill to avoid dog-related situations that are not truly dangerous. Avoidance maintains her fear by reducing her contact with dogs, and by limiting opportunities for new learning.

During *in vivo* exposure, Jill must learn that her anxiety does not reliably predict danger when it comes to dogs, and that the construct "dogs" does not have only one meaning (i.e., danger). Instead, "dogs" is an ambiguous construct that has different meanings depending on the specifics of the dog and the context in which she encounters it (Bouton & Swartzentruber, 1991). Learning shades of meaning (i.e., which dogs under what circumstances are dangerous) will enable Jill to resume a broader range of realistically safe activities and to protect herself even better than when she relied on the "most dogs are dangerous" concept. For example, Jill no longer will avoid visiting her friend, who has a friendly poodle, yet she *will* continue to avoid the large growling dog behind the "Beware of Dog" sign. Jill also will no longer run down a dark (and likely dangerous) alley trying to avoid a loose Chihuahua, which realistically can do her little harm and that Jill could (if truly necessary) kick away.

Learning cues to discriminate more precisely between danger and safety also will instill in Jill a greater sense of control, as will learning that she is able to tolerate anxiety in safe situations. For example, by thinking "I can handle this. If I just keep petting this nice dog, my fear will go away," Jill experiences an increased sense of control compared to when she thought, "I can't handle this. I have to escape before I lose it."

Learning during Imaginal Exposure

Just as safe dogs produce fear despite being safe, recalling the attack triggers intense anxiety, even though the memory cannot physically harm Jill. Similarly, just as avoiding dogs prevents Jill from refining her understanding of dogs, avoiding (or escaping) her memory of the attack (e.g., by distraction) prevents Jill from refining her interpretations of both the meaning of the traumatic event and her reactions to it. Moreover, the "story" of the attack remains fragmented, and important details are not incorporated into her interpretations. Thus, she remains "stuck" in her exaggerated negative beliefs about the level of threat in the world and her ability to cope with it (Resick & Schnicke, 1992).

During imaginal exposure, Jill learns that although thinking about the attack produces anxiety (i.e., she activates her fear), nothing happens to her (i.e., she experiences corrective information about safety; Foa & Kozak, 1986). Correspondingly, her fear decreases. Imaginal exposure also provides Jill the opportunity to assemble all of the elements of her attack memory and organize them in a logical way, so that she may draw new, perhaps more realistic conclusions about what happened.

For example, when Jill sees her scars while showering, she distracts herself from the memory of the attack by singing or counting wall tiles. As a result of her aborted recollection, she neglects pertinent details, such as her sense that something was not right with Barney, because he was not wagging his tail as usual. She also disregards the fact that Barney's owner told her that some of his teenager's friends had been teasing Barney just before she walked by. In addition, Jill forgets that she wrestled with Barney (instead of kicking him away) to prevent him from biting a child who came to see what was happening. Since the attack, Jill has believed that most dogs are dangerous. Yet the details suggest that although Barney may have had a propensity to behave aggressively, his irritated state made him more dangerous. Moreover, rather than being completely unaware, Jill detected signals that Barney was irritated, which is relevant to her perception of herself as being unable to predict danger.

Integrating this information leads Jill to modify her belief, from "Most dogs are dangerous" to "Some dogs can behave aggressively if they've been teased into an agitated state." Her belief, "I can't tell the difference between a dangerous dog and friendly dog," shifts to "I can recognize some signs of danger in certain dogs." Her belief, "I am weak—I just can't cope with bad things," changes to "I coped as best as I could, and although I was hurt, I managed to keep a bad situation from getting much worse." Her shame about running and her anger at Barney's owner, which interacted with Jill's fear and perpetuated avoidance, also may change as other thoughts are modified by exposure. Quite often, radical shifts in thinking about the meaning of the event occur during imaginal exposure, although cognitive restructuring may help facilitate these changes in many cases.

Wait! Doesn't Exposure Work by Desensitizing Fears?

The preceding description of learning during exposure may differ somewhat from explanations that you have previously encountered. Interestingly, no one knows exactly how exposure works in all cases. Several common explanations, however, have not withstood empirical scrutiny.

One early explanation, "habituation," occurs when a physiological reflex response to a stimulus, such as a tone, weakens following repeated presentation of the stimulus (e.g., when a loud tone is sounded, your body reacts to it with changes in heart rate, blood pressure, and sweat gland activity, but your body stops reacting after the tone is repeated several times). Researchers have determined that habituation alone cannot explain fear reduction during exposure, because habituation only affects automatic physical reactions we have to fears that are innate, such as our reaction to a loud noise (Mackintosh, 1987). Despite this, people continue to use the word "habituation" clinically to describe anxiety reduction during exposure, even though we understand that anxiety is far more complicated than reflex reactions.

An alternate explanation is "extinction." As noted in Chapter 2, most cognitive-behavioral models of PTSD presume that classical conditioning plays a role in trauma-related fear. Thus, fears learned through classical conditioning might be extinguished or replaced by new learning when the conditioned stimulus (dog) is repeatedly presented without the unconditional stimulus (being bitten). Extinction alone, however, does not adequately explain fear reduction, because it does not explain why the cognitive, behavioral, and/or physical aspects of fear sometimes change independently of one another (McCutcheon & Adams, 1975). Extinction also does not explain why vicariously learned fears (e.g., developing fear of flying after learning about a plane crash) still respond to exposure.

Recently, researchers have turned to cognitive factors (e.g., fear networks) to explain how acquired fears can be "unlearned." Cognitive models presume that pathological fear is due to learning incorrect associations between stimuli. For example, Jill associates dogs with danger of being bitten, and she feels particularly threatened by them at night. Foa and Kozak (1986) propose that fear is reduced when the associated fear network is activated, and, at the same time, new information about safety corrects the mistaken associations. According to this model, Jill must engage with a feared stimulus (e.g., get close to a safe golden retriever) sufficiently to experience fear and at the same time experience no actual harm (i.e., not be bitten).

Evidence supports the importance of fear activation (Jaycox, Foa, & Morral, 1998) and corrective information (Foa & Kozak, 1986). Basic research, however, does not support the suggestion that exposure weakens mistaken associations (e.g., associations between dogs and being bitten). Instead, studies of animal learning (Bouton & Swartzentruber, 1991) indicate that exposure creates new associations. Fears are not "unlearned" by exposure, but rather overwritten with more specific information that tells the person under what circumstance the stimulus is dangerous. For example, during exposure to a friendly dog, Jill learns a new, more specific association between friendly dog behaviors (e.g., calmly sitting, tail wagging, and licking, the therapist's office, and safety. The old association of dogs with danger is not erased. Rather Jill learns accurate safety cues about a particular kind of dog in a particular situation.

This finding has several implications. First, it suggests that fears may be reactivated under the right conditions, which may explain why fear sometimes returns after previous reduction. Jill never forgets that dogs bite; rather, she learns that certain dogs in certain contexts are unlikely to bite. Thus, if she is only exposed to golden retrievers on a leash in her therapist's office during daytime, Jill's fear may return when she encounters a golden retriever while strolling downtown at night. Second, this suggests that Jill may need repeated presentation of different types of dogs in different contexts to learn that the correct safety cue is a nonsnarling dog that is wagging its tail, rather than a specific breed of dog or a specific time of day.

Learning to approach dogs also likely teaches Jill another important lesson. As noted by Mineka and Thomas (1999), extensive research indicates that perceived *lack* of control is associated with persistent anxiety, and that perceived control reduces anxiety. According to this perspective, decreases in fear during exposure enhance individuals' perception of control over both the threat (i.e., the dog) and, perhaps more importantly, anxiety reactions. For example, when Jill successfully copes with her anxiety during exposure to the golden retriever, she feels more in control of her distressing anxiety reactions (e.g., the thought "I can't handle this" might change to "I can cope with my fear"). As a result, Jill feels less "crazy" and "out of control." This increased sense of control also may make it easier for her to engage in additional exposure.

> The trick is not to rid your stomach of butterflies, but to make them fly in formation.
> —OUTWARD BOUND INTERNATIONAL (2004, p. 64)

IMPLEMENTING EXPOSURE

Guidelines for *In Vivo* Exposure

There are several basic steps involved in conducting *in vivo* exposure. First, review the rationale for exposure (Handout 6.1) and help your patient identify feared stimuli to approach (Handouts 6.2 and 6.3). Next, help your patient to build a hierarchy of feared stimuli (Handout 6.4), which is a list of feared stimuli ranked according to how much fear they produce. Once the hierarchy is developed, teach your patient to engage systematically in prolonged contact with various stimuli and/or situations listed on the hierarchy (Handout 6.5). During this prolonged contact, encourage your patient to attend to and experience feelings of anxiety, so as to notice the anxiety reduction that occurs during exposure. Finally, instruct your patient in conducting repeated home practice of the *in vivo* exposure task (Handout 6.6).

Reviewing the Rationale for Exposure

You will have laid out the basic rationale when you first introduced your patient to CBT. Nonetheless, it is important to make sure that your patient fully understands the rationale before introducing them to the exposure process.

Sample Dialogue: Rationale for Exposure

THERAPIST: Today we are going to take the first steps to starting exposure. We talked about exposure previously. Do you recall what we discussed?

JILL: Wasn't it the idea that to get over my fear of dogs, I will have to go near dogs?

THERAPIST: Exactly. There are a several important details, however, that we did not get into when we first discussed exposure. I'd like to review why exposure is helpful and explain what you can expect during exposure.

JILL: OK. I am pretty nervous about all of this.

THERAPIST: And understandably so, which is why it is really important to understand as much as possible about exposure before we start. So, to start, let's think about why fear persists even though the dangerous situation is over. In other words, let's explore why you are fearful of all dogs even though it would be hard for some dogs to hurt you. For example, if we had a dog in a cage—a very secure cage that the dog could not escape—would you fear that dog?

JILL: I'd be out of this room!

THERAPIST: That is what I would have guessed. So the question is, why are you afraid of a dog that is unable to hurt you? There are two main reasons. The first is avoidance. We looked at avoidance when we reviewed common reactions to traumatic events. And, as we discussed, after surviving a traumatic event, it's completely normal to want to avoid thoughts, memories, or situations that remind you of the trauma. In fact, if we think back to the safari, it makes complete sense why you would want to avoid dogs.

JILL: Dogs are my lion.

THERAPIST: Well one dog was your lion. What are all other dogs?

JILL: My tabby cat?

THERAPIST: Correct. So now let's think more carefully about what happens when you avoid dogs, memories, or feelings that remind you of what happened. Let's say that as you are walking down the street tonight, you see someone walking a dog coming toward you. How would you feel?

JILL: Anxious, scared. I don't want to go near it.

THERAPIST: OK. I'm going to draw a picture showing your anxiety. How high would your anxiety be? Tell me when to stop. (*Draws graph—see Figure 6.1.*) And what do you do?

JILL: I cross the street. And I distract myself by counting the poles along the side of the road.

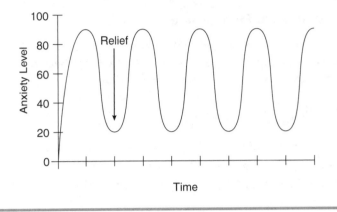

FIGURE 6.1. Avoidance "spikes."

[*Commentary: If you decide to begin with imaginal exposure for a particular patient, substitute escaping from an intrusive memory for the live stimulus, and ask the patient what happens when he or she pushes it out of his or her mind.*]

THERAPIST: And what happens to your anxiety when you cross the street and the dog is out of sight?

JILL: I feel better. My anxiety goes away.

THERAPIST: Like this? (*Draws downward line showing rapid reduction of anxiety.*) And that is what happens whenever we escape or avoid things that scare us. As we get closer to things that scare us, for example, even a dog in a cage, our anxiety goes up. And when we avoid or escape by getting away from the dog or by pushing a memory out of our heads, our anxiety goes down. And when anxiety decreases, that feels really good—relief! (*Writes "Relief" on graph.*) I think of it sort of as getting an emotional present. So, if anxiety goes away whenever you avoid, why you avoid really makes sense, doesn't it?

JILL: Yes.

THERAPIST: There is one little problem, though. Although avoiding helps reduce anxiety in the short term, what happens the next time you see a dog? What happens to your anxiety?

JILL: It goes back up.

THERAPIST: Exactly. (*Draws another peak.*) Your anxiety goes up. You avoid, and it goes down. But then it goes up again next time you are presented with the same situation. And the unfortunate thing is that your anxiety can do this forever. Up and down, forever. Though not a technical term, we have dubbed this "avoidance spikes." So, although avoiding helps you feel better in the short run, it prevents you from getting over the fear in the long term because you don't get the opportunity to learn that what you fear actually won't hurt you.

JILL: Hmm.

THERAPIST: But, if you stay in the situation, what do you think will happen?

JILL: It might go down?

THERAPIST: Right. Your anxiety will go up at first—and it may feel like it is going to go up and up forever and never go away. But, in fact, over time it will actually go down like this (*Draws Figure 6.2 overlaid on Figure 6.1.*) We call this big increase and gradual decrease in anxiety, the habituation curve.

[*Commentary: You may choose to draw Figure 6.2 overlaid on Figure 6.1 using different colors. Follow up this discussion by giving your patient Handout 6.1.*]

JILL: Hmm.

THERAPIST: Does this make sense?

JILL: It makes sense, though I am not sure it will work for me.

THERAPIST: That is understandable. I'm wondering, though, whether you have ever feared or been anxious about something in the past, where you eventually got over your fear? For example, many people who swim say that they feared diving until they got used to it. Or to go back even further, often when they first learn to swim, people are afraid to put their faces in the water to start. Also, some people who are in minor car accidents say that they are anxious when they first start driving again.

[*Commentary: It is helpful to provide evidence from patients' own lives to demonstrate that exposure has worked for them in the past. The therapist remembers that although Jill reported a minor car accident on her assessment, she also reported no problems with driving. Thus, there is a good chance that this might provide an exposure example for Jill. The therapist investigates this by asking questions. If you do not have a specific example from your patient's life, offer examples that you think might work for your patient.*]

JILL: That happened to me. I was in a fender bender years ago. And when I got my car back from the shop, I didn't want to drive it.

THERAPIST: Did you end up driving it? Or are you still taking the bus?

JILL: I had to—I didn't have a choice.

THERAPIST: What happened to your fear?

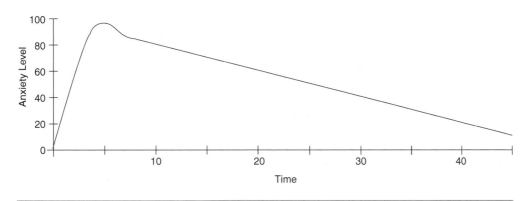

FIGURE 6.2. Habituation curve.

Jill: You're right. It went down.

Therapist: So when you were not able to avoid, over time, your fear decreased. That is the idea behind exposure. In other words, when you avoid, you don't have the opportunity to learn that the situation is reasonably safe. Yet when you don't (or can't) avoid, you are able to learn that your fear is greater than the level of danger in that situation.

Jill: It makes a lot of sense.

Therapist: Now let's consider a second factor that helps maintain anxiety, namely, unhelpful ways of thinking. For example, if you think that what happened to you was your fault, you may blame yourself, and feel guilty and depressed. Similarly, if you believe that still being afraid of dogs means that you are weak and incapable of coping with life, then you may be less likely to do the things that will help you get over your fear. Though these thoughts are understandable given what happened to you, this way of thinking is unhelpful. Very often, what we think changes during exposure. In other words, your experiences with dogs during exposure therapy likely will change how you think about dogs. However, if we notice that unhelpful thoughts are frequent, persistent, or very distressing, I will teach you how to be aware of these unhelpful thoughts and learn more helpful ways of thinking.

Building a Hierarchy

The process of building a hierarchy is fairly simple. Despite this, some patients find it confusing. Therefore, it is important to walk your patient through the steps of building a hierarchy, at least the first time. Some patients may only construct one or two hierarchies during treatment (i.e., one imaginal and one *in vivo* hierarchy). Others, however, may need to construct multiple subhierarchies to break down different types of stimuli or situations into manageable steps. Once they "get it," many such patients take the ball and run with it. Others, however, may need your guidance with each new hierarchy.

Sample Dialogue: Constructing a Hierarchy

Therapist: As we discussed, repeated exposure to a feared situation will reduce your discomfort in that situation. The first step in preparing for *in vivo* exposure is to make a plan for successive steps in approaching the feared situation. This is called a "hierarchy." If lots of different kinds of things trigger your fear, we may find it useful to have several hierarchies for your different fears. I have a worksheet that we can use to develop a hierarchy (Handout 6.4). There are four basic steps to follow when constructing an exposure hierarchy.

Step 1 involves *identifying feared situations*. The "Common Reactions" handout (Handout 5.1) is a good place to start, because you've listed some situations, places, objects, people, or animals you avoid, and you've described some of the ways you avoid these trauma reminders. For example, you've listed that you avoid going to people's homes if they have a dog, such as your sister and your friend Lisa, that you avoid watching television or reading magazines that might have pictures of dogs, and that you avoid walking within several blocks of Elm Street where Barney used to live. These provide us with a jumping off point for your hierarchy. *Step 2* in constructing a hierarchy is to *brainstorm* as many different anxiety-provoking situations as possible. So what other specific dog situations make you anxious?

[*Commentary: Using the "avoidance" section of Handout 5.1 for prompting, Jill and the therapist brainstorm a variety of situations that produce anxiety. The list does not need to be completely exhaustive. Generating a reasonably detailed list, however, can be helpful in identifying good starting points for exposure and gaining greater awareness about the full scope of your patient's avoidance.*]

THERAPIST: OK, now that we have listed quite a few situations that you are avoiding, we can move onto the next step. *Step 3* is to *rate the anxiety* you would expect to feel if you were in that situation using the Subjective Units of Distress Scale, or "SUDS." Basically, this is a way for you to rate how much anxiety you think you would feel in a given situation. The scale ranges from 0 to 100, where 0 = *no anxiety* and 100 = *maximum anxiety*.[1] One easy way to start is to look at the list and tell me which situations and objects on the list would produce the least anxiety.

JILL: They would all make me very anxious, but I guess the picture of the dog would make me the least anxious.

THERAPIST: We were not terribly specific here when we listed a picture of a dog. Your fear of dogs is quite intense—so much so that even looking at pictures of dogs is quite upsetting, right?

JILL: Yes.

THERAPIST: So is there a type of picture that would be the least anxiety provoking? In other words, what type of dog picture do you think would be the easiest to look at? For example, would a dog lying down, with no teeth showing, be easier than a dog standing, with teeth showing—or would there be no difference?

JILL: Lying down and no teeth showing would be easier. I think the important thing is no teeth.

THERAPIST: OK. So using the SUDS scale, where 0 is *no anxiety* and 100 is *maximum anxiety*, how much anxiety would you feel if you were looking at a picture of a dog with no teeth showing?

JILL: A lot—maybe a 70.

THERAPIST: OK. Now let's look at the other end of the scale. What do you think would be the most frightening?

JILL: Petting a bull mastiff on or off a leash. They are equally bad.

THERAPIST: OK. How much anxiety?

JILL: One hundred or even higher.

THERAPIST: OK. Well, 100 is as high as we can go, so let's rank these the same at 100.

---

[1]If your patient is already familiar with the 0- to 8-point scale used in many anxiety disorder treatments, you may find it easiest to continue using this scale.

JILL: You know, looking at that, I don't think the no teeth picture is a 70. It's still high, but maybe a 50. There are a lot of things that seem worse.

THERAPIST: OK. let's change that one to 50. So now let's try and fill in the middle between the lowest and highest situations. You said that a picture of a dog with teeth showing would be worse. Where would that go?

JILL: I still think that would cause a lot of anxiety. Maybe a 65.

THERAPIST: How about a small dog you know to be friendly that is on a leash or in a cage?

JILL: Sixty for the small dog in the cage and 70 for the dog on the leash.

[*Commentary: Often it is easiest for patients first to rate situations that generate the least and most fear, or vice versa, then proceed to the rest of the list. In this case, the therapist suspected that Jill might be overrating the low end of her hierarchy. Patients who have overrated low situations, however, typically will start to modify ratings on their own, just as Jill did, once they look at situations that create higher levels of anxiety.*]

THERAPIST: After you have rated all the options, the next step is to reorder your initial list of items in ascending SUDS order (from the lowest to the highest SUDS rating). Rewrite the list in the new order on the second form, wording the items as actual tasks that can be done, with specifics as to how they will be done. This will complete your initial *in vivo* exposure hierarchy [see Figure 6.3].

Using Subhierarchies to Titrate Anxiety

Many patients can complete exposure using a hierarchy like the one listed earlier. Other patients, however, benefit from converting their initial hierarchy into subhierarchies, so as to titrate their anxiety. For example, Jill rated being close to a caged,

1.	Picture of a dog with no teeth showing	50
2.	Video of a friendly dog	55
3.	Being in a room with a small dog in a crate or cage	60
4.	Picture of a dog with its teeth showing	65
5.	Being in a room with a small dog on a leash	70
6.	Being in a room petting a small dog off its leash	85
7.	Being close to a crate or cage of a large dog	85
8.	Being close to/petting a large dog on a leash	90
9.	Walk by the house where Barney lived	95
10.	Being close to/petting a large dog off its leash	95
11.	Being close to/petting a bull mastiff on its leash	100
12.	Being close to/petting a bull mastiff off its leash	100

FIGURE 6.3. Jill's initial *in vivo* hierarchy.

large dog at 85 on the SUDS. Yet it is quite possible that different types of dogs (e.g., based on size, color, or breed type) will produce different levels of anxiety. Similarly, her fear may vary based on how close the dog is, because increased physical distance often reduces anxiety. The type of cage (e.g., depending on how secure it appears) may also influence her fear. In summary, if necessary, Jill probably can titrate her anxiety by creating a specific subhierarchy that varies the characteristics of the item "large dog in cage."

In all probability, Jill will become increasingly confident that her anxiety will decrease during exposure after successfully completing lower level items, and higher level items may be easier than expected. In fact, a common analogy likens completing items on a hierarchy to climbing a ladder. As you climb each of the bottom rungs, the rungs at the top of the ladder gets closer and easier to reach. In our experience, however, completing lower level situations does not *always* make higher level situations significantly easier for patients with PTSD, even though almost all patients report increased confidence in exposure once it has worked. Thus, depending on the degree of generalization that Jill experiences, petting a large dog may still produce a high degree of anxiety and urge to avoid. In this situation, it can be helpful to create a subhierarchy. Similarly, if Jill experienced very high levels of anxiety with even her lowest rated situation (i.e., viewing dog pictures), it might be helpful to create a subhierarchy focused on dog pictures.

If it appears that a patient will benefit from creating subhierarchies, we recommend explicitly teaching the patient how to make hierarchies by reviewing the steps just listed in a slightly modified form. Step 1 involves choosing the specific feared situation (e.g., being close to an off-leash large dog). Step 2 involves brainstorming all of the ways to vary this situation (by modifying the stimulus, degree of contact, etc.). Steps 3 and 4 are unchanged, and involve rating the variations, then ordering them according to the amount of anxiety they produce. Handout 6.4 includes instructions for building a hierarchy and a model of a completed hierarchy, as well as a worksheet for constructing a hierarchy.

Selecting the First Stimulus for In Vivo Exposure

After you have constructed a hierarchy, the next step is to instruct your patient in how to do *in vivo* exposure. First, help your patient determine where to begin on the hierarchy. If possible, start at the middle of the hierarchy, with the highest rated item that your patient is willing to try. Generally, it is best to start with an item that is rated at least 50 on the SUDS. So if the hierarchy starts at 50, you may also end up starting closer to the bottom of the hierarchy in some instances.

Sample Dialogue: Selecting an Item from the Hierarchy

THERAPIST: Imagine if I were afraid of diving off the high diving board—you know—the 10-meter boards, like they have at the Olympics?

JILL: Yeah, I've seen them.

THERAPIST: I could work on this fear by first starting in a tuck position and falling into the pool. Then, I could bend at the waist into a pike position and fall into the pool. Then, from a standing position, I could push up from the edge of the pool into the air and fall into the water headfirst. Next, I might jump from the 1-meter diving board in a cannonball position, then dive from the 1 meter board. Once I have mastered diving from the 1 meter diving board, I might try jumping from the 3-meter board, then diving from it. In this way, I gradually increase the height of the diving board until I reach the 10-meter high board. This works well, but it can be tedious and take some time to work my way up the different height boards in the different positions.

JILL: Yeah, that could take a long time.

THERAPIST: Also, by starting really low and only progressing to the next step as my fear diminishes, I never really experience very much fear, so I may not learn to cope with the fear itself.

JILL: I never thought of that.

THERAPIST: Another approach is to go right to the high board and dive off. This works, too—I definitely will feel fear! And it has the advantage of helping me get over my fear quickly. The problem with this approach is that many people find it very hard to do things that evoke fear at such an intense level. I might spend a long time peering over the edge and building my anticipatory anxiety, and I might never get myself to go off the high board. This could be discouraging, and the relief I feel when I climb down the ladder of the high board would reinforce my fear. Of course, you could just push me off, but it might not help me learn to cope with my fear if I didn't make the choice to go off voluntarily—in fact, it might make me more afraid of the high board. So what would work best is for me to start somewhere in the middle—the highest board that I can get myself to dive off of—even if maybe the first time I just jump off. The point is, it should be high enough for me to feel fear, but not so high that I am overwhelmed by my fear and unable to act, or even flee the situation altogether.

Preparing Coping Self-Statements

The use of coping self-statements is optional. You may decide, however, to introduce coping self-statements to patients who show a great deal of trepidation about beginning exposure or to those who have difficulty staying with the exposure homework once it is under way. Research on phobias has shown that the use of coping self-statements may reduce the perceived intrusiveness of exposure (Koch, Spates, & Himle, 2004).

Sample Dialogue: Coping Self-Statements

THERAPIST: You may find that doing the exposure task feels unnatural at first. It may feel strange to be approaching something you have habitually avoided for so long. What you say to yourself while you are approaching a feared situation may make a difference for your success. You may find it helpful to talk yourself through it, for example, by reminding yourself that the situation you are approaching is safe. You may also find it helpful to remind yourself of what you hope to gain by approaching the very thing that you have put so much effort toward avoiding in the past. Here are examples of coping self-talk statements (*shows patient Handout 6.3*)— things that you can say to yourself to help yourself stick with your *in vivo* exposure practice situation. (Or, if you have some of your own that work for you, write them in the blanks.) Some people find it helpful to pick a few that work best for them. You can highlight them on this sheet or write them on an index card, so you have it with you in your practice situation. This will help you cope with the increase in anxiety you are likely to experience during your exposure practice.

Examples of coping self-statements are the following:

"My anxiety won't hurt me, even if it doesn't feel good."
"I'm going to stick with it and watch my anxiety go down."
"I can be anxious and still manage this situation."
"This feeling isn't pleasant, but it won't last forever."
"My fear may go up, but I can cope with it."
"This is an opportunity for me to learn to cope with my fears."
"This is uncomfortable, but it's not dangerous."

Starting In Vivo *Exposure in Session*

Once you and your patient have identified a specific starting item in a hierarchy, you are ready to begin. Most often, you conduct the first exposure in session (Handout 7.3 can be used to track SUDS scores during in-session exposure), where you can model appropriate behaviors and provide support. In some cases, however, you will have patients begin *in vivo* exposure on their own at home. For example, it often takes an entire session to review the rationale for exposure and to develop a hierarchy. If you think your patient is capable of starting independently and are concerned about anticipatory anxiety building between sessions, assign the first *in vivo* item for homework. The instructions provided after the sample dialogue are helpful for both starting scenarios (i.e., in session and at home).

In this case, Jill's mauling by Barney was very severe (i.e., she was hospitalized for several weeks after being attacked), and she was highly avoidant of anything that resembled a dog. Thus, she ended up starting with her lowest item.

Sample Dialogue: Starting Exposure

THERAPIST: Before we start, let's get a rating of your anxiety. On a scale of 0 to 100, how much anxiety are you currently experiencing?

JILL: I am pretty anxious. At least a 60.

THERAPIST: OK. To review, in a moment, I am going to show you the dog picture we agreed to begin with and ask you to rate your anxiety. Although you may feel an urge to look away, I will encourage you to keep looking at the picture for the next 45 minutes or so, or until your anxiety decreases by half. Remember, the dog in the picture can't hurt you, even if it feels scary. I will ask you to rate your anxiety again, about every 5 minutes. I am going to keep track of it here on the computer, and we'll look at a graph of the results afterward.[2] Any questions?

JILL: No, I think I get it.

[*Commentary: The therapist can keep track of ongoing SUDS ratings on a piece of paper or on a computer. We prefer a computer, because it makes it easier to produce graphs of SUDS ratings for our patients.*]

THERAPIST: OK, here is the picture of the dog. I'm going to give it to you to hold on your lap and look at. Now, how much anxiety are you experiencing as you hold the picture in your lap?

JILL: Eighty.

[*Commentary: Quite often patients experience more anxiety than anticipated when they first start in* vivo *exposure. So although Jill began with item an item rated 45 on her hierarchy, it was not surprising that her peak anxiety was 80 during her first trial. Patients' level of anticipatory anxiety often is high during the first session, because they do not know what they are going to experience.*]

THERAPIST: OK, now just stay with your anxiety and keep looking at the picture of the dog. Look at all the different aspects of the dog as you feel your anxiety. (*90 seconds pass.*) Are you still focused on your anxiety?

JILL: (*Nods.*)

THERAPIST: Good, just keep focusing on your anxiety and keep looking at the picture of the dog. Take in all aspects of the dog. Look at the color of the dog and the mouth of the dog.

[*Commentary: The therapist reminds Jill of what she needs to do so that Jill stays focused on task. This typically is needed less after the first session.*]

THERAPIST: And now where is your anxiety? On the 0–100 scale, how much anxiety are you experiencing?

JILL: It's still pretty high. Maybe 78. I really want to put it away now.

[*Commentary: The therapist keeps using the word "anxiety" to remind Jill to focus on anxiety versus global distress or an alternative emotion, such as anger.*]

THERAPIST: We can expect you will want to escape, but try to stay with it. Feel your anxiety as you focus on the picture. . . . And now where is your anxiety?

JILL: Maybe 65.

THERAPIST: OK. You are doing a good job. Just keep doing what you are doing. Stay focused on your anxiety as you look at the picture. When you feel ready you might touch the picture, or even smell it.

---

[2]Some *in vivo* exposure tasks require leaving your office. When this is necessary, take a pen and pad along to keep track of SUDS ratings.

JILL: (*Tentatively touches picture on her lap, then begins touching it more. After a moment, she looks at the therapist, then smells the picture.*) Smells like nothing—well, maybe like a calendar.

THERAPIST: Well, it is a calendar picture. So keep looking and touching the picture. Look at the dog picture and feel your anxiety ... (*4 more minutes pass.*) ... And now where is your anxiety?

When conducting *in vivo* exposure, aim to strike a balance between staying quiet, so that your patient can concentrate, and encouraging your patient to engage in meaningful contact with the object or situation. For example, sexual assault survivors may fear and avoid particular soaps if a perpetrator used a strong-smelling soap. During soap exposure, some patients initially hold the soap with just a couple of fingers or very tentatively, even if the soap is in the wrapper. Gently encouraging such patients to hold the soap firmly and rub their hands along the side of the soap to more fully expose their skin to it, or to have the soap touch other parts of their body (e.g., legs, arms, hair) increases their contact with the soap. It also may be helpful to model the behaviors by showing your patient how to rub hands together to rub the "essence of soap" more deeply into the skin, or how to run soap-"contaminated" hands through your hair.

Once your patients have completed in-session exposure, review the graph of the session, praise them for staying with the situation, and point out the change in anxiety during the session. Then, give specific instructions about home practice:

Instructions for *in vivo* exposure homework

1. Definition of prolonged exposure: Stay in the situation until SUDS rating decreases 50%.
2. Importance of record keeping: How to keep records of each exposure (walk your patient through the *in vivo* Exposure Home Practice Record [Handout 6.6]).
3. Repeat the exposure task often—at least five times in the week—preferably daily.
4. Repeat the same exposure item for the entire first week without modifying it or advancing to the next hierarchy item.

Many patients are able to complete *in vivo* exposure at home with limited instruction once they have completed in-session exposure. A sizable minority of patients make important mistakes, however. They may cut the exposure session short or race on to the next hierarchy item before completing the one below it, in an attempt to "finish" the hierarchy. It is difficult to predict who will make mistakes. Thus, it is important to give very clear instructions regarding home practice of *in vivo* exposure and use Handout 6.5 to reinforce these instructions.

Sample Dialogues: Introducing Exposure

Point 1: Defining Prolonged Exposure

THERAPIST: The most important thing about doing *in vivo* exposure is to stay in the situation. When you practice confronting a situation, you may at first experience anxiety symptoms, such as your heart beating rapidly, your palms sweating, or feeling faint; you may want to leave the situation immediately. But to get over the fear it is important that you remain in the situation until your anxiety decreases by at least 50%. Usually this will happen in 30–45 minutes, but sometimes it can take longer. Once your anxiety has decreased 50%, you can stop the exposure and resume other activities. For example, if your highest SUDS rating is 80, you should stay in the situation until your SUDS rating reaches 40. (*Draws "Habituation Curve: Staying in the Situation until Your Anxiety Goes Down by 50%" from Handout 6.5.*) If your peak SUDS rating is 60, stay in the situation until your SUDS rating declines to 30. If you leave the situation when you are very anxious, you will again convince yourself that the situation is very dangerous and that something terrible is going to happen to you. The next time you go into that situation, your level of anxiety will be as high, or even higher than before. If you stay in the situation, however, your anxiety will decrease just like in today's session, and you will eventually be able to en-counter the situation without fear.

Point 2: Importance of Record Keeping

THERAPIST: It is important to keep track of your progress. This will help you to see whether exposure is working for you and to decide when to go to the next step. Let's review how to use an *In Vivo* Exposure Home Practice Record (Handout 6.6) to track your progress. Before you start an exposure task, record the situation you will practice in Handout 6.6. Then rate your beginning SUDS. After you are done with exposure, rate your highest and your ending SUDS.

Point 3: Repeat the Exposure

THERAPIST: The more often you practice each situation on your list, the less anxiety you will experience. As a result, your urge to avoid distressing situations and people will also decline. As you can recall (*draws "Habituation Curve: Repeated Prolonged Exposure"; see Figure 6.4*), the first time you go into the situation, your anticipatory

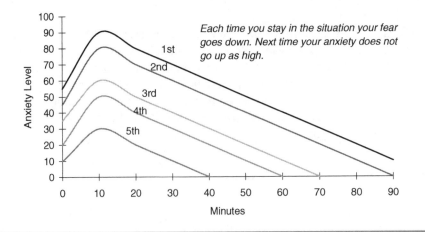

FIGURE 6.4. Habituation curve: Repeated prolonged exposures.

anxiety may be high. But with each repetition, your anxiety will diminish. Therefore, it's best if you practice exposure every day, if possible, or at least five times in the coming week.

Point 4: Maintain Consistency during the First Week

THERAPIST: It may be tempting to try to vary the exposure task or even move to the next item on your hierarchy. For the first week, however, it's best if you repeat the same exposure task each day, keeping your attention focused on the exposure stimulus and allowing yourself to feel your anxiety in the situation. You may be eager to charge ahead, but exposure cannot be rushed, and trying to move through your hierarchy too quickly can backfire. Next week, we'll look at your records together and talk about how to decide when to move to the next step.

If you are assigning your patient his or her first homework assignment without completing in-session *in vivo* exposure, you may want to create a contingency plan if the patient starts with an item that is too high on his or her hierarchy. Having patients develop mastery early improves compliance with exposure.

"Also, in some rare cases, it may be helpful to back up a step. If after staying with the exposure for more than 45–60 minutes several days in row, there is still no reduction in your fear, it may be best to switch to working on a hierarchy item that you rated slightly lower. Once you experience success with this situation, you can begin to gradually work your way up the list to approach some of the more distressing situations."

During subsequent weeks, encourage your patients to vary the ways they encounter hierarchy stimuli. The goal is to build on their experience. So, even as patients move on to different items, have them continue to expose themselves to variants of lower level items. For example, Emily was sexually molested as a child by a male dressed up as an Easter bunny. After years of avoiding all forms of the Easter bunny, she completed exposure to a stuffed Easter bunny. Subsequently, even as she moved on to other items in her hierarchy, Emily began to collect different types of Easter bunnies (e.g., different sizes and colors, some stuffed and others chocolate), lining them up in her room so that she could "once and for all get over my fear of these stupid bunnies." Ultimately, she decided to have her picture taken with the Easter bunny character at her local mall.

Sample Dialogue: Continuing Exposure Practice

THERAPIST: Now that you have completed some exposure, you need to focus on varying the situation. For example, if your task was to go into a supermarket, choose a different supermarket. This will increase the likelihood that the habituation you develop will be to supermarkets *in general*, not just to a single supermarket. Other variations may include going to supermarkets of different sizes, at different times of the day, when it is quiet and when it is busy, and so on.

TROUBLESHOOTING *IN VIVO* EXPOSURE

When So Many Things Trigger Anxiety, How Do We Decide What to Use for *In Vivo* Exposure?

There are several important considerations when designing an *in vivo* exposure assignment: safety, practicality, and clinical utility. A blend of common sense and clinical judgment helps you identifying exposure assignments that are safe, practical, and clinically useful.

Safety

In vivo exposure tasks are aimed at reducing fear in situations that are not realistically very dangerous. Therefore, situations, objects, or people that are actually dangerous should not be used. In Jill's case, there would be no need to do exposure to a vicious dog, because she would be advised to stay clear of such dogs. It also is not advisable in many cases to conduct *in vivo* exposure to childhood sexual abuse perpetrators; such individuals can present real current danger to varying degrees. For example, Jennifer's uncle, who molested her repeatedly, often showed up at family gatherings and continued to make sexual innuendos to her. In all likelihood, it makes sense for Jennifer to remain on guard with her uncle. She also became distressed, however, when looking at family photos in which he appeared. These might be useful exposure stimuli.

Similarly, exposure to guns often is ill advised, because guns can be dangerous. Under special circumstances, however, exposure to guns may be legitimately therapeutic, for example, if your patient's fear of guns interferes with recreational or vocational pursuits (e.g., hunting or police work), or if the fear interferes with legitimate gun use by family members. If exposure to guns is essential, there are several important considerations. First, consider whether your patient's history includes suicidal ideation or attempts, self-injury, or rage or homicidal thoughts toward others. If a history of acting on such urges and/or thoughts of harming self or others has been present recently, then exposure to guns may be contraindicated, because your patient may be at risk for causing harm. Second, consider consulting with another clinician with exposure experience, obtain appropriate risk management and legal consultation, and ensure that you and your patient are acting within local and state firearms regulations. Finally, if possible, conduct exposure with unloaded guns. We have yet to encounter a situation where we needed to conduct exposure with loaded guns. Supervision by a trained gun professional may be advisable during exposure if firing of a gun is required.

Exposure to knives is more commonly necessary, because the fear of knives often interferes in daily life. Yet, as with exposure to guns, knife exposure warrants careful consideration of risk for harming self or others, whether accidental or intentional. Supervising exposure prior to assigning home practice enables you to assess risk more directly.

Other safety concerns might also be raised by the nature of the stimulus. In such instances, be creative. For example, exposure to blood might be unwise, but fake blood, blood in a vial, or even ketchup might be a viable substitute. Similarly, exposure to semen may raise both safety and practicality concerns. Many patients who are afraid of semen, however, report being fearful of touching raw egg whites as well.

Practicality and Clinical Utility

Many stimuli that might be clinically useful may be practically difficult. For example, Sarah felt anxious whenever she drove by the house in which her childhood abuse took place. She was particularly fearful of the interior of the house, but because the house had been sold to another family, she could not conduct exposure to the interior. Instead, she used photographs from her childhood and similar rooms of her sister's house. Jill was quite fearful of dogs that showed their teeth. It can be difficult to get a dog to show its teeth for an extended time, so she used pictures and film. For example, she watched scenes from the movie *Cujo* repeatedly.

To be clinically useful, stimuli should be defined and concrete enough to maintain attention and facilitate habituation. We habituate most easily to stable, unchanging, or nonfluctuating stimuli or situations. When using stimuli that change over time (e.g., television shows, songs), it is important to target repetitively the key segments that are distressing. For example, in the course of 30 minutes, expose your patient to one 5-minute segment six times, rather than one 30-minute television show in which only 5 minutes are distressing.

Many patients need to be exposed to situations and stimuli that do not normally present in a continuous, stable form for 30–60 minutes. In such cases, creatively "stabilize" or prolong the stimulus to maximize the probability of habituation. A "loop" tape that continuously repeats a brief segment can be a useful tool for audio or video material, but simply rewinding and repeating a segment can be equally effective. For example, Sarah was highly anxious about watching others, including her children, vomit, secondary to watching her abusive, alcoholic father vomit frequently when she was child. She videotaped several episodes of a medical television show until she had captured half a dozen brief vomit scenes. She watched each scene, constructed a hierarchy of the scenes, then watched each scene in the hierarchy repeatedly for 5 days in a row, 30–45 minutes at a time. Later she moved on to watching her therapist simulate vomiting by taking a spoonful of chunky soup into her mouth and spitting it into a trash bin while mimicking vomit sounds. The recipe for simulated vomit can be adjusted by adding a little vinegar to enhance the vomit-like odor, or using other foods that mimic characteristics your patient finds most anxiety provoking.

Similarly, after having his car flip off a bridge, David became scared of driving over bridges. He could only drive on the short, local bridges for a couple of minutes before the bridge would end, which was not sufficient promote habituation. Instructing David to start on a bridge with little traffic and easy turnaround opportunities, however, meant that David could repeatedly drive over the bridge. Kara was terrified of the sounds of Harley Davidson motorcycles, which her abusive ex-boyfriend owned. She became very frightened when driving her car if someone rode by on a Harley. Kara's therapist created an audiotape of the sound of a Harley by visiting a dealership. Similarly, Wendy, whose childhood abuse took place in woods surrounded by dirt bike trails, conducted exposure by visiting a dirt bike racetrack. A wide variety of useful sounds for exposure also can be found on Internet websites of sound effects.

Some stimuli are such potent triggers of memories that it can be difficult for patients to maintain sustained attention to them. For example, odors sometimes can be difficult, because an odor can be potent flashback triggers. For example, Laura's perpetrator used cologne, and Laura reported flashing back whenever she smelled his brand of cologne. Research indicates that odors are particularly potent memory cues. Memories recalled using odor cues are more emotional and evocative than memories recalled using other sensory stimuli (Aggleton & Waskett, 1999; Herz, 2004). Thus, it may be difficult to slow or prevent the onset of a flashback, which can render the exposure unhelpful, because patients do not experience corrective information about safety while flashing back (see below). Rather than begin with smelling the cologne, Laura started with the bottle in its box. Similarly, if the stimulus is a food, it may be necessary to separate the odor, touch, and/or taste of the food from its appearance in building the hierarchy. Sometimes using photos of the stimulus can be helpful as a first step.

Patients with abuse or assault histories frequently identify "people" and "conflict" as the only things that trigger anxiety. *In vivo* exposure should be to specific people (e.g., men who look like the perpetrator) or specific situations with people (e.g., speaking to a small group, sitting next to people on a bus, or being in a crowded café). Sometimes patients say they are fearful of people, when in fact they have difficulty trusting people in relationships. This is not an appropriate stimulus for *in vivo* exposure. Difficulty trusting others is best handled by using cognitive restructuring and behavioral experiments aimed at building trust in relationships gradually, and testing beliefs about trust. Although *in vivo* exposure can have a role in this, *in vivo* exposure tasks must be more specific to be clinically useful.

Exposure to "conflict" also may not be clinically useful. Patients raised in abusive environments often say that they are sensitized to yelling. Exposure to yelling might reduce their discomfort, but it is important to ask whether becoming desensitized to yelling serves an adaptive function for a given patient. If your patient is fearful of conflict to the point that lively debates elicit fear, then exposure to conflict, possibly using film, may be appropriate. Yet, in other situations, you may prefer your patient to insist that family members learn to resolve conflicts without yelling. Moreover, if by "conflict" your patient means that he or she cannot tolerate any disagreement with others, assertive communication skills training may be more helpful than exposure.

If We Have Constructed Several Different Hierarchies, How Do We Choose a Hierarchy to Start?

If a patient has several hierarchies outlining different classes of stimuli, a good practice is to start with an *in vivo* hierarchy related to the first memory addressed in imaginal exposure. Another consideration in selecting a hierarchy is how avoidance of that class of stimuli is affecting your patient's life. For example, Gretchen constructed two hierarchies: one related to police uniforms, which triggered flashbacks to her sexual abuse, and the other related to her aunt's house, where her sexual abuse took place. Her aunt, who was an important support in her life, still lived in the house, and avoidance of the house limited Gretchen's ability to make use of this support. Thus, she decided to start by reducing avoidance of her aunt's house.

What If We Cannot Identify a Stimulus for *In Vivo* Exposure?

With probing and creativity, it is usually possible to identify a stimulus that is appropriate for *in vivo* exposure. Probing can be as simple as providing a copy of the Ways I Avoid Worksheet (Handout 6.2) to patients who have difficulty with the avoidance section of Common Reactions to Traumatic Experiences (Handout 5.1). In other instances, however, you may have to work a bit harder. For example, Lisa, a highly aroused physical assault survivor, was unable to identify any objects or situations for *in vivo* exposure. Lisa also did not believe that exposure would work for her. Thus, her therapist wanted to start with a simple *in vivo* task. The therapist and Lisa scheduled an out-of-the-office appointment, during which they walked in and out of stores to see if anything scared Lisa. When Lisa walked into a sporting goods store, she realized she was terrified of fishing poles, which her husband had used to beat her. In this case, it was helpful to have Lisa's therapist accompany her, because she had been unable to complete a similar homework assignment. Some patients, however, can hunt for triggers on their own.

In instances where you find that nothing is evident, simply begin with imaginal exposure. Inform your patient that many people have difficulty identifying cues for *in vivo* exposure and that together you will continue to look for cues, because including *in vivo* exposure may improve outcome. It is rare that cues for *in vivo* exposure do not become apparent once you start imaginal exposure, and details of the memory often point to possible stimuli. For example, Carrie could not think of any concrete cues that made her anxious, but during imaginal exposure she described the perpetrator of a sexual assault in great detail, including the fact that he wore a green work shirt and smelled like soap. After a little discussion, she noted that in the medical center she avoided a hallway where painting was being done, because the painters wore similar shirts. Similarly, she never purchased his brand of soap. Barbara could not think of any *in vivo* stimuli, but when she described her memory of sexual abuse by her uncle, she described how he took his penis out of the opening in his boxer shorts. After the exposure session the therapist asked her how she felt about boxer shorts. Barbara told the therapist that when her son was in junior high school, he asked her to buy boxer shorts because all his friends had them, and she flew into a rage. Barbara used boxer shorts as her next *in vivo* exposure stimulus.

It is important to plan carefully how to obtain *in vivo* exposure stimuli. Whenever possible, it is best to encourage patients to obtain the item, because this normalizes the activity (e.g., buying a bar of soap) and encourages mastery over the stimulus. Quite often patients can purchase an item, such as the bar of soap, from a store on their own and bring it home in an opaque bag. For some patients, however, obtaining the object (i.e., handling it for 15 minutes in the store, carrying it home in a bag, and bringing it to session) may produce significant anxiety, and they may be unable to do this as the first step. In such cases, you may need to obtain the item for them. For example, Susan was molested by her grandfather when he was drunk. During the molestation, she would stare at the empty cans of beer, and she was terrified both of the can and the smell of beer; thus, the therapist obtained the stimulus, and also informed the clinic directors before the next session, so that they could approve the action of bringing beer cans into the clinic.

What If the Patient's Anxiety Does Not Go Down?

Sometimes, anxiety reduction may be so slow that it is difficult to detect, particularly if the exposure sessions are not long enough. For example, Carmen began *in vivo* exposure on her own to music that she associated with her abuse. She returned several days later, reporting that she had done it three times for 10 minutes each, and her anxiety stayed at 100 the entire time. As a result, her therapist opted to initiate an in-session exposure, first coaching Carmen on the importance of focusing on the music rather than on any memories that might be triggered by it. During her first exposure to listening to the 4-minute segment of music repeatedly for 45 minutes, Carmen's anxiety decreased from 100 to 95 within 30 minutes. She had a very hard time continuing but with encouragement, she did, and her anxiety went down to 80 after an additional 15 minutes of exposure (see Figure 6.5).

Following such a gradual reduction in anxiety, it might have been easy for Carmen and her therapist to conclude "It's not working." Instead, her therapist praised Carmen for focusing on the music for this long and noted that although the reduction in anxiety was slow, it did go down. The therapist emphasized that Carmen likely would experience further reductions with continued repetition, and also drew the repeated habituation graph again for Carmen (see Figure 6.5). In the subsequent session, Carmen's anxiety continued to show gradual within- and between-session habituation. In the middle of the second session, the therapist showed Carmen her graph (Figure 6.5). Carmen said, "Oh, I see this how it works," then asked, "How long do I have to do it?" The therapist reminded Carmen that optimally she should stay with the exposure stimulus until her anxiety was reduced by half. The therapist encouraged Carmen to extend her home practice to achieve the 50% goal, even though this was not possible in the first session, because they had been unable to extend that exposure session beyond 50 minutes. The therapist also reviewed a graph of Carmen's homework practice data and pointed out that the between-trial reductions in anxiety at home were limited, because the sessions were too short. Finally, the therapist reminded Carmen that she might experience more anxiety at home, because she was doing *in vivo* exposure in the environment where her abuse took place. Patients often experience higher anxiety levels during home practice, which may be due to both the change in environment and the absence of the therapist, who may be a signal for safety.

Sometimes, when a patient's anxiety does not go down within or across trials, you need to do some troubleshooting to figure out why habituation is not occurring. Several factors may account for this. First, your patient may be altering the hierarchy items

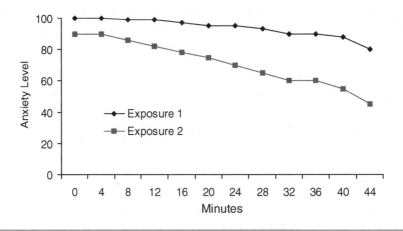

FIGURE 6.5. Carmen's *in vivo* exposure to ragtime jazz: sessions 1 and 2.

between trials. For example, John was afraid of basements, because he was abused in a basement. His hierarchy involved successively approaching the basement of his sister's house (John built his own house without one). His first step was to sit on the basement steps with his sister nearby in the kitchen. His Exposure record showed that his anxiety went down during the first trial, and that peak anxiety was reduced between Trials 1 and 2. But on Trial 3, peak anxiety was higher than that on the two previous trials. When the therapist asked John to describe more precisely what he had done, he revealed that the third time, he did not wait for his sister and started on his own. Sitting on the steps alone was actually the fifth item on John's hierarchy. When asked why he did this, John stated, "I wanted to get through this, and I just thought I should be able to do this on my own." The therapist validated John's eagerness to see progress and his desire to do things on his own. She also pointed out that the changes John made explained why his anxiety went up rather than down.

Sample Dialogue: Patient Skips Hierarchy Items

THERAPIST: I see that you are really hoping to get through the exposure quickly, and it's frustrating to feel so dependent on your sister. This explains what we are seeing on your graph. It makes sense that your anxiety was higher on the third trial, because what you did that day was actually something you had rated much higher on your hierarchy.

JOHN: Yeah, I guess so. I thought I could do it.

THERAPIST: And you did do it! Good for you. At the same time, you can expect your anxiety to be higher when you change to a new situation. We generally recommend sticking with your first item until your peak SUDS rating is no higher than 20. Your peak SUDS rating on the third trial was 75. I would recommend that you return to that item before advancing on your hierarchy. That way, you will get to see what it feels like when your anxiety goes down to a greater degree, and you will develop more confidence in exposure.

A second reason why anxiety may not decline is because the task selected may be inappropriate (e.g., dangerous, unhealthy, or fluctuating/not sufficiently stabilized). For example, Sarah wanted to overcome her distress at being around her mother, even though her mother remained married to her stepfather, who had repeatedly abused Sarah sexually. Although Sarah's stepfather no longer sexually abused her, neither he nor her mother had ever acknowledged the abuse. Moreover, whenever Sarah visited her mother, her stepfather would make inappropriate and sexually suggestive remarks about Sarah's appearance and her relationship with her boyfriend. Doing exposure to being around her mother was not appropriate. Instead, Sarah's treatment needed to address setting boundaries with her stepfather and assertively communicating her needs to her mother.

Similarly, Jennifer, a physical abuse survivor, was distressed by her inability to watch movies out of fear of violent scenes. Jennifer did not initially admit to her therapist that her boyfriend was pressuring her to watch violent pornography as a prelude to sex, and that this was her primary motivation for wanting to habituate to movie violence. Completing exposure to violent pornography was not the most appropriate way for Jennifer to manage her boyfriend's pressure. Instead, Jennifer's therapist focused on assertive communication.

Finally, when Jill initially completed exposure to 5-minute sections of the movie *Cujo,* she showed very slow habituation. After viewing the clip, the therapist noticed that there was a brief break in the dog attack, approximately 1 minute into the clip. Jill confirmed that her anxiety decreased during this section, then increased again when the dog resumed the attack. Shortening the clip to the disturbing 3 minutes after the less tense section produced better results.

A third reason that anxiety may not decrease during exposure is because your patient is not sufficiently focused on feelings of anxiety. This might mean that your patient is either attending to other emotions, such as anger, guilt, or shame, or is simply focused on another external stimulus as a means of distracting attention away from the associated anxiety. The research literature regarding the effects of distracting attention from the stimulus during *in vivo* exposure for phobias has been mixed. Yet studies of exposure for PTSD have found that attending to anger during exposure is associated with poor outcome (Foa, Riggs, Massie, & Yarczower, 1995). No similar studies of guilt and shame during exposure are available. There is, however, evidence that patients with high levels of guilt or shame do not have as good an outcome from exposure alone (Smucker et al., 2003). We also have observed that patients fail to habituate when they focus on shame and guilt during exposure, or vacillate between focusing on anxiety and other emotions. Ideally, patients should focus on anxiety during exposure and, to the extent possible, "shelve" other emotions, which can be addressed more directly after exposure, using other methods, if necessary. Lack of focus on anxiety tends to be less of a problem during *in vivo* exposure, and when it does happen, it may mean that the patient is attending to the memory rather than just the *in vivo* stimulus (see below). In some instances, if your patient is unable to focus on anxiety, you may find it useful to work on the anger, shame, or guilt-related thoughts using cognitive restructuring (see Chapter 8) first, then return to exposure after you have observed reduction in these emotions.

Finally, if your patient does not attend to the *in vivo* stimulus during exposure, anxiety may not go down. It also may decrease abruptly, which may indicate that you started too high on the hierarchy. For example, Paul appeared highly anxious during in-session exposure to a nightgown that resembled the one his mother wore when she sexually abused him. At 15 minutes, Paul's anxiety had not decreased from his initial report of "100." After a while, the therapist noticed that Paul's voice became more monotone; he stopped trembling, his expression flattened, and his gaze looked far away. The therapist asked, "Paul, are you with me? Please look at me." Paul blinked, looked up and said, "What?" Questioning revealed that approximately 20 minutes into exposure, after thinking "I don't think I can do this. This is too much," Paul started thinking about sailing his boat, something he often did when he felt stressed. Switching to an item that produced less anxiety improved Paul's confidence in his ability to stay with his anxiety, and he subsequently completed exposure to the nightgown.

At times, patients may be able to complete in-session exposure but experience difficulty at home. For example, Lucia was able to complete in-session exposure successfully to an empty wine bottle that reminded her of her physically abusive mother. During exposure at home, however, she reported becoming overwhelmed and dissociating.

If your patient reports dissociative responses during *in vivo* exposure practice at home but did not show such behavior in your office, its possible that conducting the exposure task at home (vs. in the office) is higher on the hierarchy for them. It may be helpful to drop to a lower hierarchy item for initial home practice sessions.

What If the Patient Does Not Experience Much Anxiety during *In Vivo* Exposure?

Occasionally you may find that your patient experiences surprisingly little anxiety during exposure. There are three primary reasons for this. First, patients who have very high levels of anticipatory anxiety occasionally misjudge how much anxiety the actual object or situation will provoke. In such cases, your patient may report a very rapid decline in anxiety and state that exposure to the item is nowhere as bad as expected. In such cases, just move up the hierarchy or on to imaginal exposure.

Second, some patients report minimal anxiety because they "numb out" or dissociate. This might indicate (as in the case of Paul) that you have started too high on your patient's hierarchy. In such cases, moving to a lower level item may be all that is needed. In other cases, this might indicate that your patient does not have the requisite emotion skills needed for exposure (e.g., an ability to stay present while experiencing anxiety). In these cases, we typically turn to dialectical behavior therapy (DBT) methods (see Chapter 9), such as mindfulness, distress tolerance, and emotion regulation skills training, then return to exposure. The aim is to teach patients to be aware in the moment and to accept and be present with unpleasant emotions. Once your patients have developed skills for staying present, you can prompt them to use these skills to stay present with their anxiety during exposure.

Finally, your patient may be relying on safety behaviors to reduce anxiety. Safety behaviors include a wide range of coping strategies that patients develop to manage anxiety. For example, Carol carried around a picture of her father, who had removed her from her mother's house after learning that Carol had been abused by the mother's boyfriend. Carol reported "feeling better" whenever she had the picture, and she carried the photo anytime she needed to do something that provoked anxiety. Carol did not experience significant anxiety during exposure until the photo was removed from the office. Safety behaviors can include carrying objects, a change in breathing, counting, and so forth. If a patient does not experience significant anxiety during exposure, carefully observe your patient for possible safety behaviors and inquire whether there are things he or she does to minimize distress. Engaging in safety behaviors during exposure tends to result in a less satisfactory outcome (Clark, 1999; Kim, 2005; Salkovskis, Clark, Hackmann, Wells, & Gelder, 1999).

What If the Patient Flashes Back during *In Vivo* Exposure?

Some patients reexperience the memory vividly during *in vivo* exposure, even to the point of "flashing back." Flashing back during exposure is undesirable, because it means that, to some extent, your patient has lost awareness of reality and feels as though the trauma is actually happening. Therefore, your patient may not experience safety or the necessary corrective feedback. Even if your patient does not flash back, vivid recollection during *in vivo* exposure can be undesirable if the memory is so vivid that *in vivo* exposure becomes an unsystematic imaginal exposure. As a result, anxiety reduction may not follow the expected pattern, and your patient may not gain confidence in the exposure process. For example, in discussing her exposure to Toby, her sister's golden retriever, Jill told her therapist that exposure went as expected at first (see Figure 6.6). Despite high anticipatory anxiety, Jill's anxiety peaked at 70 during her first trial and dropped off quickly. During the next two trials, her anticipatory anxiety reduced and her peak anxiety was lower than in the previous trial. During her fourth trial, however, Jill's anxiety level peaked at 95. Jill believed this meant that exposure would not work for her. Jill also reported that her sister's cat had entered the room and Toby snarled. This snarl led her to recall vividly the attack by Barney. As a result, the exposure became imaginal exposure to the memory of the attack, and the shift in focus from Toby to the memory interfered with learning that Toby was a safe dog. After discussing what had transpired, Jill agreed to continue *in vivo* exposure practice with Toby. If her attention were drawn to the memory of the attack again, she would remind herself that (1) she would work on the memory of Barney separately during imaginal exposure, (2) Toby was not Barney, (3) Toby's reaction to the cat did not mean he would attack a person, and (4) she needed to refocus her attention on Toby. This worked well in Jill's case. Some patients, however, find that they cannot expose themselves to the trauma reminder without becoming immersed in reliving the memory. In such cases, use the strategies for titrating anxiety during exposure, described in Chapter 7. In some instances, it may be necessary to teach mindfulness skills (see Chapter 9) and prompt your patient to use these skills to maintain awareness of the present environment when returning to exposure.

For example, Elizabeth, a survivor of childhood sexual abuse, identified raw egg whites and brown beer bottles as *in vivo* exposure items. Attempts to initiate *in vivo* exposure with these stimuli inevitably led to full immersion in the trauma memory. As a result, her therapist decided to conduct imaginal exposure first, and introduce *in vivo* exposure to egg whites and beer bottles after imaginal exposure had been completed.

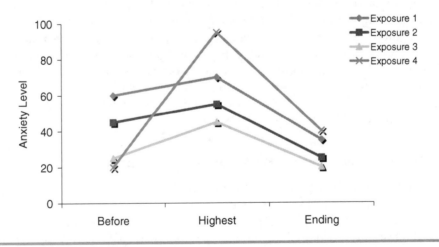

FIGURE 6.6. Jill's *in vivo* exposure to Toby: home practice.

Even after having fully habituated to the associated memory, Elizabeth experienced a high degree of anxiety in reaction to both egg whites and beer bottles. This reaction highlights the importance of returning to or starting *in vivo* exposure if relevant stimuli have been identified.

CONCLUSION

Exposure is a remarkably powerful clinical tool in the treatment of PTSD. Many patients experience marked relief surprisingly quickly using this strategy. Thus, we encourage you to consider using it with most of your patients with PTSD. The majority of these patients who begin exposure are likely to complete it and reap its benefits. With careful analysis, creativity, and perseverance you can help those with atypical reactions during exposure to engage successfully in exposure to achieve the desired results.

WHY DOES MY FEAR PERSIST EVEN THOUGH THE DANGER IS PAST?

Fear and arousal are natural reactions to danger. Fear becomes a problem when it continues even after the danger is past. In this program, we focus on the fears and negative thoughts that you experience as a result of your traumatic experience(s). Although most of the symptoms we have talked about gradually decline with time, some symptoms endure for many trauma survivors and continue to cause marked distress, sometimes for many years. By understanding what causes your reactions to continue, it is possible for you to recover from the effects of your traumatic experience(s). Two main factors are involved in prolonging posttrauma difficulties.

Avoidance

The first factor is avoidance of situations, memories, thoughts, and feelings that remind you of your traumatic experience(s). It is quite normal for people to want to escape or avoid memories, situations, thoughts, and feelings that are painful and distressing. You may have found that avoiding thoughts, memories, and reminders of trauma helped you to survive, both physically and emotionally. However, although the strategy of avoiding painful material works in the short run, it actually may prolong posttrauma reactions and prevent you from "getting over" your trauma-related difficulties.

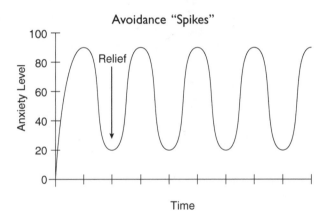

When you confront the painful material rather than avoid it, you will have the opportunity to process the traumatic experience(s). For example, if you avoid trauma-related situations that are objectively safe, you do not give yourself the opportunity to get used to being in these situations. Unless you confront the situations, you may continue to believe that they are dangerous, and your anxiety in these situations will remain indefinitely. However, if you confront these situations, you will find out

(continued)

that they are not actually dangerous, and your anxiety will diminish with repeated exposure. As a result of this process your symptoms will decline. The same is true for painful memories. For this reason, treatment typically involves repeatedly thinking about your traumatic memories and confronting safe situations that you are now avoiding.

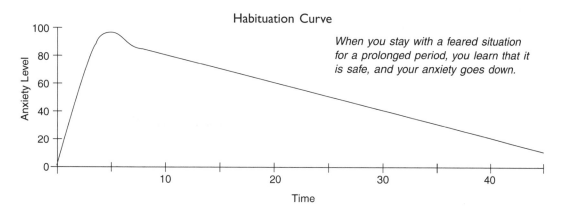

Unhelpful Ways of Thinking

The second factor that maintains your posttrauma distress is the presence of unhelpful negative thoughts. After the traumatic experience(s), you may have learned to expect bad things to happen in your life. Given your experience(s), it makes sense that you would adopt a negative outlook on life. Such an outlook may be unhelpful in that it may foster excessively negative thoughts and expectations that tend to maintain posttrauma distress. For example, if you think that your experiences were partially your fault, you may blame yourself, and this may contribute to overwhelming guilt and depression. Similarly, if you were assaulted by a man, you may think that all men are dangerous and may expect to be hurt by men. This would understandably lead you to avoid being around men; thus, you would limit your opportunities to interact with men who are not dangerous. Likewise, if you believe that experiencing flashbacks is a sign that you are losing control, you may try very hard to push the memories out of your mind. However, the more you try to push these memories away, the more they intrude on your consciousness and the less control you actually have over the memories. In this program, we help you overcome your posttrauma difficulties by identifying your unhelpful thoughts and expectations, and teaching you how to think in more helpful ways.

TREATMENT BY EXPOSURE AND COGNITIVE RESTRUCTURING

There are three main parts to cognitive-behavioral treatment for PTSD that your therapist may include in your individualized plan. In the first, *in vivo* exposure, you approach safe situations that you usually avoid because they remind you of the traumatic event. In the second part, imaginal exposure, you safely recall the trauma repeatedly in your mind. In the third part, cognitive restructuring, you learn how to evaluate whether the ways you think about yourself and the world are accurate and helpful. You also learn to challenge views that are not helpful to you.

(continued)

Exposure Therapy

Imaginal and *in vivo* exposure work in similar ways. Many people who have experienced a traumatic event try to avoid thoughts, feelings, situations, and activities that remind them of their trauma. Because such reminders can be very distressing, you may find yourself trying to avoid them. However, although avoiding can make you feel more comfortable in the short run, it actually can make the problem worse in the long run by preventing you from overcoming your fears. When you decide to confront your fears in a systematic way, under relatively safe circumstances, you learn that you can manage anxiety. You learn that your fear gradually decreases when you repeatedly approach things that you have avoided, and that you can become relatively comfortable in these situations again. We call this *habituation*.

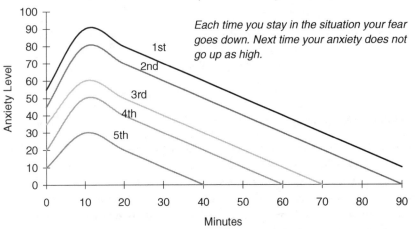

Habituation Curve: Repeated Prolonged Exposures

Each time you stay in the situation your fear goes down. Next time your anxiety does not go up as high.

Habituation is the process by which anxiety decreases on its own. When you stick it out and stay in a frightening situation for a long enough time, and go back to that same situation often enough, you simply become less frightened of the situation. In a way, it is similar to getting back on a bicycle after falling off: If you refuse to try again over time, you become more and more frightened of riding bicycles. But if you persuade yourself to ride them despite your fear, you eventually become less afraid. Habituation works the same way with frightening memories. Allowing yourself to engage with the traumatic memories rather than avoiding them helps you remember the trauma with less distress. Exposure (e.g., reliving the trauma in imagery) allows you to gain control over the memories, so that they will be less likely to pop up at unwanted times. Thus, the flashbacks, nightmares, and intrusive thoughts that you and many trauma survivors may experience are less likely to occur after you recall the trauma repeatedly; when the flashbacks and intrusive thoughts do occur, they will be less upsetting.

(continued)

Cognitive Restructuring

Following traumatic experiences, people may adopt views about themselves and the world that are unrealistic and unhelpful. For example, you may look at the world as a scary place or you may view yourself as a helpless, worthless person. These kinds of thoughts may reflect the bias in your thinking that we discussed previously. Remember, that after an encounter with a lion, it is wise to be on the lookout for danger. So, it makes sense that after the lion attack you feel a chill go down your spine when the tabby cat prances across the street. However, your being attacked by a lion does not make tabby cats dangerous. Cognitive restructuring (CR, for short) is a method for learning to be aware of what you are thinking when you feel distressed, and to evaluate your thoughts. CR also enables you to change thoughts that are not helpful to you. Most importantly, by helping you to recognize the reality of a situation, CR empowers you to take back control of your life.

Treatment by imaginal exposure, *in vivo* exposure, and CR may seem difficult at first, but with time, these tools work to help you conquer your fear, guilt, shame, and depression, allowing you to feel better about yourself.

HANDOUT 6.2. Ways I Avoid Worksheet

Make a list of some of the ways that you avoid being reminded of your traumatic experiences. These could be situations, places, or people you avoid; ways you've organized your life to avoid certain reminders or memories; changing the topic of conversation; using alcohol or drugs; "numbing out" in certain situations; and so forth. You may find you need to come back to this task several times as other ways you avoid occur to you. Below is an example of such a list:

1. Avoiding basements
2. Only seeing people when it is unavoidable
3. Not watching the news or reading newspapers
4. Drinking alcohol when I get home to avoid thinking about it
5. Avoiding men in work shirts
6. Getting angry when people try to talk with me about what happened
7. Canceling or not showing up for therapy
8. Not letting my husband touch my breasts during sex
9. Not going to grocery stores alone
10. Worrying about other people's problems instead of dealing with my own

Use the space below to make your own list.

1. _____
2. _____
3. _____
4. _____
5. _____
6. _____
7. _____
8. _____
9. _____
10. _____

DECIDE TO FACE YOUR FEAR

One way you may cope with distress related to traumatic experiences is to avoid situations, people, and things that remind you of the traumatic events. By now you have begun to recognize how this avoidance plays a role in maintaining your fears. Also, it is likely that you are becoming more aware of the ways that you avoid reminders of past traumas and the consequences of your avoidance for your life. In some instances you may decide that the negative effects of your avoidance in the long run outweigh the short-term benefits, such as temporary anxiety reduction.

Once you have made a decision to change a particular avoidance, the next step is to plan how you may begin to approach what you have been avoiding. Implementing your decision to change your avoidance may be "easier said than done." The short-term benefits of avoidance may continue to exert influence over your decisions about how to respond. You may continue to feel a strong urge to avoid, perhaps because you prefer the short-term benefit (relief) over the discomfort of approaching what you fear. As you move forward in this process, you may find it useful to continue to remind yourself of the long-term consequences of your avoidance and potential long-term benefits of reversing this avoidance.

APPROACH WHAT YOU FEAR

The *in vivo* exposure part of this treatment program involves helping you to systematically approach situations that trigger fear. This does not mean that you should go into unsafe situations. The goal is to reduce your avoidance of situations that are *realistically* safe—*not* that you should learn to view truly dangerous situations as safe. Repeated exposure to anxiety-producing situations almost always results in an eventual decrease in anxiety. As you learned before, we call this process *habituation*. Habituation takes place when you expose yourself repeatedly to situations that make you anxious, until your anxiety gradually decreases. Below is an example that illustrates how habituation works:

> When Adrienne was a little girl at the zoo with her mother, a tiger in a cage let out a big roar. This frightened Adrienne so much that the next day, when she went to her cousin's house for his birthday party, she was reluctant to go in because she was afraid of her cousin's cat. When Adrienne entered the house and saw the cat, she started to cry and ran to the door. Her uncle took her hand and reassured her that the tabby cat was friendly and would not hurt her. She stayed through the entire party and the next day came to visit again; this time, her uncle helped her to move closer to the cat. Then they gradually moved closer to the cat and eventually Adrienne's uncle demonstrated to her that he could pet the cat safely, and he encouraged her to do the same. Because she didn't escape the house and instead, with her uncle's encouragement, approached the cat, Adrienne's fear of the cat diminished and eventually she was able to enjoy visiting her cousin and even began to play with the cat again.

Many people fear that if they stay in a situation that is frightening, their anxiety will remain high indefinitely. The graph below shows what actually happens when you stay in an anxiety-provoking situation for a long time. Gradually, your anxiety goes down.

(continued)

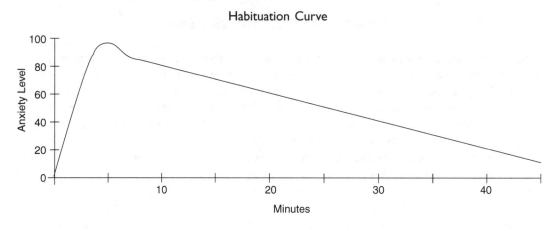

TALK YOURSELF THROUGH IT

You may find that doing the exposure task feels unnatural at first. It may feel strange to be approaching something you have habitually avoided for so long. What you say to yourself while you are approaching a feared situation may make a difference for your success. It may be helpful to remind yourself why you are approaching the very thing that you have put so much effort toward avoiding in the past. You may also find it helpful to remind yourself of the positive changes you expect will come from *not* avoiding.

The following are examples of coping self-talk statements—things that you say to yourself to help yourself stick with your *in vivo* exposure practice situation. (Or, if you have your own self-talk items that work for you, write them in the blanks.) You may find it helpful to pick a few of these and write them on an index card, so that you have it with you in your practice situation. This will help you in coping with the increase in anxiety you are likely to experience during your exposure practice.

- My anxiety won't hurt me, even if it doesn't feel good.
- I'm going to stick with it and watch my anxiety go down.
- I can be anxious and still manage this situation.
- This feeling isn't pleasant, but it won't last forever.
- My fear may go up, but I can cope with it.
- This is an opportunity for me to learn to cope with my fears.
- This is uncomfortable, but it's not dangerous.

- _____
- _____
- _____
- _____

Repeated exposure to a feared situation will reduce your discomfort. In preparation for *in vivo* exposure, make a plan for successive steps in approaching the feared situation, a "hierarchy," using the worksheet on p. 114.

- **Step 1: Choose a Feared Situation.** Look over your list of triggers and things you avoid on your Common Reactions to Traumatic Experiences handout (Handout 5.1) and your Ways I Avoid list (Handout 6.2), if you have one. These lists help you identify situations, places, or people you avoid, or ways you've organized your life to avoid certain trauma reminders. Choose one of the situations you avoid from this list for this exercise.
- **Step 2: Brainstorm.** Write down as many aspects of the situation you can think of that you are presently avoiding (use additional paper, if necessary).
- **Step 3: Rate.** Evaluate each item in terms of expected anxiety on the SUDS scale to reflect how much anxiety you would likely feel if you were in that situation. SUDS, which stands for Subjective Units of Distress Scale, is a scale from 0 to 100, where 0 = *no anxiety* and 100 = *maximum anxiety*.
- **Step 4: Rerank.** Rank-order your initial list of items, this time in ascending SUDS order. Rewrite the list in the new order on the second form, wording the items as actual tasks that can be done, with specifics as to how they will be done. This completes your *in vivo* exposure hierarchy.

MODEL FOR *IN VIVO* EXPOSURE HIERARCHY

Sample Situation: <u>Going to the supermarket</u>

Aspects of feared situation	SUDS
Going to the supermarket by myself	100
Going to the supermarket with a friend, but we get separated	50
Being dropped off at the supermarket and having to go in alone	70
Going to the supermarket with my friend	20
Aspects rewritten as hierarchy of *in vivo* exposure exercises	SUDS
My friend accompanies me to the supermarket and we walk around.	20
My friend accompanies me to the supermarket and stays in a specific area in the store, while I walk around alone.	50
My friend drives with me to the supermarket and stays in the parking lot, while I walk around the supermarket alone.	70
I go to the supermarket by myself, and my friend waits by the telephone at his or her home or office.	90
I go to the supermarket by myself, without telling my friend.	100

(continued)

How Do I Plan a Hierarchy? *(page 2 of 2)*

IN VIVO **HIERARCHY WORKSHEET**

Step 1: Choose your feared situation: _____

Step 2: Brainstorm as many aspects of your feared situation that you can list.

Step 3: Rate each item on the 0–100 SUDS.

Object or situation	SUDS

Step 4: Rank-order your list from lowest to highest SUDS ratings.

Hierarchy for *in vivo* exposure exercises	SUDS

Now that you have developed your hierarchy for your first exposure task, where do you begin? In the first week, begin with a situation from your hierarchy that you rated about 50 on the SUDS. If, after trying several times for more than 30 minutes, you are unable to approach this situation, pick an item that you gave a slightly lower SUDS rating and start from there. Once you experience success with this situation, you can begin to work your way gradually up the list to approach some of the more distressing situations. If you prefer, your therapist may help you get started by doing the *in vivo* exposure task with you.

STAY IN THE SITUATION

When you practice confronting a situation, you may initially experience anxiety symptoms, such as your heart beating rapidly, your palms sweating, or feeling faint, you may want to leave the situation immediately. But to get over the fear it is important that you remain in the situation until your anxiety decreases. You should *remain in the situation for 30–45 minutes, or until your anxiety decreases by at least 50%*. If, by the time 45 minutes has passed, your SUDS rating has not decreased by at least 50%, then remain in the situation until that point. Once your anxiety has decreased by 50%, you can stop the exposure and resume other activities. For example, if your highest SUDS rating is 80, you should stay in the situation until your SUDS rating reaches 40. If your peak SUDS rating is 60, stay in the situation until your SUDS rating declines to 30. If you leave the situation when you are very anxious, you will again convince yourself that the situation is very dangerous and that something terrible is going to happen to you. The next time you go into that situation, your level of anxiety will again be as high, or even higher. If you stay in the situation, however, your anxiety will decrease, and you will eventually be able to encounter it without fear. The more frequently you practice each situation on your list, the less anxiety you will experience. As a result, you will feel less of an urge to avoid situations and people that are now distressing for you.

Habituation Curve:
Staying in the Situation until Your Anxiety Goes Down by 50%

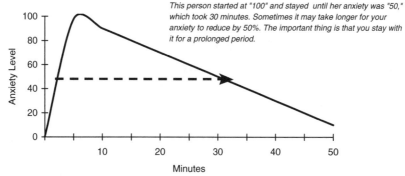

This person started at "100" and stayed until her anxiety was "50," which took 30 minutes. Sometimes it may take longer for your anxiety to reduce by 50%. The important thing is that you stay with it for a prolonged period.

(continued)

Keep Track of Your Progress

Keeping a record of your experiences with *in vivo* exposure exercises will help you and your therapist monitor your progress and plan your exposure tasks. Before you start an exposure task, record the situation you will practice on the *In Vivo* Exposure Home Practice Record (Handout 6.6). Use the instructions on the form to assist you in keeping records of your practice.

Vary the Situation

Once you have completed your entire first *in vivo* exposure hierarchy, you may find it helpful to try to vary the exposure situation slightly. For example, if your task was to go into a supermarket, next choose a different supermarket. This will increase the likelihood that the habituation you develop will be to supermarkets in general, not just to a single supermarket. Other variations may include going to supermarkets of different sizes, at different times of the day, when it is quiet and when it is busy, and so on.

Name _____ Date _____

Situation practiced _____

- *In vivo* exposure is exposure to a situation, object, or activity in real life.
- Ideally, you should practice *in vivo* exposure every day. The more often you practice, the quicker you will notice results and feel more comfortable in the situation.
- Pick an item from your hierarchy and describe it very specifically.
- Note your beginning (preexposure) anxiety level using the 0–100 SUDS.
- Watch your anxiety (it may go up). Record your highest SUDS rating for the exposure.
- Remain in the situation for 30–45 minutes, or until your anxiety decreases to at least 50% of its highest level.
- Record your ending SUDS rating.
- To track your progress, graph the Beginning, Highest, and Ending SUDS ratings below. (*Hint*: Use a different color or symbol for each exposure practice.)
- Repeat this exposure daily until your highest SUDS rating is 20 or less (as it is for "5th Time" on the third graph, "Habituation Curve: Repeated Prolonged Exposures" in Handout 6.1). Then you may move on to the next item on your hierarchy.

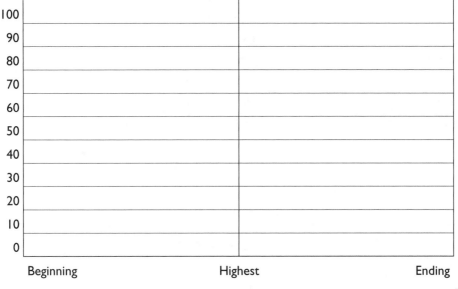

0	10	20	30	40	50	60	70	80	90	100
None		Mild		Moderate		Severe		Very severe		Extreme

Subjective Units of Distress Scale (SUDS)

(continued)

Subjective Units of Distress Scale (SUDS)

0	10	20	30	40	50	60	70	80	90	100
None		Mild		Moderate		Severe		Very severe		Extreme

Situation Practiced: _____

1. Date:_____   Beginning SUDS   _____
   Situation:_____   Highest SUDS   _____
   Duration:_____   Ending SUDS   _____

2. Date:_____   Beginning SUDS   _____
   Situation:_____   Highest SUDS   _____
   Duration:_____   Ending SUDS   _____

3. Date:_____   Beginning SUDS   _____
   Situation:_____   Highest SUDS   _____
   Duration:_____   Ending SUDS   _____

4. Date:_____   Beginning SUDS   _____
   Situation:_____   Highest SUDS   _____
   Duration:_____   Ending SUDS   _____

5. Date:_____   Beginning SUDS   _____
   Situation:_____   Highest SUDS   _____
   Duration:_____   Ending SUDS   _____

6. Date:_____   Beginning SUDS   _____
   Situation:_____   Highest SUDS   _____
   Duration:_____   Ending SUDS   _____

7. Date:_____   Beginning SUDS   _____
   Situation:_____   Highest SUDS   _____
   Duration:_____   Ending SUDS   _____

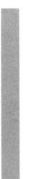

SEVEN

Imaginal Exposure

Like *in vivo* exposure, imaginal exposure seems straightforward. Your patients recount a traumatic event from start to finish and imagine it as if it were happening again. They also experience the feelings they felt at the time, while recognizing that they are currently safe, and that the event is now just a memory. They do this again and again and again. With repeated exposure, patients' anxiety diminishes as they learn that no harm occurs in the present, even when they think about what happened and feel the associated emotions.

Despite the apparent simplicity of the task, implementing imaginal exposure can be challenging. Imaginal exposure is a critical element of treatment for many patients, yet it is often a feared element. In addition, although some patients easily complete imaginal exposure "by the book," others require adjustments to benefit from it. The therapist's challenge lies in making adjustments that facilitate imaginal exposure instead of undermining it. With too much adjustment, you risk fostering avoidance and counterproductive behavior; too little, and your patients may remain "stuck"—either unwilling or unable to engage effectively with their traumatic memories in a therapeutic way.

Two factors appear critical in learning to make useful adjustments. First, you need a solid understanding of the process of imaginal exposure, as well as options for adjusting the process. Second, you must stay the course and not give up, which can be difficult if it appears that your patient is struggling or not habituating. Thus, you need complete confidence that the process works. Imaginal exposure is a like a sailing trip between two islands. By the time you realize that sailing is not smooth, you may be too far from the first island to return. You cannot stand on the boat and say "Let's just give up," because that leaves you floating midocean. Being fearful of starting the trip also does not get you to your destination island. Instead, you need to rely on your skills and commitment to reach your goal. Similarly once you start with imaginal exposure, it is best that you not turn back, if at all possible.

PREPARING FOR IMAGINAL EXPOSURE: THE RATIONALE

You will have explained some of the rationale for imaginal exposure to patients at the start of treatment. Review the rationale again, however, before initiating imaginal exposure, and let your patients know that you plan to audiotape the exposure to facilitate home practice (see "Preparing Patients for Home Practice" for more details). Preparing for imaginal exposure is simpler when your patients already have begun *in vivo* exposure, because patients who have experienced fear reduction during *in vivo* exposure understand the process. Thus, the rationale for imaginal exposure is straightforward. You explain that imaginal exposure reduces anxiety associated with thinking about trauma memories in the much same way that exposure to *in vivo* stimuli reduces anxiety related to those stimuli. You also review the notion of "processing" the memory; this sets the stage for addressing other aspects of the memory, including those associated with guilt, shame, or anger. In the sample dialogue, we demonstrate the use of a movie metaphor to explain processing to patients.

In addition, help your patients build commitment to imaginal exposure. This helps them to persist if difficulties arise and the urge to avoid increases. One strategy for enhancing commitment involves constructing a list of reasons for doing exposure. To use humor in this process, we construe this task as a "Top 10" list, which is included in Handout 7.1. Figure 7.1 is a sample of a completed "Top 10 Reasons to Do Imaginal Exposure."

TOP 10 REASONS TO DO IMAGINAL EXPOSURE

Many people realize when they start treatment for PTSD that at some point it will involve thinking about what happened. You and your therapist have talked about imaginal exposure, and you have read about it in this handout. You may have some experience with *in vivo* exposure under your belt that has influenced your thinking about it. Everyone has their own reasons for doing imaginal exposure—without good reasons, you probably would decide *not* to do *it*! If you have some good reasons for doing imaginal exposure, now is a good time to list them. You may find it helpful to refer back to this list later in treatment, if you feel the urge to avoid taking over.

10. Helps get it out of your system.

 9. If you understand your fear, you own it.

 8. Learn to look at it and evaluate it with adult emotions.

 7. If you stay with it, you become more comfortable; you learn it can't hurt you anymore if you're not there. It's just a memory.

 6. Break the cycle for self and family.

 5. Become less volatile.

 4. Improve social relationships.

 3. Gives you courage to live the life you wanted.

 2. Have more control over your thoughts and reactions.

 1. If you can get through one memory, you can get through the next.

FIGURE 7.1. Example of "Top 10 Reasons to Do Exposure."

Sample Dialogue: Introducing Imaginal Exposure to Your Patient

THERAPIST: Jill, you've done some terrific work on your fear of dogs. When you stayed with the dog pictures, your anxiety went down, and you are on your way to progressing through your hierarchy. We are going to continue working on your *in vivo* hierarchy so that you continue to feel comfortable around dog pictures and also around actual dogs that are friendly and safe, as well as other situations that you have been avoiding. Our next step in your treatment is to begin to address your distress about the memory of the attack. You may recall that we briefly talked about imaginal exposure as one of the important components of treatment.

JILL: Yeah, I've been dreading it!

THERAPIST: It's natural to feel anxious about starting imaginal exposure.

JILL: Do I really have to do it?

THERAPIST: You don't *have* to do anything that you don't decide to do yourself. Every step of this treatment is up to you. To help you decide, let's review the ways that imaginal exposure can be helpful and then talk about some of your reasons for doing imaginal exposure and your reasons for not wanting to do it. Then, you can decide what's right for you.

JILL: OK.

THERAPIST: As I've said, in the same way that *in vivo* exposure has resulted in less anxiety about pictures of dogs, imaginal exposure can reduce the fear you feel when you think about the attack.

JILL: I guess that makes sense.

THERAPIST: In addition, imaginal exposure will also help you to process the memory of the attack. You've said before that, deep down, you sort of knew that if you came to therapy, it would probably involve talking about what happened, and that's why you waited so long to come. Since the attack, your friends and family have said things to you like "Let's not dwell on it . . . " and "It happened, you survived; now, put it behind you and get on with your life!" You've told me how you also have felt ashamed and weak, and therefore tried not to think about the whole ordeal. As a result, your avoidance has prevented you from carefully thinking through the whole experience and sifting through the details of what happened. This is a lot like sifting through the details of a mystery movie to make sense of it when you leave the theater. Doing this helps you to understand the story in its entirety instead of the bits and pieces of the memory that pop into your mind. By putting all the pieces together, you can start to make sense of it, so you can put it away for good. Quite often, when we review a memory in depth, we come to appreciate many details that we had forgotten, and some of these details may be important for understanding what the event means about you. Imaginal exposure can not only reduce your fear but it also gives you the opportunity to think through all the different parts of the memory, some of which you may have forgotten. Does that make sense to you?

JILL: Yeah. I know its weird, but I'm just scared. And I've been having nightmares all week.

THERAPIST: That's understandable. You've avoided it for so long, it makes sense that you'd feel scared of facing the memories. As I said before, it can be helpful to remind yourself of your reasons for doing this work. What are you hoping imaginal exposure might do for you?

JILL: Will it get rid of my nightmares?

THERAPIST: Well, at first, you might notice an increase in your nightmares and daytime intrusions. But most people eventually find that as their anxiety goes down, their intrusions diminish. The good news is that if you do experience an increase in nightmares or other symptoms in the beginning, that doesn't mean you won't benefit from the treatment. Is there anything else you are hoping to change in your life by doing imaginal exposure?

JILL: Well, it would be great if I wasn't putting so much energy and time into avoiding reminders. Maybe I could go back to doing some of things I liked to do, like taking my kids places and going for long walks. I could also watch new movies again without constantly being afraid that a dog will show up. I also just want to feel better and to really put this behind me. I want to get on with my life.

THERAPIST: Those are good reasons for doing exposure. It will be helpful to remind yourself of these reasons if there comes a time when you don't want to do the exposure or feel an urge to avoid it.

If your patient has not started imaginal exposure, you need to combine material from the rationale for *in vivo* exposure in Chapter 6 with the rationale for imaginal exposure. Typically, first you sell the broad concept of exposure in a manner more akin to that in Chapter 6. Then, draw a parallel between an *in vivo* stimulus and a memory (i.e., "Lets think again about the trauma of being attacked by a lion. Just as *in vivo* exposure to an orange tabby cat can help you feel less afraid of cats, it also is important for you to learn to be less afraid of your memory of the lion chasing you. When you think about the lion attack, you learn that the memory is not the same as *actually* being attacked by the lion, and your fear diminishes.") Finally, expand into the movie metaphor or develop your own way of explaining the need to process memories. You may find the information on processing in Chapter 2 helpful in developing alternative ways to explain this to your patients, if the movie metaphor does not work for you.

Some patients find it helpful to think of their memories as a feared object with a strong smell. They have put their memories/object in a box, taped the box tightly, and put it in a trunk in the attic. Then they put chains around the trunk, lock it up, pile blankets on the trunk, and lock the attic. Despite all of their efforts, though, they can still detect the smell in the house, because the smell can escape the box and the trunk and the attic. The goal of imaginal exposure is for patients to unlock the trunk, get the box, take out the object, and discover that if they face their fear of the object, they can hold it, study it, and even hand wash the smell out of it. They also discover that the object/memory does not hurt them. Finally, they can put it on a shelf in the main part of the house. At this point, the object is just like any other object in the house, just as the memory is like other memories.

PREPARING FOR IMAGINAL EXPOSURE: CONSTRUCTING A HIERARCHY AND SELECTING THE FIRST MEMORY

As with *in vivo* exposure, you typically need to identify and organize the critical memories into a hierarchy before starting imaginal exposure. You do not need to do this with all patients, though, because some patients report only one disturbing memory. Many of these individuals experienced only one traumatic event. Others, however, may have experienced multiple events but report that only one memory continues to be disturbing. At times, however, you might not discover that only one memory is disturbing until you go through the process of constructing a hierarchy of traumatic memories.

Construct the hierarchy immediately after you present the rationale for imaginal exposure. Constructing a hierarchy should be a brief process, 15 minutes or less, if possible. The goal is to identify the key memories, while preventing your patient from becoming so immersed in a single memory that it becomes an exposure in itself. To construct the hierarchy, ask your patient for a brief description of the memories that have been most distressing in the past month and write them on the List of Trauma Memories (Handout 7.2). The description should include a concise overview of what happened (e.g., "We were driving on the highway and this huge truck hit us. The car flipped. My brother died by the side of the road"). If possible, obtain the age the patient was at the time, who else was involved, and other brief details that will facilitate communication about the memories during exposure. Then ask patients to rate how anxious they felt describing that event. This sample of anxiety is your best representation of what the anxiety level may be like during exposure, although many patients experience more or less anxiety once they begin exposure.

Constructing the Hierarchy of Traumatic Memories: The Case of Mikala

Mikala, a 35-year-old female, reports an extensive history of childhood sexual abuse by an uncle. Mikala's father died when she was young, and she often stayed with her aunt and uncle while her mother worked to support Mikala and her three siblings. Mikala also reported a history of physical assault by a boyfriend.

THERAPIST: To get started with imaginal exposure in our next session, I want to have a clear idea of which memories are bothering you the most, so we can decide where to begin. I realize quite a number of distressing things have happened in your life. Can you tell me which events have been most distressing for you lately?

MIKALA: It's all just awful. I don't know where to begin. Whenever I think about all of this, it is just so overwhelming. I can't deal with it.

THERAPIST: Well, think about just the past week. When you have had unwanted memories of events from the past, what did you remember?

MIKALA: Well, like last night when I was watching my 6-year-old daughter playing with her cousin, it reminded me of the way things were for me when I was that age.

THERAPIST: What do you mean? What specifically did you think about?

MIKALA: Well, you know, what my uncle did to me.

THERAPIST: Was there a specific memory of the sexual abuse that you remembered?

MIKALA: Well, I'm not sure exactly. It happened so many times that it all blurs together. Also, when I remember it, I get really upset, so I usually try to get it out of my mind as fast as I can—like last night, I turned on the TV and watched a game show for a while until I calmed down.

THERAPIST: Well, let's see if we can nail down a memory of one time when it happened. For example, many people who have been sexually abused find that certain times it happened stand out the most in their memories. For example, sometimes the first time the abuse happened will stand out in a person's memory.

MIKALA: Well, I was so young when it started, I don't think I really remember the first time.

THERAPIST: That makes sense. You might find then that the memories that stand out are the first time he did something in particular, like the first time there was penetration, or a time that was particularly frightening. For example, you mentioned that although the abuse started when you were about 5 years old, there was no penetration until you were quite a bit older. Do any memories from this period stand out for you?

MIKALA: Well, yeah.

THERAPIST: What comes to mind?

MIKALA: Well, first he started putting things inside me, and it hurt. He said it wasn't going to, but it did hurt. I wanted him to stop, but he wouldn't.

THERAPIST: How old were you when he did this?

MIKALA: Well he did it many times.

THERAPIST: Well, when you think about it lately, which time do you think about?

MIKALA: Well, I guess usually I remember lying on the couch in my aunt and uncle's house and hurting down there.

THERAPIST: What happened?

MIKALA: I'm not sure exactly, but I think he put the handle of a screwdriver inside me. I remember taking a nap while other people were around, but when I woke up, everyone was gone except my uncle. Then he was touching me, and then it really started to hurt as he put the handle inside of me. It was a big screwdriver.

THERAPIST: Do you have any idea how old you were?

MIKALA: Maybe 10.

THERAPIST: OK, and how anxious were you as you told me about this memory?

MIKALA: Really anxious, like 95.

THERAPIST: What other memories stand out.

MIKALA: I hate this.

THERAPIST: I know it's hard, but you are doing a good job. Let's keep going and get through this, though.

MIKALA: OK. I also really remember the first time he raped me, you know, himself. I remember him on top of me, and he smelled of beer and sweat, and I just wanted him to stop. It really hurt.

THERAPIST: And how old were you then?

MIKALA: Probably around 11.

THERAPIST: And how much anxiety did you feel telling me about this?

MIKALA: One hundred.

THERAPIST: OK. Let's keep going. You are doing great. What other memories really keep bothering you?

MIKALA: When I was older, there was this time I tried to fight back. You know, to stop him. He slapped me really hard and told me it was going to have to hurt this time, so that I learned to be good. (*Laughs.*) Like it didn't always hurt. But he was really rough that time. He was right. It really hurt, and he kept pinching me too.

THERAPIST: And how old were you then?

MIKALA: Around 15. I was just starting high school and thought that now that I was in high school, maybe I could make him stop.

THERAPIST: How much anxiety did you feel telling me about this memory?

MIKALA: Maybe a little less than the others—85.

THERAPIST: Any other particularly disturbing uncle memories?

MIKALA: No, I think those are the ones that bother me the most.

THERAPIST: Now you mentioned at your assessment that you had a violent boyfriend right after high school.

MIKALA: Yeah. He was older. I went to live with him to get away from my family.

THERAPIST: Any memories of him?

MIKALA: The first time he beat me. . . .

Probe until you patient has identified all or a significant number of key memories and rated them. The list of memories serves as a preliminary map for your exposure sessions. The amount of detail on the map, however, varies from patient to patient, and diversions are likely and expected. For example, often is not necessary to conduct exposure for every memory. Also, some patients will add memories to the list later in treatment. Thus, the list does not need to be exhaustive.

If your patient has many memories, it can be helpful to develop short names for the memories. For Mikala, the first memory might come to be known as the "screwdriver memory." The next memory might be the "first uncle rape." Having short names for the memories facilitates discussion of the hierarchy items (e.g., which memory to tackle next) without requiring patients to think intensively about each memory. For example, after eliciting additional memories, including one in which Mikala's boyfriend slammed her head against a brick wall, the therapist noted, "It seems that your boyfriend memories are somewhat less anxiety provoking than your uncle memories. And the brick wall memory seems to produce the least anxiety at 75. So I think that would be a good starting point. What do you think?"

What If the Patient Is Unable to Pinpoint a Specific Memory?

Some patients have had so many instances of a similar event that the memories merge together, and a single memory is hard to delineate. This often happens for sexual or physical abuse survivors, or those with extended war zone exposure. Encourage patients to identify specific memories for imaginal exposure. For example, ask whether they recall the first time it happened, the last time, or some other significant feature of one instance of the event. If a patient cannot identify a specific memory, you may need to work with a "composite" memory that includes different instances of the event. If you do this, be sure that the memory stays consistent across exposures, because changes in the memory may interfere with between-session habituation.

What If the Patient Has Only Very Fragmented Memories?

Some patients may report very fragmented memories that do not fit together coherently. For example, Gabrielle reported only a few disjointed images, such as being in a dark place, accompanied by a suffocating feeling and a strong odor. In such instances, patients often feel that their recollections are insufficient for exposure and that they must recall more for the memory to be useful. It is common for patients to flesh out some details of a memory during exposure or even to recall entire events that they previously could not verbalize. This is not an explicit aim of exposure, however, and it important to communicate this to patients, because exposure does not involve "recovering" memories. You do not want to inadvertently create false memories by encouraging patients to generate details they cannot readily recall. Thus, if patients report fragmented memories, tell them that it is OK if they do not recall anything further. For example, Raul reported a memory of standing near basement stairs and hearing rustling noises. The memory produced extreme anxiety, and Raul said he "knew" that his father was torturing his older brother in the basement. Raul did not know how he knew this, what age he was in the memory, or why he was at the top of the stairs. He had no other memories that confirmed what occurred in the basement, and, because his brother committed suicide and Raul was estranged from his parents, no external sources of confirmation. In this case, Raul completed exposure to the memory fragment and habituated to the memory. Cognitive restructuring and radical acceptance, a skill drawn from dialectical behavior therapy (DBT; Linehan, 1993a), helped Raul accept that he might never recall more information.

Segmenting Very Involved Memories

Some patients also may have experienced events over a long period of time or that had distinct segments. In this case, you may need to treat each segment as a separate memory. For example, Dasha was abducted and raped over a period of 3 days. Dasha and her therapist divided the 3 days into 10 memory segments. If you anticipate the need to segment memories based on your assessment, do so during construction of the hierarchy.

Selecting a Memory for the First Exposure

Once you have the hierarchy, select a starting memory. Ideally, as with *in vivo* exposure, your patient will have some memories rated between 50 and 65 on the SUDS, and you can choose one of the moderately rated memories to start. Some patients, however, may rate all memories very high (e.g., ranging from 90–100). In such cases, pick a starting memory from a selection of closely rated, very anxiety-provoking memories.

When choosing among closely rated memories, consider the clarity of the description and the extent to which it meets the DSM-IV definition of a traumatic event (American Psychiatric Association, 1994). It is best to choose a memory that has a relatively clear description and appears to meet both the A1 (threat to physical integrity) and A2 (fear, helplessness, horror) definitions of a traumatic event. Some survivors may list disturbing memories that do not meet Criterion A1. For example, child abuse survivors may include memories of adults yelling at them and/or calling them names. Other patients may include memories of sad, extended events, such as watching a family member dying of cancer. These may not be suitable for exposure if they lack a prominent anxiety component. Some patients' reported memories are so fragmented that they lack sufficient detail to determine whether they fit the definition of a traumatic event. For example, Rose described a memory of feeling uncomfortable sitting on her grandfather's lap when she was 4.

Some memories also may not clearly meet Criterion A2. For example, Lindy reported a memory of her ex-boyfriend coming home drunk, yelling at her, and throwing dishes. She primarily reported anger and disgust during this situation. If it is clear that a memory is primarily associated with anger and not anxiety, it is not a good starting memory; in fact, it may not be an appropriate memory for exposure at all. Similarly, primarily shame- or guilt-based memories are not ideal starting memories. Trista reported two memories of sexual assault: one of being coerced by her boyfriend into performing oral sex on his friend, and another in which a man violently raped her in the parking lot of her apartment. The later memory, rated 80, was more clearly fear based, whereas the former, rated 65, involved mostly shame. Thus, her therapist suggested that they begin with the latter memory, even though the SUDS rating she reported for it was higher than that for the former memory.

You can conduct exposure to anger-, shame-, or guilt-based memories. Doing so may not have the desired outcome, however, because these emotions do not decrease as reliably as anxiety does during exposure. If there is a choice among memories that are based mostly in guilt, shame, or anger, and others that are clearly based in fear, it is best to start with fear-based memories. Doing so increases the likelihood that distress will diminish during exposure and that the patient will experience success. Early success helps increase willingness to pursue exposure and stick with difficult exposure sessions. Other memories can be addressed later in therapy.

Once you have chosen a starting memory, suggest it to your patient. For example:

"Mark, in looking over the list of distressing memories that we made last week, I noticed that you rated the memory of your stepfather hitting you with the razor belt when you were 6 years old as 60, whereas the other memories were rated quite a bit higher. I wonder if this might be a good place for us to start. What do you think?"

CONDUCTING IMAGINAL EXPOSURE: THE BASIC STEPS

In conducting imaginal exposure, remember that the goal is for patients to be exposed to the memory of the trauma, not actually to relive the trauma. Although some therapists advocate a "reliving" approach with respect to exposure, we do not concur with this. You do not want to expose patients to feeling as if they are actually being raped, mugged, and assaulted again. You want them to learn, via exposure, that their *memories* of these events are not dangerous. Thus, patients should be aware that they are currently in a safe environment, conducting exposure to a memory. If patients believe that the event is actually happening again and lose awareness of their surroundings, new learning is unlikely to occur. As such, manage the exposure process so that your patients experience the emotions associated with the event but do not become so overwhelmed by them that they lose awareness of reality. You also need to reinforce patients' willingness to experience the memory and associated affect, so that they will engage in continued exposure at home and in future sessions.

During the first exposure, ask patients to recount the memory of the event from the start. They need to describe the event as if it were happening again, and in sufficient detail to enable them to experience "emotions that you felt at the time." Do not be overly directive in shaping how patients carry out the initial exposure; rather, focus on using feedback strategically to reinforce willingness to recall the event, and engagement with the memory and associated emotions. Standard instructions for the first exposure include telling patients to close their eyes and describe the event in the first person, present tense. These strategies appear to facilitate engagement.

Imaginal exposure requires that patients describe memories over and over again. Many patients, however, stop talking after describing the first memory the first time. Thus, you may need to instruct them to do it again. Repetition is the key to habituation. For example, the first time Steve described watching his father shoot someone, tears poured down his face. When he finished his description, he stopped talking. His therapist asked him to "take me through what happened again." Steve responded, "I don't think I can." His therapist quietly said, "Take me through it again." As Steve repeatedly told the story he became calmer. He later noted that he could not believe that his anxiety began to plummet around the sixth time through the description. He stated, "It became something in the past, just a memory. . . . I never thought that could happen."

Length of Exposure Sessions

Plan to spend 60 minutes conducting exposure during the first exposure session, so that patients can repeat the memory for a full 60 minutes, or until their anxiety has declined to below 20. This means scheduling a 90-minute session, if at all possible. Occasionally, a patient may habituate quickly, and you will not need 60 minutes. Generally, however, this is not the case, and patients need to repeat the memory many times. If you have started with *in vivo* exposure and you know that a patient habituates very slowly, you may plan an even longer session for the first exposure (e.g., 75–80 minutes of exposure). Obviously, this may not be possible for some patients due to logistical or insurance reasons.

Tracking Anxiety Levels

Typically, you will ask your patients for a SUDS rating at 5-minute intervals during exposure. Keep track of this information during every in-session exposure (see Handout 7.3). We also recommend graphing this data. By keeping exposure data on a computer, you can add data each session and produce colorful graphs that your patients can take home. Many patients find graphs highly reinforcing and often post them in a conspicuous place (e.g., their refrigerator) to remind themselves of the results of their efforts. Graphs of exposure sessions help patients to continue exposure even when progress feels negligible, and may be used as evidence when patients challenge hopeless thoughts about the possibility for change (see Chapter 8). Graphs also provide important information about exposure (i.e., you can track trends in habituation).

Sample Dialogue: The First Imaginal Exposure

THERAPIST: OK, Jill, lets get started. What I'd like you to do first is get comfortable in your chair, then, if you feel you can, it will be helpful if you close your eyes. Closing your eyes will help you to recall the memory vividly. What you want to do is to recall the memory as vividly as you can, as if its happening again now, but at the same time realize that it is not *really* happening—that you are actually just recalling a memory—and that you are safe here in my office. If you become so immersed in the memory that you lose connection with reality—if you forget that it is a memory and that its not actually happening again, then I'll have you open your eyes. Of course, you can always open your eyes yourself anytime you wish. Do you feel comfortable starting with your eyes closed?

JILL: Yes, I think so.

[*Commentary: Patients who are unable to start with their eyes closed may start with their eyes open.*]

THERAPIST: OK. So I'd like you to start from the beginning of what you remember happening that day and review what happened in as much detail as you can. Allow yourself to feel all the feelings that you felt at the time it was happening. I'd like you to recount the events if as they are happening now, so use the first person and tell the story in the present tense, if you can.

Feedback after Imaginal Exposure

After patients stop repeating the memory, discuss their reactions to the first imaginal exposure and review the graph of data from the exposure session. This gives your patients a chance to process the experience, and you a chance to verbally reinforce them for completing a difficult task. You can also use the graph to highlight success.

Preparing Patients for Home Practice

After providing feedback, instruct patients in home practice. Patients conduct home practice by listening to an audiotape of their exposure session. You will have briefly explained home practice during the rationale to explain why you audiotape the imaginal exposure sessions. Preparing patients in advance for the idea that exposure includes homework also makes home practice easier to accept. Nonetheless, the first session can be draining. As a result, many patients are more focused on being relieved that it is over than on thinking about doing it again. Thus, you typically need to remind them about home practice.

Basic Instructions

Getting patients to adhere to home practice is critically important, because studies indicate that repetition is key to achieving success with exposure. You can use the graph of repeated anxiety reduction to highlight the importance of repetition by showing your patients that between-session anxiety reduction leads to the memory becoming less disturbing (see Figure 6.4).

It often is helpful to integrate a motivational pep talk with *very specific* instructions for home practice. Advise patients to listen to the exposure tape every day, if possible, or at least five times per week, for optimal treatment effects. Discuss the best time of day to do this, taking into account other life demands (work, child care, etc.). Remember to tell patients not to listen to the tape while doing other things, particularly driving. Such activities may distract patients from the memory and experience of anxiety. This can interfere with between-session habituation, particularly if the activity is cognitively demanding (Kamphuis & Telch, 2000; Telch et al., 2004). In addition, activities such as driving may be unsafe to do while listening to the tape. Instructions also should include walking patients step-by-step through Handout 7.4, which includes recording SUDS ratings at three points during each home practice, the duration of the home practice (e.g., at least 30 minutes or until the SUDS rating drops by 50%), and, if helpful, any other details (e.g., eyes open or closed, where the practice took place). Finally, assess obstacles patients may face, such as finding a time, a place, and/or a tape player.

Environmental Factors to Consider

You need to understand the environment in which your patient will carry out exposure homework. For example, children should not be nearby during home practice, because they should not overhear the content of tapes, and they may interrupt home practice. Their mere presence also may be distracting for some patients. Child concerns may warrant explicit discussion with some patients.

At times, it is useful to include partners in a session, so that they can learn the rationale for exposure and ask questions, and you can enlist partners as a source of support. Partners who do not understand or accept the rationale sometimes sabotage treatment by discouraging patients from doing exposure home practice because it is upsetting. Conversely, when they understand the treatment rationale, spouses or partners can be an important source of support.

Sharing the Content of the Tape with Support Persons

Another consideration is whether patients listen to tapes with other adults present. Many patients fear doing exposure at home alone at first. We advise most patients *not* to share tapes with family members or others, unless there is a specific purpose for doing so. Listening to the contents of an exposure tape may induce secondary stress symptoms in family members that you may not be able to address, because they are not patients. Using a headset is a good way to ensure privacy and allows support people to be nearby without hearing the tape.

Another possible negative outcome of others hearing a tape can be invalidation. For example, Jerry was listening to a memory of sexual abuse that involved his being fondled by his teacher. When his wife, a survivor of a violent assault, heard the tape, she was surprised by the relatively less threatening nature of his trauma. This led her to think that Jerry was overreacting. She made statements such as, "That really wasn't as bad as I thought" and "You shouldn't really be *this* upset." She also began pressuring him to "get done" with therapy. It is hard to predict how others will respond if they know the contents of the tape. Thus, we typically encourage patients not to share tapes with others. Instead, patients should ask support persons to be present nearby when they are doing the work, and to help comfort or spend time with them afterwards.

There are instances, however, where sharing a tape appears beneficial. If a patient decides to do this, it is not necessarily cause for alarm. For example, Bridget found that sharing her childhood abuse memory with her husband increased intimacy in their relationship. And Henry, whose daughter died in a plane crash, found that sharing the tape with his wife stimulated discussion about the grief they had kept buried for many years. Henry did not report any disturbing effects for his wife. He also felt that sharing the tape benefited them both and increased his feeling that he was supported in his therapy.

Use of Self-Soothing and Activity Planning after Exposure

Some patients benefit from explicit instructions regarding what they should do after completing home practice (or even after returning from in-session exposure). For example, Veronica felt proud after completing exposure to a very anxiety-provoking tape. As a result, she decided that she could tackle just about anything; when she confronted a brother who owed her money, she quickly became overwhelmed by feelings of anger and guilt. The confrontation was not a success, and she experienced urges to self-injure. Upon reviewing the incident, her therapist suggested that Veronica might not have had the emotional resources to face her brother immediately after completing difficult home practice. Veronica admitted that, in addition to feeling proud, she also felt exhausted and angry.

Many patients benefit from explicit instructions to engage in pleasant or soothing activities after completing exposure. Such activities prevent patients from attempting difficult tasks when they are emotionally depleted. Pleasant activities also can moderate nonanxiety negative emotions that fail to change during a specific session of exposure. Finally, such activities can be used to reward patients for completing something they find difficult and unpleasant. Interestingly, many patients with PTSD have to be taught to reward themselves with pleasant activities, and to soothe themselves after emotionally challenging events. Explicit plans and preestablished lists of possible activities are often helpful for such patients.

STRATEGIES TO TITRATE ANXIETY
DURING IMAGINAL EXPOSURE
AND FACILITATE ENGAGEMENT AND HABITUATION

Procedural variations can affect the intensity of anxiety during exposure, and facilitate habituation and engagement. If anxiety is so high that patients are unable to participate in exposure, use strategies that reduce the amount of anxiety experienced. Conversely, if patients are not fully engaging with the memory, use strategies that increase engagement.

Using the First Person and Present versus Past Tense

As noted earlier, typical instructions include using the first person and speaking in the present tense. Occasionally patients ignore the first person instruction and use the third person ("He pushes her on the bed and she is lying there feeling helpless"). This likely serves to distance patients from their emotional experience of the event. Some patients state that during the event, they felt as if they were watching themselves, and this is why they describe themselves in the third person. Using the first person is important, because patients need to experience events as they happened to them, rather than artificially distancing themselves.

Regarding use of the present tense, no research has determined whether the effectiveness of exposure is affected by the verb tense used. Patients often use the past tense, regardless of your instruction. Many patients experience quite intense anxiety describing their memories in the past tense, and, unlike using the third person, the past tense is a natural way of thinking about one's past experiences. Recalling a memory in the present tense is more akin to having a flashback and can be viewed as less "healthy." If doing so increases the vividness so much that your patient is unable to stay with the memory (i.e., disconnects or dissociates) or does not habituate, then it makes sense to encourage use of the past tense.

Timing: How Quickly Should I Increase Anxiety
or Correct a Patient Who Is Doing It Wrong?

Many patients engage quickly, regardless of whether they recall the memory in the past tense, or using the third person. In the first session, be supportive and nonjudgmental of any effort to describe and experience the trauma memory. Thus, unless a patient is not engaging with the affect (e.g., is reporting a SUDS rating substantially lower than expected, or a SUDS rating below 50), limit your correction of procedural variations during the first exposure session. Patients who are very sensitive to perceived invalidation sometimes respond with self-invalidation and discouragement (e.g., "I can't even do this right!" or "It's too hard. I won't be able to do it").

Once a patient has experienced anxiety reduction with the initial exposure sessions, you can encourage modifications that increase anxiety further and correct procedural mistakes that might be reducing anxiety. In addition to using the present tense and speaking in the first person, this also might include closing the eyes or describing particular details, sensations, or thoughts in greater detail. For example,

Daphne was only able to complete her first exposure session by keeping her eyes open. Yet her anxiety reduced to zero within 20 minutes during her second exposure session, with her eyes open, so her therapist suggested that she continue the exposure during this session with her eyes closed. Not surprisingly, this resulted in an increase in her anxiety, followed by a return to a 0 SUDS rating at 45 minutes. In the next session, her anxiety peaked again, yet it followed an expected pattern of habituation.

Should Patients Use Distraction to Titrate Anxiety?

We do not use distraction during exposure. Although distraction during exposure can be viewed as a strategy to titrate anxiety, we generally find that we can titrate anxiety using other methods. In addition, the literature is unclear as to whether using distraction to titrate anxiety during exposure is detrimental to treatment outcome for PTSD.

We explicitly encourage patients to focus on their anxiety, to the exclusion of other emotions, during exposure. One way to do this is to ask them to rate their anxiety ("Where is your anxiety now on a 0- to 100-point scale?") versus the more general SUDS rating ("What is your SUDS rating, 0–100?"). Our rationale is simple. Compared to other anxiety disorders, we find that exposure for PTSD appears to more reliably elicit a range of negative emotions beyond anxiety, which may or may not change during exposure. Thus, we encourage patients to focus on anxiety, so that they can be reinforced by the relatively reliable decrease in anxiety as a result of exposure.

Structuring the Memory to Modulate Anxiety and Facilitate Habituation

It often is necessary to guide patients in delineating segments of memories that are of appropriate length and intensity for exposure. For example, some patients will have difficulty describing memory fragments in coherent ways, or they may be reluctant to articulate them at all. Other patients describe memories with great detail leading up to and following the worst part of the event, but they race through the worst part. For example, Morgan provided a detailed description of the events leading up to and following her rape. But she described the actual rape very briefly, stating, "Then he pushed down my panties and raped me." Traumatic memories also may consist of multiple segments that are separate traumas. For example, the memory of an accident might consist of several segments, such as the moments leading to the accident, awaiting rescue, being extricated from the vehicle, riding to the hospital, and being treated.

Each of these scenarios produces memories that are not optimally structured for exposure. An ideal memory is one that has sufficient detail and can be repeated a number of times in a 60-minute session, because, as noted earlier, repetition is the key to habituation. Simple math tells you that patients who have 5-minute memories will have the opportunity to repeat them twice as many times as those with 10-minute memories. The exact length of the memory is dependent on the features of the memory. Yet, in the end, you will be able to structure many (though not all!) memories to fall within a 4- to 10-minute time frame.

Structuring Long Memories

Very lengthy memories can take 30 minutes to 1 hour to recount the first time through. In such situations you have a few options. You know that in-session exposure is unlikely to provide sufficient repetition to result in substantial anxiety reduction. Nonetheless, your first option is not to interfere with your patient's initial approach and simply to reinforce his or her willingness to engage with the memory and associated affect. This gives you a chance to develop a template of the memory, so that you can determine how to structure it. This approach is useful when you need to hear the entire story to determine why the memory is so long and/or how you might structure it. For example, you may need to hear the entire memory to realize that a patient is focusing on the less emotionally relevant parts of the memory to avoid the more emotionally difficult parts.

Recounting the entire story at this stage also likely promotes cognitive processing of the memory. In later sessions you can segment the memory or encourage your patient to skip less important parts of the memory. Figure 7.2 shows how Jill's therapist worked with segments of her traumatic memory. During the first session, she allowed Jill to tell the entire story of her mauling, which took 30 minutes. Thus, Jill only repeated the story twice. In the second session, the therapist prompted Jill to stop after the first segment, and repeat that segment. Greater within-session habituation was achieved during the second session. In the third session, when Jill showed rapid anxiety reduction to the first segment, the second segment was reintroduced.

At times, it may become clear during the first recounting that a patient is finishing a segment. In such cases, you may decide to stop the patient and have him or her repeat that segment. You can do this by quietly saying, "OK, let's stop there for the moment and go back through that part of your memory." Usually the patient will hesitate when he or she comes to the end of the segment the second time through. You can easily encourage repetition by saying, "Take me through that portion again." The patients quickly learns to repeat the segment. Once the exposure is completed, you can explain why you stopped him or her. The advantage of this approach is that patients are more likely to experience a significant reduction in anxiety during the first session. The difficulty is identifying a coherent segment without hearing the entire memory in detail.

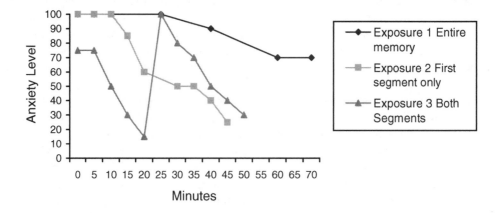

FIGURE 7.2. Jill's imaginal exposure: segmenting a lengthy memory.

Structuring Short Memories

Some patients describe memories very succinctly with minimal detail, yet report extremely high anxiety levels. Brief memories of this sort typically are stated within a minute or so. Often it is best not to push for more detail until patients have attained some anxiety reduction to the memory in its rough form. Some patients add detail on their own as their anxiety reduces to a more manageable level. But if they do not, you can later encourage them to describe sensory or emotional features in greater detail. When the memory description is very brief, the early exposure sessions involve many repetitions of the initial description. For example, in her first exposure session, Daniela's initial preexposure anxiety rating was 90, indicating tremendous anticipatory anxiety about starting exposure. Daniela's first account of her sexual abuse excluded any detail about the actual sexual contact, yet it was associated with very high anxiety.

DANIELA: I was lying in bed. He came in the room. He pulled my pajamas off and got on top. He smelled bad. There's a crack on the ceiling and I held my doll. I want him to go away. And then he was done and he told me not to tell anyone or he would hurt my sister, and he got up and left. That's all.

THERAPIST: OK, good job. What is your anxiety level now?

DANIELA: It's 100. I don't want to do this.

THERAPIST: It's good that you are letting yourself feel the anxiety. You are doing a good job. Let's keep going with it. Remember, it's important to stay with the memory for a prolonged period for your anxiety to go down. This is the hardest part, so it's best if we keep moving forward.

DANIELA: OK. I was in bed and he came in and pulled my pajamas off and got on top. He told me not to tell anyone, and then he left.

THERAPIST: You are doing a good job. Just keep letting the feelings come. Let's keep going.

Daniela's therapist asked for her anxiety rating after the first description of the memory, even though it only took a little over 30 seconds. This was because he wanted to gauge her degree of affective engagement. If Daniela's SUDS rating had been lower, her therapist might have encouraged more detail. If the SUDS rating had been extremely low, her therapist would have assessed for the presence of possible dissociation or numbing. Given that the SUDS rating suggested a high degree of engagement, her therapist decided to proceed without expanding the level of detail. Her therapist reinforced Daniela's willingness to think about what happened and encouraged her to continue. Some of her subsequent descriptions reduced the detail even further; her therapist did not remark on this, but just continued to reinforce Daniela's willingness to allow herself to feel her anxiety. In the end, Daniela repeated this brief description approximately 70 times in her first exposure session. After the first retelling, Daniela's therapist asked for her SUDS rating approximately every 5 minutes, or after every 10th repetition of the memory. By the end of the first exposure, her anxiety had decreased to 55.

Some patients have only a very brief description of the traumatic event. Although doing exposure with a very short memory may feel odd and repetitive, it can serve the same purpose as exposure to a longer memory. Remember that the purpose of exposure is to reduce anxiety that a person feels about the memories they have, not to recall memories that are not disturbing. Nonetheless, some patients may persist in their efforts to recall more, or they may berate themselves for not being able to recall important parts of what happened. Validate and normalize their difficulty with recalling the event, and remind them that it is not necessary to recall more to benefit from the treatment. Rather, the goal is to reduce distress related to the parts they do recall. Sometimes the information about the event was not encoded and stored by patients at the time of the event, and in such cases, their efforts to recall more are futile.

Targeting "Hot Spots"

After the first week of home practice you may need to target "hot spots" of the memory. In most cases, a memory of a traumatic event has one or more emotional climaxes, a point during the event that evoked the most fear or other emotional arousal, typically referred to as hot spots. Hot spots often correspond to the elements of traumatic memories that intrude during nightmares, unwanted memories, and flashbacks (Holmes, Grey, & Young, 2005). If your patient's memory is already very short (e.g., taking a few minutes or so to describe), there may be no need to do this. But, in cases where the original memory takes longer than 5–10 minutes or so to describe, targeting hot spots is often necessary.

You can identify hot spots by noting changes in SUDS rating over the course of the memory description, observing your patient's facial expressions and behavior, or simply asking your patient which parts of the memory were most distressing. Many memories include details of preliminary and subsequent events that typically are not as emotionally relevant as the hot spots. Once you identify a hot spot, instruct your patients to bypass the preliminary aspects of the story and fast-forward to the period just prior to the hot spot. At the conclusion of the hot spot, cut off further detail and ask them to "rewind" back to the start of the hot spot. Typically, a hot spot segment should be brief, no more than 5 minutes. Repeating the hot spot for the remainder of the session reduces anxiety pertaining to this very emotionally relevant aspect of the memory.

For example, Yolanda's imaginal exposure focused on her memory of being mugged. In the first session, she told the story four times, taking approximately 15 minutes each time. After her first session, Yolanda practiced exposure six times. In the second session, her therapist quickly noted that her anxiety was markedly lower than in the previous session, and was on a trajectory for continued reduction. Her therapist decided that Yolanda was ready to work on hot spots. After the first time through the story, the therapist instructed Yolanda to start at the point when she was approaching the man on the street. This instruction deleted detail about Yolanda leaving her office, what she was thinking about on her way home, and the sights along the way. Then, her therapist encouraged her to elaborate about her experience of the actual attack, the thoughts that went through her mind when she saw the perpetrator's knife, and how she was feeling at that moment. After the hot spot, her therapist asked her to stop and return to that same point, rather than to proceed with the description of how she was found and taken to a hospital. Targeting the hot spot initially increased Yolanda's anxiety. As she repeated this hot spot over and over, however, she experienced a subsequent reduction in anxiety.

Asking questions helps patients to elaborate hot spots. Morgan, who had initially described her hot spot as "Then he raped me," was reluctant to describe any details about the actual rape. To target the hot spot, Morgan's therapist asked her, "What did it feel like when he pushed inside of you?"; "What were you thinking?"; "Where were his hands?"; and "Where were your hands?" and "What did he smell like?" Morgan eventually began to describe the rape in great detail, and her anxiety rating increased from 50 for the entire memory to 100.

Initially you might feel that you are being mean when you ask patients to elaborate on hot spots in exquisite detail. The level of detail is uncommon in many other forms of therapy. Yet this detail is needed for patients to process their traumatic experience fully and to benefit fully from exposure. Moreover, in doing so, you communicate to patients that you can hear exactly what happened and still care about them. Morgan later reported, "When it was time for me to open my eyes, I was afraid you would see me differently. But when you looked at me just the same as you always have, and treated me just the same, my shame about what happened got less."

Combining Imaginal and *In Vivo* Exposure

If your patient habituates rapidly in session, you may find it useful to combine *in vivo* exposure and imaginal exposure. Molly showed rapid habituation in session, and her homework records also showed habituation. Therefore, Molly brought her *in vivo* exposure material, safety pins, to this session. Once she had habituated to the memory alone, her therapist had her hold the safety pins in her hands as she proceeded with the imaginal exposure (see Figure 7.3). In Molly's case, it was necessary for her to open her eyes to experience the *in vivo* stimuli fully.

When to Move to a New Memory

In most cases, you need to conduct exposure with more than one memory. Therefore, you should have a plan for deciding when to conclude exposure to one memory and

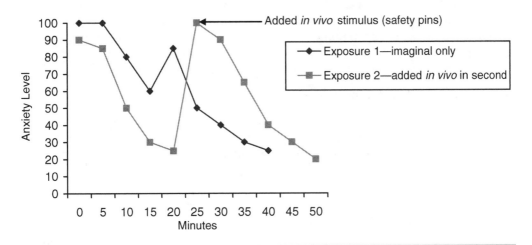

FIGURE 7.3. Molly's exposure: combining *in vivo* and imaginal exposure.

move to the next. We bring many memories down to a 0 SUDS rating. You know you are done with a memory when your patient has previously engaged and experienced significant anxiety but now reports "Nothing, I am not anxious at all," even at the start of the exposure. Patients may also report being bored with the memory. Some patients, however, continue to report SUDS ratings of 10 or 20 at the start of the exposure and do not show much further habituation. Even at this level, patients may report being bored with the memory. For example, Yoel rated his anxiety at 15 after 3 weeks of exposure to his memories of childhood sexual abuse. He reported that he was bored with the memory, and that his feeling of anxiety was substantially lower than he could ever remember it being. He also noted that whenever he stopped concentrating on this memory, his anxiety actually increased as he started noticing different anxiety-provoking stimuli to a greater degree. In this case, the therapist hypothesized that Yoel's rating of anxiety was more strongly related to his inability to completely tune out other anxiety-provoking stimuli. Thus, the therapist decided to move on to another memory. If you reach a point where there are no hot spots and it appears that the memory has been fully processed, it is probably time to move on to a new memory.

TROUBLESHOOTING

Responding to Things Patients Say during Exposure

Requests to Stop

Patients periodically ask for permission to stop. For example:

> "I wish this were over."
> "Do I have to keep doing it?"
> "I've had enough, can I stop now?"
> "How long do I have to keep doing this?"

Your goal is to encourage them to continue, while you reinforce their sense of control over the process. For example, you tell them that it is good for them to keep going, because they will get the most out of treatment by staying with the exposure, even though it is hard. At the same time, remind them that no one is forcing them to do this, and that it is their decision to continue.

Believing That They Cannot Do Exposure

Some patients are doubtful that they can complete exposure. They may express this as either a question, "What if I can't do it?" or a statement, "I can't do this." In either case, communicate to them that their concerns are understandable, but that they still should try exposure.

LYNETTE: I don't think I can do this. Maybe you should give up working with me.

THERAPIST: You've avoided thinking about the accident for so many years, it's natural to wonder if you can let yourself think about it and feel the feelings. Most people who start this work are quite fearful of these feelings. Yet once they get started, most people find that they are able to do it. During the assessment, you were able to tell me quite a bit about what happened, and it was fairly upsetting for you, yet you got through it all right. So I believe you will be able to describe it again. As you repeat it and stay with it, it will get easier.

LYNETTE: But what if it doesn't?

THERAPIST: Well, I really think it will work. But if it doesn't, we'll work together to figure out why and change the procedure to make it work for you. It's extremely rare that a person is just unable to do it, and I haven't seen any indications that that would be the case for you.

Trying to Prevent an Event That Has Already Happened

Exposure involves accepting the traumatic event. Some patients resist acceptance, and occasionally their resistance appears to influence habituation. Brenda's moderately elevated anxiety did not diminish substantially within or between trials of exposure. During each session, about 30–45 minutes into the exposure, she held her hands in front of her face and shook her head saying, "No, No." Shortly thereafter, Brenda's anxiety increased and she asked to stop. After the third session, her therapist asked Brenda if she knew what she was thinking while she was shaking her head and saying "No." Brenda stated that she "didn't want him to do it" and that she "wanted him to go away." It appeared that Brenda was so immersed in the memory that she felt that she could somehow stop it from happening rather than accepting it as an event that had already happened in the past. Brenda's therapist had taught her to use the DBT skill of radical acceptance of events in her life (see Chapter 9). She encouraged Brenda's radical acceptance of her childhood sexual abuse during imaginal exposure. Brenda then began to habituate.

Expressing Responsibility for the Traumatic Event

Patients sometimes express responsibility for their traumatic event during exposure. If this happens, although you may have an urge to stop imaginal exposure, in general, we do not recommend it. Many patients continue to experience anxiety reduction, even though their expression of responsibility may elevate guilt. Other patients also may reduce their sense of responsibility via exposure. Thus, until it becomes clear that an expression of responsibility is completely blocking habituation, continue with exposure. If the patient still feels responsible at the end of exposure, address the matter by using cognitive restructuring. For example, in the midst of describing his childhood sexual abuse during exposure, Gary said, "I could have fought him off." Gary's therapist made note of this and encouraged him to continue and complete the full 45 minutes of planned exposure. Afterward, she initiated cognitive restructuring to examine the noted thought.

Unable to Speak/Refusal to Disclose

Occasionally, patients who have agreed to do exposure are nonetheless unable to speak when prompted to begin exposure. A patient who does not verbalize the memory is unlikely to benefit from treatment. Proceeding by having a patient imagine the memory (without verbalizing it aloud) is not advisable, because you cannot determine the extent to which the patient is focused on the memory. Lack of verbalization also prevents patients from learning that you can hear their horrible experience(s) and still support them. If a patient does not speak, validate him or her, be patient, and use gentle prompts, such as "You've never said it before, so it's understandable that it's hard to start talking about it"; "What's the first thing you remember happening?"; or "It's safe here; you can tell me what happened and you will be OK."

If after 10–15 minutes of validation and prompting, the patient remains silent or utters only a few words, consider whether modifications may be helpful to get started. Some patients find that writing the memory first is easier than saying it out loud. In fact, we have had patients who preferred to write rather than to speak during the first exposure to every memory. In the next session, they verbalized the memory after a week of writing it daily at home. Writing also can be useful for patients who are unable to verbalize details of hot spots. No matter how much she was prompted, Katy would not elaborate on her childhood physical abuse. However, she was able to write in great detail and was also able to read repeatedly what she had written.

On rare occasions, we have had patients who appeared to have little verbal memory of the events secondary to being very young at the time of the trauma; some of these patients started by drawing their trauma. The drawings were used as a stepping-stone to writing and then to verbalizing. If patients with clear memories from older ages are reluctant to verbalize or write a memory, we might also have them begin by drawing the disturbing images. The goal, however, always is to progress as quickly as possible to standard exposure.

Dissociating and Numbing

Patients who dissociate and/or numb out during exposure do not benefit, because they are not experiencing the required elements of successful exposure. Dissociated patients are either too immersed in the memory (i.e., having a flashback) and are unaware that they are safe, or they are no longer engaged with the memory and their emotional response. Similarly, patients who "numb out" are not experiencing their anxiety. You have several options when you encounter patients who dissociate or numb out during imaginal exposure. First, if dissociation during exposure leads you to discover that your patient is *highly* dissociative (e.g., living much of life in a dissociated state), you may decide that the patient needs a brief, or not-so-brief, course of DBT/mindfulness training before proceeding with exposure (see Chapter 9). A short course of mindfulness training may also help some less dissociative patients.

A second, often successful option is to use strategies from the section of this chapter on titrating anxiety to reduce the intensity of patients' anxiety while recounting the memory. For example, have patients open their eyes. Titrating anxiety levels is appropriate for patients who can tolerate moderate levels of anxiety but who dissociate or numb out if the memory becomes too vivid and the anxiety too intense. Sometimes you need to be creative in finding ways to titrate anxiety. For example, inviting a safe person, such as partner, to the session can make exposure tolerable for some patients.

Third, you can return to or start with *in vivo* exposure. Many patients appear less prone to dissociation and numbing during *in vivo* exposure, possibly because objects and situations are more concrete than memories. *In vivo* exposure also typically involves patients keeping their eyes open, and the safety of the situation may be more obvious. Patients can more readily use cognitive strategies to help them stay with their anxiety and not dissociate. For example, during *in vivo* exposure to a T-shirt left behind by her abusive husband when he moved out, Justine kept repeating to herself, "There is no way a T-shirt across the room can hurt me. I can stay present." In addition, you can more easily adjust the intensity of *in vivo* stimuli, for example, by moving an object farther away, which gives patients a chance to learn how to stay present during exposure.

A fourth strategy involves grounding techniques to help patients stay present. One strategy is to use sensory stimuli, such as touching cold objects (e.g., a soda can or the metal arms of a chair), that can help patients maintain present awareness. Your voice can also serve this purpose. Maintaining a patter of supportive direction can help patients stay connected and in the present (e.g., "You are safe here, you can touch the shirt and no one is going to hurt you. . . . Just let yourself feel the fear, knowing that nothing bad will happen and anxiety cannot hurt you. . . . Allow yourself to approach the shirt whenever you are ready"). When using your voice during imaginal exposure, however, be careful to not interrupt patients' recounting of the memory. Asking for more frequent SUDS ratings is usually a safe way to use your voice to remind patients that they are in a safe setting. Often it is helpful to discuss and agree on strategies ahead of time, particularly with such things as a gentle tap on the arm or, as we have used in a few extreme cases, smelling salts.

A fifth strategy is to discourage dysfunctional behaviors. Some patients display very clear retreating behaviors as they begin to dissociate (e.g., curling up into a ball on the chair, moving into a fetal position on the floor, covering their ears). Such behaviors likely reduce their interaction with the world. Instructing such patients to engage in more functional behaviors may help interrupt the dissociation. For example, if a patient starts to curl up during imaginal exposure, gently say, "Why don't you put your feet back on the floor while we continue? And maybe you could also sit back against the chair, like you were earlier." One way to ease into such instructions is to ask first for a SUDS rating. Be alert to and assertively interrupt any patient's potentially dangerous behaviors, such as curling under the corner of a table or stabbing him- or herself with a pen. Even highly dissociated patients often respond appropriately when safety issues are pointed out.

A sixth strategy involves engaging the assistance of a prescribing provider, because some patients are able to complete exposure after medication changes or additions. If possible, identify a psychiatrist who is (1) familiar with medications that may help in such situations and (2) understands exposure. Medication changes (combined with other strategies in this section) can help some patients with severe dissociation and psychotic symptoms proceed with exposure. For example, Margot was prone to dissociative flashbacks in daily life. Following these episodes, she typically had little recollection of her behavior or the situation. Each time that Margot attempted *in vivo* exposure, she immediately numbed out, so that her SUDS ratings never rose above 0. After the first exposure, she also reported, "My grandfather came to me last night and beat me up and then threatened to hurt you if I keep telling you his business. I woke up under a table with a bloody nose." Because Margot's grandfather was dead, the therapist contacted Margot's psychiatrist, who was supportive of CBT. After an increased dose of antipsychotic medication, Margot was able to proceed with exposure. Similarly,

we have observed that medication changes help patients who report that after exposure sessions, they felt they were "in a fog" and unable to function for days afterward.

Typically, the goal of medication adjustments at this stage is to attenuate sympathetic nervous system arousal that may trigger dissociation and to reduce psychotic
phenomena, not specifically to block anxiety. It is important to note that benzodiazepines (e.g., lorazepam, alprazolam) have not shown efficacy for PTSD symptoms
(Braun, Greenberg, Dasberg, & Lerer, 1990; Gelpin, Bonne, Brandes, & Shalev, 1996) and
usually are not complementary to the goals of exposure. If a patient is already taking a
benzodiazepine at a stable dose, the medication need not be changed during the beginning phase of exposure. However, discourage patients who ask to increase their use of
benzodiazepines (e.g., by taking one during or prior to exposure practice) from doing
so by reminding them that they need to experience anxiety during exposure, and that
things that dampen anxiety, such as taking medications or engaging in safety behaviors
(see Chapter 6), interfere with its effectiveness. If your patient is taking medication during exposure, keep in mind that new learning that occurs in the drug context may not
generalize to nondrug contexts, so further exposure may be necessary for generalization when the medication is discontinued (see Chapter 10). Also discuss any significant
medication issues with the prescribing clinician.

In many cases, you need to combine strategies to reduce dissociation. For example,
Justine was able to start exposure successfully and stop dissociating by switching to *in
vivo* exposure with the T-shirt, keeping her eyes open, having her therapist provide a
fairly steady stream of instructions, having her best friend attend the session, and by reminding herself aloud that she was safe. After she habituated to the T-shirt in session,
she and her therapist devised a careful T-shirt hierarchy for her to start at home. Part of
the process for Justine was learning to engage with her anxiety while practicing skills
aimed at keeping her present. As these skills improved, she was able to return to
imaginal exposure.

Responding to Complications Reported after the Session

It's a good idea to plan a follow-up call within a few days of the first exposure session
with patients who appear at risk for difficulties. Most patients do not have much difficulty during this period, particularly if they experienced substantial within-session
anxiety reduction. Some, however, experience a worsening of symptoms, difficulty carrying out exposure homework, and/or a reemergence of maladaptive coping, such as
drinking, drug use, purging, or self-harm. Be prepared to respond to such patients and
to assess safety, if it becomes a concern. For example, despite a substantial reduction in
anxiety, Carla disclosed at the end of the first imaginal exposure session that she had
increased urges to cut herself. This was not surprising, because Carla had a history of
cutting. Her therapist also noted that Carla stated, "I feel so dirty," several times during
exposure, which suggests that urges to cut might be related to shame. The therapist
used the remainder of the session to do cognitive restructuring of this thought and
made a plan with Carla for strategies to resist urges to cut.

Laura's therapist called her several days after her first exposure to a memory of being mugged. Laura stated that she had not listened to the tape since the session, because she felt too frightened. When Laura thought about doing exposure, she found

herself overwhelmed by fear, and her vigilance increased to the point that she was unable to sleep. As a result, Laura's therapist decided to schedule another session of imaginal exposure that same week. This is a good example of the importance of approaching rather than retreating from exposure when symptoms worsen. In the second session, Laura experienced more anxiety reduction, after which she agreed to start home exposure by writing a description of her assault during daylight hours. After her third exposure session a week later, Laura started doing exposure with the audiotape at home.

Li Mei had been physically abused by her boyfriend for several years. In the week following her first exposure session, Li Mei reported that she was feeling increasingly depressed and her Beck Depression Inventory score increased from 21 at intake to 37. Several factors appeared to contribute to her depression. First, Li Mei reported feeling responsible for the abuse, because she believed it was her responsibility to please her boyfriend. Also, she stated that her need for help meant that she was a failure and a burden to others. Finally, Li Mei had few leisure activities or outside social contacts. Li Mei's therapist created a two-pronged approach to address the depression without interrupting exposure. First, she worked with Li Mei to identify and to engage in pleasurable activities. Second, she used cognitive restructuring to target beliefs that she hypothesized might be contributing to Li Mei's depression.

Reluctance to Do Exposure or Exposure Homework

Some patients are so fearful and reluctant to do exposure and home practice that they produce a variety of reasons for not doing so. For example, patients may try to convince you that it will not work. Other patients' anticipatory anxiety about exposure actually exceeds the anxiety they experience when they begin. Respond to reluctance by validating patients' concerns and fears. At the same time, emphasize that the best thing your patients can do is to move forward with exposure, so that they start to reap its benefits. In addition, stress the importance of repetition. Also encourage them to adopt an experimental, "Let's see" approach to treatment. With respect to homework, use problem-solving strategies to help patients find a way to start home practice.

Occasionally, patients report that they simply do not want to hear themselves on the tape. For example, Glenda, a survivor of childhood sexual abuse, had a strong reaction to the idea of listening to herself on tape.

GLENDA: You mean you are going to make a tape of my voice and you want me to listen to it? I don't think I would like that!

THERAPIST: Yes. Home practice is critical for success of exposure therapy, because it increases the amount of repetition. Remember, exposure works when it is repeated. Most people find it hard to just repeat the memory out loud at home. The tape is used to guide you through your memory of the assault during your home practice.

GLENDA: But I hate hearing my voice on tape—I sound awful.

THERAPIST: Well, another option is that you can say the memory out loud without a tape at home, or if that doesn't work, you can begin writing it. The key is that if you write it or say it, you should do it for the same amount of time that we spend on it today. What we can do is go ahead and make the tape. That way you can decide later how you'd like to conduct your home practice. Would that be all right with you?

GLENDA: Sure. I don't really care about you recording me; it's listening to myself that makes me so uncomfortable.

In some cases, a patient's discomfort with listening to an exposure tape might be part of an overall tendency to invalidate his or her emotional reactions. This may be particularly likely in patients with borderline personality disorder (BPD). For example, despite significant within-session habituation in her first exposure session, Deirdre reported the next week that she could not listen to the tape in which she had recounted a memory of her mother breaking her arm. Deirdre said, "I sounded so whiny, I couldn't stand hearing myself be such a baby." The therapist noted that rather than mindfully participate in the exposure exercise while listening to the tape, Deirdre adopted a judgmental, invalidating stance toward herself. Thus, rather than experiencing anxiety, she became mired in her secondary reaction (primarily shame) and escalated in her self-invalidation. The intervention in this case was simply to educate Deirdre about the importance of mindful participation in exposure, and about what self-invalidation is and how it interferes with experiencing anxiety during exposure. The therapist also suggested that an active task, such as writing about the memory, might work better and preclude Deirdre's judgmental observation of her reactions. Though Deirdre responded to this brief intervention, some patients might require a lengthier focus on mindfulness before being able to engage in exposure productively.

Slow or No Habituation, or Erratic SUDS Ratings

Very slow or no habituation may occur for a number of reasons. Poor habituation might also be expressed via an erratic SUDS pattern, in which SUDS ratings spike and drop repeatedly throughout the exposure session. When you determine that a patient's habituation process is not proceeding as you would like, you need to determine the problem, typically by hypothesizing possible reasons, then exploring these reasons with your patient.

Interference from Other Emotions Such as Anger and Shame

As noted throughout this book, among emotions, anxiety habituates most reliably during exposure. Optimal conditions for anxiety reduction include steady engagement with the anxiety-provoking stimuli and the emotion anxiety. Repetition in imaginal exposure is the mechanism for creating this steady engagement. When patients focus almost exclusively on other emotions, such as anger or shame, they are not experiencing the optimal conditions for exposure and may show less than satisfactory habituation. Similarly, if patients ricochet between anxiety and anger, or anxiety and shame, they may not experience ideal habituation. This pattern may produce erratic SUDS ratings patterns as well.

If other emotions interfere with patients' experience of anxiety, you have two primary options. First, attempt to instruct them to focus on their anxiety to a greater degree, and let them know that you will address residual emotions with cognitive restructuring. Some patients can do this. One patient described this as "shelving" her other emotions during exposure, and taking them off the shelf after exposure. Some patients, however, first have to be taught to identify and label different emotional states. The need to identify and label different emotional states occurs with both exposure and cognitive restructuring. Handout 8.5 is useful for teaching patients how to do this. It is beyond the scope of this book, however, to extensively detail strategies for teaching emotion recognition. We typically rely on strategies from DBT. Interested readers are referred to DBT resources (Linehan, 1993a, 1993b).

Other patients experience nonanxiety emotional responses as too intrusive to shelve during exposure. Cognitive restructuring is a good tool for addressing these emotions prior to returning to exposure. For example, Laurie reported very erratic SUDS ratings that were tied to surges in anger at her rapist. She and her therapist used cognitive restructuring to resolve her anger. Laurie subsequently proceeded successfully with exposure.

Intermittent Numbing or Dissociating

Some patients may intermittently shut down or become numb during imaginal exposure. This reduces habituation and, again, may produce erratic SUDS ratings. Shutting down and numbing are usually a sign that patients are attempting to recall a memory that is too difficult for them. The strategies described earlier to titrate anxiety and increase grounding are often effective.

Missing Hot Spots

Poor habituation or erratic SUDS ratings may also indicate that a hot spot needs to be addressed. Look for the signs described in the section on hot spots to determine whether the patient has an unaddressed hot spot.

Exposure Context

The environment in which patients conduct home exposure practice also may interfere with habituation. As noted in Chapter 6, exposure enables patients to learn a new meaning (safety) for a stimulus that was previously associated with danger. The new meaning may, however, be fairly specific to the context in which the new learning occurred. Therefore, learning that takes place in your office may not apply to situations outside the office, which is why fear may return in another context, and why home practice is very important for generalization of fear reduction. Although there is still much we do not know about how contexts influence fear reduction, attending to context may help when you are not observing between-session fear reduction.

Carmen was physically abused by her husband for 20 years. When she came for PTSD treatment, she still resided in their home, which she won in her divorce settlement. Carmen's therapist observed that although her anxiety was going down slowly within each session, there was minimal anxiety reduction between the first three sessions of exposure (see Figure 7.4). Carmen was highly motivated and persevered with exposure despite her very high distress levels. Nonetheless, the minimal between-

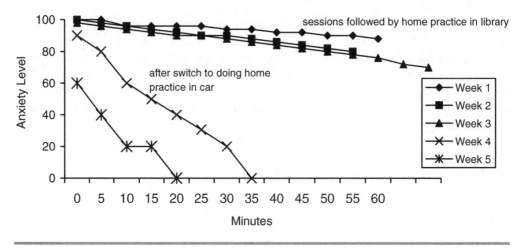

FIGURE 7.4. Carmen's imaginal exposure sessions: 1 week apart.

session habituation was of concern, because between-session habituation is associated with treatment outcome in randomized trials (Jaycox et al., 1998).

Upon discussion, Carmen disclosed that she had been listening to her exposure tape in the library of her home, where much of the abuse took place. Carmen's therapist hypothesized that conducting exposure in the context in which the abuse took place would result in an increase in fear. Consistent with this hypothesis, Carmen's home practice imaginal exposure records (Figure 7.5) showed little between-trial habituation. Carmen's therapist suggested that she listen to the tape in a location outside the house. Carmen decided to listen in her parked car. Figure 7.6 shows the results of exposure conducted in the car. Conducting exposure outside the abuse context resulted in reduction of Carmen's anxiety during the exposure in her therapist's office (greater between-session habituation), as shown in Figure 7.6. After Carmen's anxiety had diminished in the car, her therapist had her return to doing the exposure practice in the house, first

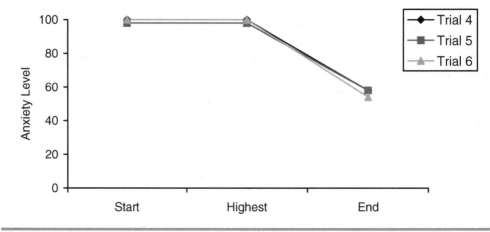

FIGURE 7.5. Carmen's imaginal exposure home practice: second week—in library.

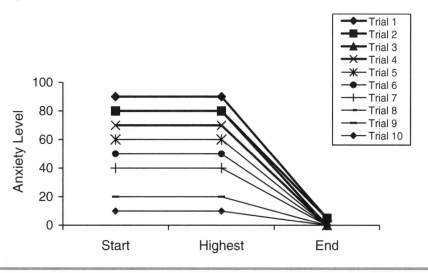

FIGURE 7.6. Carmen's imaginal exposure home practice: third week—in car.

beginning in the living room, which was a less frequent location of abuse, then moving to the library (Figure 7.7). Upon moving to the living room, Carmen's initial anxiety rating was higher than in the car, but lower than it had been in the library. When she returned to the library, where the abuse most frequently took place, her anxiety again increased. Yet after attaining habituation in a different context, Carmen began to habituate in this environment as well. This example illustrates the importance of attending to context in exposure therapy, particularly when you observe an absence of between-session habituation in sessions and in home practice records. It also demonstrates how careful record keeping and the use of graphs can help to identify problems and assess progress.

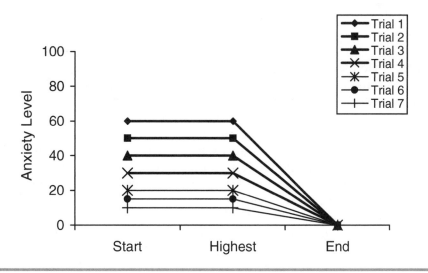

FIGURE 7.7. Carmen's imaginal exposure home practice: fifth week—in library.

UNUSUAL REACTIONS

Sexual Arousal during Exposure

Some patients experience sexual arousal during imaginal exposure to a memory of sexual abuse, even abuse that was violent, painful, and forced. They may also recall being aroused at the time of the abuse. Be forewarned of this possibility. You do not want to be caught off guard by such a disclosure, because it might lead you to inadvertently express surprise or disdain. Such responses may not only be countertherapeutic but also harmful. Although sexual arousal is uncommon, it is typically a source of tremendous shame. Patients often interpret sexual arousal to mean they are perverse or abnormal. Sexual arousal is confusing for such patients, and to resolve the dissonance, they conclude, "Well, I must have wanted it," or "I'm abnormal." It is very important to respond to sexual arousal disclosures in a nonjudgmental way, and communicate unconditional positive regard, acceptance, and validation.

Some patients who feel aroused by their abuse memory also believe that their arousal indicates that they, like their perpetrator, are prone to sexually abuse children. Importantly, some patients may in fact have a history of perpetration that will need to be addressed in treatment. Be sure to assess fully for perpetration history *before* making a comment such as "Even though you are aroused, that doesn't mean that you are going to assault children." For example, if a patient forced sexual acts on her sibling as a child, your statement obviously is unlikely to be persuasive. Even if the patient's behavior is abnormal and/or must stop because it is illegal or harmful, it is still possible to communicate that it is understandable. Other tactics also will be necessary to reduce the distress related to guilt (see Chapter 8).

Vomiting

Vomiting, or fear of vomiting, is another reaction that patients may have to their trauma memories or the associated anxiety. It is not uncommon for patients to fear vomiting during exposure, or to report vomiting during exposure practice at home or in the parking lot after an exposure session. Interestingly enough, although we have had dozens of patients report being fearful of vomiting during session or having vomited outside of session, we have never observed patients *actually* vomit in a session, even when they were certain that they would.

Fears of vomiting like other fears, tend to be exaggerated (i.e., patients overestimate the likelihood of the event occurring and how bad it would be if it did occur). Many patients expect that you will be discouraged from proceeding with exposure once you know about their urge to vomit. They assume that you would be either too disgusted or that you would realize the extent of their anxiety and not want them to proceed. Some also fear that if they vomit, you will vomit. In their minds, what could be worse than making your therapist lose control and get sick? For this reason, if you have discomfort or fear of vomit, you should treat your own fear prior to initiating exposure with patients who are likely to express this fear.

When patients state that they expect to vomit, the most helpful response is, "I know that it's unpleasant to feel the nausea, although it is understandable that you feel like vomiting when your anxiety is so intense. It's OK with me if you need to vomit" or "I can see why you'd feel like throwing up—what he did to you really was revolting. If you need it, the trash can is right here." This communicates several important things. First, it shows patients that you are not afraid of their reactions, even reactions that many people find distasteful, such as vomiting. Second, it normalizes vomiting. This is important because for some of these patients, a sense that vomiting is "disgusting" can add to their shame around the events. Third, you decatastrophize vomiting by communicating that vomiting is *not* dangerous, though it is unpleasant. Fourth, and perhaps most important, it sends the message that you will not be derailed or deterred from exposure by patients' reactions to the memory, nor should they. Although vomiting is one of the more extreme kinds of reactions, it is important to communicate similar messages regarding other reactions to the exposure that your patient might fear.

CONCLUSION

We cannot emphasize enough how powerful a tool imaginal exposure is in the treatment of PTSD. Unfortunately, research indicates that it is an underutilized tool in clinical practice (Becker, Zayfert & Anderson, 2004; Rosen et al., 2004). Our purpose in this chapter was to provide you with information needed to proceed with imaginal exposure. Many patients who are often viewed as unacceptable candidates for exposure can complete exposure using the strategies discussed in this chapter. Thus, we encourage you to persevere in teaching patients that their memories cannot hurt them, and that facing these memories will help them recover from their trauma.

HEY, IT'S WORKING . . .

From your practice with *in vivo* exposure, by now you have begun to understand that exposure therapy involves repeatedly approaching what you are afraid of for an extended period of time. You have learned that when you stay with the thing you are afraid of, after many repetitions, you feel more comfortable in its presence. So, if you were afraid of tabby cats because of your encounter with the lion, you practiced *in vivo* ("in real life") exposure to tabby cats. You made a hierarchy (a graduated list). Perhaps you started with your friend's kitten, which she held in her lap across the room from you. At first you were frightened, but, after half an hour or so, your anxiety went down. Then, after a week of this, you found that you were no longer anxious, so you moved closer to the kitten. After several sessions at close distance, as your comfort increased, you decided to pet the kitten. Next, you decided to move to a full-grown cat, eventually working your way up to an orange cat (but not a lion!). Your *in vivo* exposure work might also include looking at pictures of lions in magazines or watching them on television shows. We hope you have been able to start this work and have experienced what this feels like. It is important that you learn (1) how to stay in the situation, (2) how to use the exposure principles to plan your exposure work, and (3) to trust that exposure works—that you will feel more comfortable in the situation after repeated practice.

BUT, I STILL CAN'T STOP *THINKING* ABOUT THE LION

All this exposure to cats has been very helpful: You are no longer afraid of cats, so you visit friends who have cats and are able to walk down the street without watching over your shoulder for a cat. Yet despite success in overcoming your fear of cats, you are still bothered by memories of the lion attack. Sometimes, without warning, when you are busy going about your day, the image of the lion's teeth and claws just pops into your mind, and you suddenly feel frightened. You might find yourself trying to stay busy, so that your mind won't "idle" and there won't be room for the memory to pop up. The lion attack is still very vivid and the feeling of being unsafe still haunts you. You may worry a lot about your safety, and the safety of those you love. So you are still watchful for danger around you. And when you sleep at night, you may still dream about running from the lion. To make matters worse, it's frustrating that you can't get the lion out of your mind, because realistically, you *know* that you are no longer in Africa, and that you are quite safe from the lion now. You might even feel ashamed that you can't get over it, or angry that it has taken over your life for so long. So you try even harder to push away the memories and get back to your life. But the harder you try, the more the memories keep coming back, causing fear, confusion, and exhaustion.

SO, WHAT IS *IMAGINAL* EXPOSURE?

As we have said before, the harder you try to not think about something, the more it comes back into your mind. If you try not to think about a pink elephant, what are you thinking of? The more you sweep things "under the rug," the more they come out the other side. By this time you know that avoidance often does not produce the hoped for results. This applies not only to avoidance of reminders of the lion attack, like tabby cats, fur coats, and lions on television, but also to the memories

(continued)

of the lion attack themselves. Imaginal exposure works just like *in vivo* exposure, except that you expose yourself to the memory of the lion attack instead of a reminder of the attack. You do this with your therapist by telling the story of the lion attack step-by-step, moment-by-moment, and recounting all that happened, what you felt, and what you were thinking and doing at the time.

IT SOUNDS AWFUL—WHY WOULD I WANT TO DO IT?

Yes, imaginal exposure can be very scary. Most people with PTSD feel reluctant to bring back memories they have been suppressing for a long time. After all, it was bad enough to live through it when it happened! You are lucky to have survived, so why on earth would you want to think about the awful things that happened? Some people believe that thinking about what happened is like actually reliving it again: The first time was bad enough, so why go through it again? Some people fear that they might "have a nervous breakdown" or "go crazy," but as you will learn, that is very unlikely. In fact, although it's true that people's emotions can be very intense when doing this work, most people find that they gain an increased sense of control from doing imaginal exposure. When you allow yourself to think about it, you learn that a memory is just a memory, and it can't hurt you. You also have the opportunity to think through the details of what happened through "new eyes." You get to see things through the eyes of who you are now rather than who you were at the time of the trauma. This allows you to "process" the memory and come to new understandings about the meaning of what happened. Being able to "finish" the "unfinished business" allows you to put it away for good.

TOP 10 REASONS TO DO IMAGINAL EXPOSURE

When they start treatment for PTSD, many people realize that at some point treatment involves thinking about what happened. You and your therapist have talked about imaginal exposure, and you have read about it in this handout. You may have under your belt some experience with *in vivo* exposure that has influenced your thinking. Everyone has his or her own reasons for doing imaginal exposure. Without good reasons, you probably would decide *not* to do it! If you have some good reasons for doing imaginal exposure, now is the time to list them. You may find it helpful to refer back to this list later in treatment, if you feel the urge to avoid taking over.

10. _____

9. _____

8. _____

7. _____

6. _____

5. _____

4. _____

3. _____

2. _____

1. _____

(continued)

UNDERSTANDING THE PARADOX OF EMOTIONAL CONTROL

Traumatic experiences can make you feel that you have lost control of your life. During a traumatic event you may feel out of control of things happening to you. After the event, you may feel that you have lost control of your mind. Thoughts, memories, and emotions related to the trauma may intrude in your daily life. Sometimes these emotions can feel very overwhelming. Survivors of trauma commonly try very hard to control thoughts and feelings, to feel more in control of life. We often think that feeling certain emotions is a sign of weakness, or that it is unsafe to feel emotions. Yet efforts to control emotions by suppressing them often backfire. The more you try to control such thoughts and feelings, the less you may feel in control of them.

If you tend to see your emotions as "the problem," and experiencing emotions as a sign of weakness, it is understandable that you would try hard *not* to feel them. In fact, emotions have a useful purpose in our lives (see the table "Understanding Your Emotions" in Handout 8.2) and understanding that purpose may help you to respond constructively to events in your life. Also, when you understand the purpose of your emotions, you may be less frightened by them.

Regaining control of your life may mean allowing yourself to feel certain emotions, even if they sometimes lead you to feel "out of control." Challenging your thoughts about controlling emotions may lead you to discover more helpful ways to think about emotions.

Client _____   Date _____

Dates of exposure	Description	SUDS
	(1)	
	(2)	
	(3)	
	(4)	
	(5)	
	(6)	
	(7)	

Exposure Session Record

(For therapist documentation of in-session exposure)

Name _____ Date _____

Memory/Stimulus No. _____ Exposure Session No. (for this memory or stimulus)_____

Description of memory/stimulus: _____

_____

_____

_____

		SUDS	Vividness ratings, notes on cognitions, etc.
Baseline 0	min	_____	
_____	min	_____	
_____	min	_____	
_____	min	_____	
_____	min	_____	
_____	min	_____	
_____	min	_____	
_____	min	_____	
_____	min	_____	
_____	min	_____	
_____	min	_____	
_____	min	_____	
_____	min	_____	
_____	min	_____	
_____	min	_____	
_____	min	_____	
_____	min	_____	
_____	min	_____	
_____	min	_____	

Name _____ Memory No. _____ Date _____

Description of memory for exposure _____

_____

- Ideally, you should practice imaginal exposure every day. The more often you practice, the quicker you will notice results and feel less distressed by the memory.
- Find a quiet and safe place to listen to your entire exposure tape. (For safety reasons, do not listen to the tape while driving a car.)
- Enter your SUDS rating before you start the exposure.
- Do not distract yourself by doing other things while listening to the tape. Allow yourself to experience the feelings as intensely as you did when the event happened, without the distraction of other thoughts, images, or activities.
- Follow any special instructions provided by your therapist.
- When you are done, enter your highest SUDS rating while listening to the tape, and your SUDS rating at the end of the exposure.
- To track your progress, graph the Beginning, Highest, and Ending SUDS ratings below. (*Hint.* Use a different color or symbol for each exposure practice.)

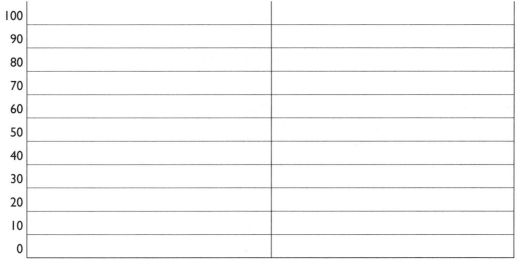

Subjective Units of Distress Scale (SUDS)

0	10	20	30	40	50	60	70	80	90	100
None		Mild		Moderate		Severe		Very severe		Extreme

(continued)

Subjective Units of Distress Scale (SUDS)

0	10	20	30	40	50	60	70	80	90	100
None		Mild		Moderate		Severe		Very severe		Extreme

1. Date:_____   Beginning SUDS   _____
Location:_____   Highest SUDS   _____
Duration:_____   Ending SUDS   _____

2. Date:_____   Beginning SUDS   _____
Location:_____   Highest SUDS   _____
Duration:_____   Ending SUDS   _____

3. Date:_____   Beginning SUDS   _____
Location:_____   Highest SUDS   _____
Duration:_____   Ending SUDS   _____

4. Date:_____   Beginning SUDS   _____
Location:_____   Highest SUDS   _____
Duration:_____   Ending SUDS   _____

5. Date:_____   Beginning SUDS   _____
Location:_____   Highest SUDS   _____
Duration:_____   Ending SUDS   _____

6. Date:_____   Beginning SUDS   _____
Location:_____   Highest SUDS   _____
Duration:_____   Ending SUDS   _____

7. Date:_____   Beginning SUDS   _____
Location:_____   Highest SUDS   _____
Duration:_____   Ending SUDS   _____

EIGHT

Cognitive Restructuring

Emilia, a 22-year-old female, was referred for treatment of nightmares. Emilia grew up in a loving and protective Catholic household. For example, her parents did not allow any of their daughters to date or drive. A strong student in high school, Emilia was permitted to apply to residential colleges only after a concerted campaign of begging her parents. During Emilia's first semester of college, she was invited by a fellow student, Daniel, to attend an exclusive party held by the basketball team. Emilia was very flattered and decided to attend, even though she knew that her parents would have forbade her to do so had she consulted them. Emilia also lied to her mother before going to the party, stating that she had to end their phone conversation so that she could study. Daniel picked Emilia up in his car and took her to the party. He complimented Emilia, telling her how pretty she looked. When they arrived at the apartment where the party was being held, Emilia discovered that she was the only female invited. Emilia, a virgin, was violently gang raped by six male students that night. She also was sodomized both orally and anally. When the male students were done, Daniel told Emilia to "clean yourself up in the bathroom" and then drove her home. He dropped her off at her dorm and said, "Thanks for the good time; you were wonderful. Welcome to college." Emilia wore clothing that concealed her body and makeup over the next few weeks to hide her bruises, and she never told anyone what had happened. Several times she encountered her perpetrators, and three complimented her for being "such a good fighter." Emilia dropped out of college over Christmas break, returned to living with her parents, and enrolled in her local community college. Emilia's parents told her they were glad that she "came to her senses before anything bad happened."

Several years later, Emilia was invited to visit her former college roommate, with whom she had remained friendly. The roommate was engaged and wanted Emilia to meet her fiancé. She also wanted Emilia to be a bridesmaid in her wedding. When Emilia arrived at her friend's apartment, she discovered that her friend's fiancé was one of the students who had raped her. After vomiting in the bathroom, Emilia told her friend that she thought had developed food poisoning and needed to return home. That night, Emilia began having nightmares.

WHY SHOULD I USE COGNITIVE RESTRUCTURING?

You use cognitive restructuring to help your patients alter the meaning of their traumatic events (Resick & Schnicke, 1993). Research indicates that cognitive restructuring alone can effectively treat PTSD (Marks et al., 1998). However, to address emotions and accompanying beliefs not resolved by exposure and psychoeducation, we typically use cognitive restructuring as an adjunct to exposure. Many patients experience changes in nonanxiety emotions during exposure secondary to changes in nonanxiety beliefs. For example, Keisha was raped by a former marine. During exposure she realized that because her attacker was much stronger than she, she likely would have been hurt even more had she fought her rapist; this resulted in a reduction of her guilt. Some patients, however, do not alter such beliefs during exposure. Such patients often benefit from cognitive restructuring aimed at beliefs that drive nonanxiety emotions, such as guilt, shame, and anger (Jaycox, Zoellner, & Foa, 2002; Kubany et al., 2004; Kubany & Watson, 2002).

We also use cognitive restructuring to address unhelpful beliefs prior to starting exposure, or when there are good reasons to postpone exposure. For example, sometimes we reduce the intensity of a nonanxiety emotion before starting exposure. You may choose this path if it seems that a nonanxiety emotion is impairing a patient's ability to complete exposure, or if the emotion interferes with his or her experiencing anxiety during exposure. Emilia was so focused on her extreme shame and guilt about being raped that they appeared to limit her experience of anxiety. Some research suggests that cognitive restructuring may be more effective in reducing emotions such as shame and guilt (Resick et al., 2002). Thus, Emilia's therapist attempted to reduce these emotions before starting exposure. Suzy, in contrast, started exposure treatment for her rape but was unable to stay focused on her anxiety. Instead, she vacillated between anxiety and intense rage. Research and published case studies indicate that severe anger can hinder exposure (Foa et al., 1995; Jaycox & Foa, 1996). Thus, the therapist stopped exposure and targeted thoughts related to Suzy's rage with cognitive restructuring. Then, Suzy successfully completed exposure.

Starting with cognitive restructuring, or *in vivo* exposure plus cognitive restructuring, also may be warranted when a patient reports very few reexperiencing symptoms and/or limited memory of the event. Ursula complained of chronic low self-esteem, dysthymia, and worry. She reported that she had always known that she had been sexually abused by her uncle when she was 3 years old, although her memory for the actual abuse was very sparse. After her uncle died, she briefly experienced nightmares. Upon entering therapy, the only reexperiencing symptom she reported was moderate distress upon hearing a song that reminded her of the abuse. Her most prominent PTSD symptoms were avoidance, anhedonia, numbing, detachment, poor concentration, and irritability/anger. Given the nature of Ursula's symptoms, her therapist decided to begin with *in vivo* exposure and cognitive restructuring. Kaya's therapist also chose to start with cognitive restructuring, because Kaya did not have a clear memory of her rape. The police believed that Kaya was given the rape drug Rohypnol. Kaya was fearful of certain stimuli that appeared to be related to the rape; thus, her treatment also included *in vivo* exposure.

As an aside, when you notice that you are inclined to start with cognitive restructuring, we advise that you ask yourself whether you are colluding with your patient in avoiding exposure. For example, given the brutal nature of Emilia's rape, before starting cognitive restructuring, Emilia's therapist asked herself whether she was making excuses to avoid exposure. Several clinicians have admitted to us that they sometimes want to avoid PTSD exposure because it seems unkind. Therapists may be more likely to experience an urge to avoid exposure when traumatic events seem particularly horrific. During her evaluation, Emilia noted that she was "smeared in blood," "horribly torn," and that there were "penises everywhere." Emilia's experienced PTSD therapist was disturbed by the evaluation alone. Given that many patients with equally horrible traumas have benefited rapidly from exposure, the therapist rightly questioned her motivation for postponing exposure. In Emilia's case, however, the therapist decided there was a legitimate reason to postpone exposure in favor of cognitive restructuring, because she suspected that Emilia's guilt would impair her ability to experience anxiety during exposure.

Finally, cognitive restructuring can facilitate processing of traumatic events and resolution of unhelpful beliefs in patients who are unable or unwilling to complete exposure. For example, Harry became extremely anxious, then emotionally numb, every time he tried to complete imaginal exposure to his memory of being shot. Harry's therapist tried many strategies to titrate the exposure task, but nothing worked. Harry was able to write about his experience in small segments, however. He and his therapist used his stream-of-consciousness writing to identify unhelpful trauma beliefs. Harry processed his traumatic experience by challenging his beliefs about the meaning of his trauma.

WHAT IS COGNITIVE RESTRUCTURING?

Cognitive restructuring teaches patients to systematically replace unhelpful thoughts with more helpful and realistic thoughts (see Handout 8.1). Based on the cognitive model of depression developed by Beck (1976), cognitive restructuring presumes that the way we interpret events in the world influences our emotional responses to those events. For example, if your friend Gary was 45 minutes late for a dinner date, you might think, "Gary must have been in an accident." Alternatively, you might think, "Gary is so inconsiderate that he thinks it is OK to be 45 minutes late. He really should have called." Another thought might occur: "I must have told Gary to go to the other restaurant. He is probably waiting there. This mix-up is my fault." If you interpreted Gary's lateness using the first example, you would probably be anxious. The second interpretation would likely produce anger, and the third, guilt. The objective situation has not changed, but your emotional reaction varies based on your interpretation.

Given the assumption that what we think directly influences our emotional response, it follows that making *meaningful* changes in our thinking will change how we feel. Changing thinking meaningfully, however, is often difficult. Many people also assume that cognitive restructuring teaches people to think positively (e.g., "I'm sure everything is all right with Gary, and there is no reason for me to be upset"). CBT therapists often label this type of thinking as "Pollyannaish," and this is not your goal. Rather, you want to teach your patients to use cognitive restructuring to create more balanced and accurate conclusions that generally are more helpful, and often more complex, than their habitual ways of thinking.

As we noted in Chapter 2, different cognitive theories and therapies utilize different terminology and constructs (thoughts, beliefs, schemes, appraisals, etc.) to describe patients' cognitive processes. All models of cognitive processes are to some degree metaphorical (Hertel, July 2002, personal communication). Thus, it is not clinically essential to delineate between models and varying terminology. In this chapter, we largely use the terms "thoughts" and "beliefs." We prefer to describe thoughts that contribute to negative affect or the maintenance of PTSD as "unhelpful," "biased," or "problematic" instead of "irrational," "dysfunctional," "erroneous," "maladaptive," or "distorted." Some patients who are sensitive to being invalidated seem to find the terms such as "unhelpful" or "problematic" less invalidating.

At times, we find it helpful to distinguish between thoughts and beliefs (Beck et al., 1979; Foa & Rothbaum, 1998). "Thoughts" may be conceptualized as the actual thoughts that your patients have during specific situations. "Beliefs" are more general assumptions (or more pervasive thoughts) held by your patients. Usually you do not need to determine whether an interpretation is a thought or a belief. The distinction is mostly helpful in recognizing that basic beliefs about the world and the self may provide the supporting framework for specific thoughts. Thus, challenging an easily identified thought sometimes is fruitless, because the patient needs to address a more fundamental belief that supports the initial thought. For example, Emilia had difficulty challenging the thought, "I'm dirty." Questioning revealed that Emilia believed that bad things happen to people who are not virtuous. Thus, Emilia not only believed that the rape had "dirtied" her, but also that she was raped because she was already "unworthy," "immoral," and "unclean" for being attracted to Daniel and flattered by his attention.

Six Steps of Cognitive Restructuring: Overview

Cognitive restructuring consists of six main steps (see Handout 8.2). In the first step, patients identify a situation in which they were distressed. Next, patients attempt in the second step to identify the specific emotions elicited by the situation and rate the intensity of those emotions on the same 0- to 100-point scale used in exposure. The third step involves identifying thoughts associated with the negative emotions and rating the degree to which patients believe each thought. Often these are described as "automatic thoughts," which are rapid thoughts that occur with little intention or awareness (Beck et al., 1979). Identifying automatic thoughts can be challenging. You may find it helpful to provide an example (e.g., Gary's lateness), so that patients understand how thoughts contribute to negative emotions. After the appropriate thoughts have been elicited, you and your patient select one thought to challenge and change. It also can be helpful for some patients to start with a homework assignment that just focuses on identifying thoughts (vs. identifying *and* changing thoughts; see the Automatic Thoughts Log in Handout 8.3) as the initial step in teaching cognitive restructuring.

The fourth step involves gathering evidence that supports the thought (i.e., *evidence for*) and evidence that does not support it (i.e., *evidence against*). It may also include identifying alternative interpretations of the situation, asking whether the patient would have the same interpretation if someone else were in the same situation, and investigating the consequences of the thought. After you have gathered all of the available information, your patient generates a rational or helpful response in the fifth step. Many patients have difficulty doing this at first and find that using a formula helps to get started. The formula that we use involves starting with some fact from the *evidence for* section (often prefaced with the words "Even though" or "Although") and connecting it with information from the *evidence against* section, often via the words "yet" or "in fact." During this step, patients rate the degree to which they believe the response. Finally, your patients rerate all of the negative emotions in the sixth step.

Some patients need to conduct a behavioral experiment to elicit evidence that supports or refutes their thoughts. The rational response also might include recognition of the need for a behavioral experiment, which for patients involves doing something to find out what happens as a result of their actions. Exposure can in part be conceptualized as a behavioral experiment that demonstrates that patients are able to tolerate thinking about the event and that their anxiety decreases. Other behavioral experiments may also be helpful. Kaya believed that her father would reject her if he knew that she had been raped. During cognitive restructuring, Kaya decided that the available evidence was somewhat ambiguous regarding her father's potential reaction. She concluded that she would rather find out how he would react, as opposed to continuing to ruminate about his possible reaction.

Many patients who learn cognitive restructuring find it frustrating. Indeed, for all of the clinical concern regarding the difficulty of completing exposure, many patients with PTSD have equal difficulty with cognitive restructuring. Thus, it can be helpful to forewarn patients of the challenges associated with learning to think differently. Some patients respond well to either sports or musical instrument metaphors. For example, in explaining cognitive restructuring to Kaya, the therapist built on Kaya's experience as a dancer. Specifically, she asked Kaya whether she had ever had a new dance instructor who wanted to change her dancing (e.g., how she placed her feet or moved her body). After Kaya responded "yes," the therapist asked if Kaya initially found it awkward and slow to dance the new way compared to the old way. Kaya again agreed. The therapist told Kaya that she might experience that same type of awkwardness and slowness in learning to think differently.

Even with this preparation, many patients return after their initial efforts at cognitive restructuring with blank homework sheets. Often this frustration can fuel self-invalidation; your patient may say, "You see this proves how stupid I am" or "I should be able to do this. It shows what a failure I am." When this happens, immediately use these thoughts for the next example of cognitive restructuring; such thoughts tend to be relatively easy to challenge, and the result is to formulate a self-validating response.

The Case of Emilia: Sample Dialogue of the Six Steps

As noted earlier, Emilia's therapist decided to start with cognitive restructuring because of the extremity of Emilia's guilt and shame. Emilia came to this session very distressed after receiving a call from her former roommate, which triggered an intrusive memory of her rape.

Introducing Cognitive Restructuring

Prior to starting cognitive restructuring, provide an overview of the rationale.

THERAPIST: It sounds like you had a really difficult week after that phone call.

EMILIA: Yes. I feel so gross, so dirty. I can't stop thinking about what happened. I wish I hadn't been so stupid and gone to that so-called party. If I had just done what my parents wanted, I would have been OK. None of this would have ever happened. I wish I could go back and make a different choice. I would do it so differently this time. I would listen to my parents.

THERAPIST: I can see that it has been really hard. So let's see if we can start to help you deal with what happened. Do you remember when we talked about learning to change how you think? We talked about this when I reviewed what we would do in therapy.

EMILIA: I remember.

THERAPIST: This seems like a good time to start this. We are going to use a strategy called "cognitive restructuring." You will find it helpful in managing some of these feelings you have as a result of your rape. Now, the first thing to remember with this strategy is that the goal is to help you change your thinking, which will help you change how you feel. I want to clarify that we are not looking to make all of your thinking positive, or to have you start to think like Pollyanna.

EMILIA: Good, I don't think that would work too well. There is no way I am going to believe that everything is sunshine.

THERAPIST: You're absolutely right. The positive thinking approach doesn't work very well. What we are going to do instead is have you learn to think in ways that are as realistic and helpful as possible. Let me use an example to explain. Imagine that your best friend—I think you said her name was Amanda—didn't call you for 3 weeks. How would you feel?

EMILIA: Really worried.

THERAPIST: Why? What would you be thinking?

EMILIA: That something happened to her. Amanda's parents are scatterbrained, and they would never remember to call me. She could be in the hospital.

THERAPIST: OK. So, in this case, you think that something bad has happened to her and then you feel worried. How do you think you would feel if you had the thought that Amanda has found new friends and doesn't want to be your friend anymore?

EMILIA: I would feel really sad, really hurt.

THERAPIST: And how would you feel if you thought that Amanda's new boyfriend was purposely cutting her off from her other friends?

EMILIA: I would feel really mad at him. And mad at Amanda for being so stupid.

THERAPIST: Right. And what if you thought, "Amanda has a lot of work right now. If she isn't calling, she must be really busy with work. She'll call me as soon as she has time."

EMILIA: I guess I would be OK. Not feel much of anything.

THERAPIST: Now, in all of these examples, the situation stays the same. Amanda hasn't called you in 3 weeks. Yet your emotional response varies depending on how you interpret the situation. Thus, if we change how you think, we change how you feel.

EMILIA: I get it. Good luck, though, changing how I think about what happened to me.

THERAPIST: It may feel impossible to change your thoughts about your rape. They may seem to be just the truth about what happened. Even so, your thoughts about the rape may not be helpful to you in coping with what happened. And you may not have had much opportunity to stop and look at them, and see how well they reflect reality. After all, if you've been thinking that the rape was your fault, it can be very unpleasant to feel the guilty feelings that come with that. Thus, you may try to push these thoughts from your mind. Yet by paying attention to our thinking, we can learn to notice problems in our thinking and replace unhelpful thoughts with more helpful ones.

EMILIA: I really can't imagine how I could think differently.

THERAPIST: Well, let's try to walk through the steps of the technique and see how it works.

EMILIA: OK. I'll give it a shot.

Figure 8.1 lists some points to include in your rationale. The point of the rationale is to convince your patients that learning to challenge unhelpful thoughts is worthwhile. To enhance the persuasiveness of the rationale, make it interactive and tailor it to each patient. It is not necessary to include all the points in Figure 8.1 for your rationale to be persuasive. If you sense that a patient is not sold on cognitive restructuring, however, consider whether some essential points for that patient were left out, or if there are other ways of making these points. Handout 8.1, which summarizes the rationale for cognitive restructuring, is not a substitute for discussing the rationale. Having patients review it, however, reinforces your discussion. You also may find it useful to return to some of the rationale points throughout cognitive restructuring. For example, if patients have trouble recognizing their thoughts, validate how thoughts can be hard to notice, because they are so automatic.

Steps 1 and 2

You typically will find it easiest to teach cognitive restructuring by walking your patient through the strategy (as outlined in Handout 8.2). Handout 8.4 is a sample

1. How you think affects how you feel and act.
2. A traumatic experience can affect your thoughts about yourself and the world.
3. We are not usually aware of our thoughts.
4. Many thoughts are automatic and habitual.
5. We often are not aware of these thoughts, and they can contribute to distress.
6. Believing a thought is true does not automatically mean it is.
7. Thoughts related to your trauma are prone to be unhelpful.
8. You may prefer to avoid focusing on automatic thoughts.
9. Paying attention to your thoughts enables you to detect problems in your thinking.
10. You can learn how to think in more balanced and helpful ways.

FIGURE 8.1. Points to include in a rationale for cognitive restructuring.

worksheet for cognitive restructuring (modified from Beck et al., 1979, p. 403). We prefer this version, because it provides the more detailed instruction patients with PTSD find helpful when trying to complete the form on their own. It also provides ample space to specify evidence for and against a thought, or other challenges to the thought. Writing down facts and relevant information facilitates the construction of a helpful response to an unhelpful thought, because writing keeps the information organized and accessible for review. Writing also helps patients stay focused on the task.

Some patients may be resistant to practicing cognitive restructuring in writing first. We recommend using Handout 8.4 for at least several weeks, however. Inform patients that the goal is eventually to carry out the process in their heads, but that initially, writing helps most people organize and learn the process, until they get the hang of it. Handout 8.2 reviews the steps of cognitive restructuring in detail and can be used to reinforce points made in session.

THERAPIST: OK. Let's start at this first box. This is the situation that triggered your distress. What was the situation that really made this a bad week for you?

EMILIA: That phone call from my old roommate and then the memories.

THERAPIST: OK. So why don't you write that down right here in this first box.

[*Commentary: Typically you will want your patients to write the information down during cognitive restructuring. Writing forces patients to be more active participants in the process. Also, when patients practice restructuring at home, they will need to write. Only in rare cases do we write. For example, if a patient is* extremely *reluctant to participate in cognitive restructuring, we occasionally find it helpful to start the writing, then turn it over to our patient.*]

THERAPIST: Now, what emotions were you feeling after you got the phone call—mad, sad, glad, guilt, shame, anxiety?

[*Commentary: You may find it helpful initially to cue your patients regarding possible emotions. If your patient has particular difficulty recognizing and labeling various emotions, you may find it useful to take time to review the table "Understanding Your Emotions" in Handout 8.2.*]

EMILIA: Really ashamed and guilty. I guess I was also anxious.

THERAPIST: OK. So write down "shame, guilt, and anxiety" in this box. On a scale of 0–100, how much shame did you feel?

EMILIA: Oh, 95.

THERAPIST: And guilt?

EMILIA: That's 100. It was all my fault. I never should have gone.

THERAPIST: How about anxiety?

EMILIA: That was pretty bad, but not as bad as the other two. Maybe 45.

Steps 1 and 2 are straightforward. Despite this, be aware of potential problems associated with these steps, particularly Step 2. As implied earlier, certain types of thoughts typically give rise to specific emotions. Thoughts about danger or something bad happening give rise to fear. Because guilt is driven by beliefs that one should have behaved differently in some way, Kubany and Watson (2003) distinguish between shame and guilt, although they are often viewed as closely related (Foa & Rothbaum, 1998, p. 177). Shame involves thoughts that devalue the individual. Such thoughts are often expressed as "I feel" statements (e.g., "I feel dirty," "I'm tainted," "I feel like a nobody"; Kubany & Watson, 2003, p. 70). Anger beliefs typically focus on the unfairness or wrongness of a situation. Finally, thoughts about loss and the improbability of things improving often produce sadness and hopelessness. Understanding the link between particular thoughts and their accompanying emotions is important, because challenging an anger belief may or may not alter shame. Yet a single situation, such as Emilia's phone call, may trigger a host of emotional responses driven by a range of different thoughts. This raises two possible problems.

First, patients who expect massive reductions in all negative emotions based on challenging a single thought, may be disappointed, and this can reduce compliance. Thus, it is important to elicit *specific* emotions, along with their intensities, so that patients can see their rage plummet after successfully challenging a thought about the unfairness of the situation, even though their shame does not decrease. The need to connect specific types of thinking with specific emotions may be more important for patients with PTSD than for patients with other anxiety disorders or depression. For example, although patients with panic disorders may experience shame about lack of functioning, the primary cognitive restructuring task in panic treatment is to challenge anxiety-related thinking. Rarely does a single incident simultaneously elicit very intense anxiety, anger, shame, and guilt in patients with panic. Yet this commonly happens with patients with PTSD and can pose problems for unaware therapists. We have observed experienced CBT therapists who are new to PTSD stumble with cognitive restructuring, because they were unprepared for the vast range of intense emotions and thoughts elicited by a single situation. Consequently, they sometimes failed to help their patients connect shame-related thinking to the emotion shame, and so forth. As a result, when patients experienced a reduction in only one emotion and still experienced others intensely, they thought that cognitive restructuring did not work even when it did. Handout 8.5 is a useful tool to help many patients learn to identify the types of specific thoughts that may underlie their specific emotions.

Second, patients also may have difficulty identifying reductions in specific emotions when they report the intensity of their global distress, which may be conceptualized as the sum of all negative emotions. Thus, they may not experience the benefit of successful cognitive restructuring when the challenged thought is linked to only one emotion. For example, Joel successfully challenged the belief "The car accident was all my fault," and replaced it with "Although I might have reacted in time if I had been driving slower, 16 other drivers had an accident on that stretch of road because of the ice. Even if I had done everything right, I probably would still have had an accident." Although Joel reported believing his new thought 100%, he did not experience any reduction in his guilt. Questioning revealed that Joel had blended anger and sadness into his initial SUDS rating of "guilt" at 100. When he separated guilt and anger, he discovered that his guilt SUDS rating had markedly decreased to 20, but his anger rating was still 100, secondary to his belief that the city should have posted warnings, salted the road, and done a better job of clearing snow. His sadness about his dead dog also had not changed.

Many patients with PTSD, particularly those with histories of childhood abuse, appear to have difficulty identifying and labeling specific emotions. Rarely do such patients spontaneously articulate this difficulty, and they may pretend to understand when you discuss specific emotions as a matter of habit. In such cases, you may not identify their inability to distinguish between different emotions until they fail to respond to either cognitive restructuring or exposure.

Some of these patients can learn about specific emotions by linking emotion names to their corresponding urges (Linehan, 1993a, 1993b; see Handouts 8.2 and 8.5). For example, teaching Joel that guilt is associated with the urge to repair (e.g., Joel had a strong urge to apologize to his wife, who was badly injured in the accident) and that anger is associated with the urge to attack (e.g., Joel reported a desire to "beat the fool that didn't keep track of the ice on the road") helped Joel separate anger from guilt. Some patients, however, may need more work on this issue. Strategies from DBT (see Chapter 9) can be helpful in such instances.

Step 3

Step 3 involves identifying the thoughts that were generated in the situation.

THERAPIST: Let's figure out what thoughts led to those emotions. What were you thinking?

EMILIA: Well, what I just said. It was all my fault. I should have listened to what my parents would have said and stayed home.

THERAPIST: OK. Let's start there and write that down. Why don't you write "The rape was all my fault" so that we are being really specific. Good. And now write down "I should have listened to what my parents would have said and stayed home." What else did you think?

[Commentary: Therapist models how thoughts are articulated for the purpose of challenging.]

EMILIA: I'm dirty, and I'll never be clean again.

THERAPIST: OK. So write each of those down as well. What else?

EMILIA: I can't go to that wedding, because it isn't safe. And I feel upset about not telling my roommate. What if he hurts her? I'm so weak. I should be able to tell her.

THERAPIST: OK. Let's get that all down as well. You said, "I can't go to the wedding because it isn't safe." Let's also write down that "I should tell my roommate what happened so that he doesn't hurt her." Does that sound right to you?

[Commentary: The therapist hypothesizes that the thought driving Emilia's distress with respect to her roommate is a thought that she should tell the roommate. She checks this with Emilia to make sure that she has not misinterpreted.]

EMILIA: Yes, I should tell her for her safety.

THERAPIST: OK, there was one last thing that you said. Do you remember?

EMILIA: No.

THERAPIST: Wasn't it "I'm so weak"?

EMILIA: I am. I'm weak. I'm so weak I gave in to temptation instead of listening to my parents. And I got raped because of it. I'm so pathetic.

THERAPIST: So let's write "I'm weak" down as well, also "I'm so pathetic."

This section highlights the utility of writing the thoughts on paper. Emilia displays a common tendency to roll rapidly from one negative thought to another, then back again. Writing her thoughts on paper helps to pin the thoughts down, so that the thoughts can be carefully dismantled, one at a time.

The therapist noted that Emilia stated that the rape was "my fault" numerous times throughout each session. She decided that Emilia needed to challenge that thought as soon as possible. She also noticed that Emilia's interpretation about the rape being her fault seemed connected with her belief that she should have done what her parents would have wanted her to do. Emilia almost always linked these two statements. Based on Emilia's history (i.e., her strict upbringing), the therapist hypothesized that Emilia believed that she should have done what her parents would have wanted her to do not only because of the rape but also because she had an underlying belief about the importance of listening to one's parents. The therapist also hypothesized that this belief provided a portion of the infrastructure supporting the *my fault* thought. Thus, dismantling the infrastructure might help Emilia challenge the *my fault* thought. Despite having this hypothesis, however, the therapist still had not decided which thought seemed to be the best starting thought (i.e., Emilia might benefit from challenging a different thought or two before tackling the *my fault* thought). Thus, she decided to explore Emilia's beliefs with respect to her parents so that she and Emilia could make a more informed decision.

THERAPIST: Now, I would like to return to one of your earlier statements. You said that you should have done what your parents would have wanted you to do. Why?

EMILIA: Well, in the first place, if I had done what they would have wanted, I wouldn't have been raped. I would have just studied more. I really should have listened to them.

THERAPIST: Should you only do what your parents want you to do if doing something else produces a bad outcome? In other words, let's say that you went to the party and had a good time. Would you still think that you should have done what your parents would have wanted?

EMILIA: Well. I probably wouldn't feel quite as strongly, but yeah. I would still have felt guilty about lying to my mother and not following her teachings.

THERAPIST: So it sounds like this goes beyond just this situation. It sounds like you have a belief about the importance of following your parents' teachings.

EMILIA: Yes. Your parents are your authority figures. They teach you values. I should always do what my parents say or what they would want me to do.

THERAPIST: OK, let's write that down. What does it say about you, that you didn't do what your parents would have wanted you to do?

EMILIA: It means I'm weak and not a person of good values. I'm not a good person.

THERAPIST: OK. So let's sort of sum this up. "To be a good person, I must do what my parents would want me to do." Is that an accurate statement for you?

EMILIA: Absolutely.

THERAPIST: OK, let's go back and rate how much you believe these thoughts. We got so caught up in identifying thoughts that we forgot to rate them. Let's start with your thought, "It was my fault." How much do you believe that is true?

It can be difficult to identify which thought is a good first thought to challenge. Several factors help you to decide this. First, early in treatment, it can be helpful to target thoughts that seem relatively easy to challenge. Success with cognitive restructuring helps motivate patients to follow through with this sometimes difficult task. You typically also do not want to start challenging thoughts that are heavily supported by evidence. Such thoughts are predominantly challenged by focusing on the consequences of holding the thought, a more difficult strategy for most patients to learn. In addition, at the start of cognitive restructuring, ideally you want patients to discover that some thoughts are very clearly not supported by facts.

Second, you may want to target critically important thoughts that you think will give you the "most bang for your buck." Third, consider challenging underlying beliefs, because patients sometimes think that a given thought makes complete sense, because it logically follows from a deeply held belief. Finally, use the ratings to help you choose a thought. For example, if a patient reports that he or she rates belief in four thoughts on a relatively low level and one thought very strongly, you may decide to challenge the strongly held thought.

Use these same guidelines to decide whether you need to identify underlying beliefs. If it is difficult to challenge automatic thoughts because of underlying beliefs, identify and challenge those beliefs. In other situations, however, you may be able to successfully challenge more obvious thoughts, and doing so may be easier and faster than challenging underlying beliefs. Deeply held beliefs also sometimes shift on their own because of behavior changes that result from challenging automatic thoughts. For example, George believed that he was only a good person if he never angered anyone. As a result of challenging his specific thought, "I shouldn't disagree with my boss," George gradually changed his behavior, and this behavioral change modified his underlying belief.

Emilia's therapist now faced a choice. Emilia identified a series of important thoughts and beliefs, many of which she used to support one another. Emilia's therapist identified two paths that might be very helpful. First she could challenge the *my fault* thought from the perspective of trying to elicit *evidence against* the notion that Emilia alone was at fault. In other words, she could try to help Emilia shift some blame to her rapists. Alternatively, she could tackle Emilia's beliefs about obeying her parents, because Emilia used that belief as evidence that she could have prevented the rape. Ultimately, the therapist chose the former path first, because she thought she could change Emilia's *my fault* thought, even without challenging her parental belief, and that this might alleviate some guilt relatively quickly. In addition, she hypothesized that the parental belief was going to be harder to challenge.

There are no right answers in choosing a thought to challenge, although at times you may conclude that you picked the wrong answer. For example, when your patient is struggling, or when the thought seems more convoluted the more you work on it, you have two choices. You can continue challenging the original thought and replace it with a slightly more functional thought. Alternatively, you can tell your patient that it would be better to address a different thought first. In other words, admit that you did not choose the best path first, and that another path might work better. Then return to the original thought.

The therapist could have guessed Emilia's underlying parental belief. Instead she sought to elicit the belief using questions. Cognitive restructuring is best conducted in a Socratic style, in which you use questions to help your patients discover new meanings and beliefs. Use of the Socratic style helps you avoid arguing with your patients, even when their beliefs seem illogical and unfair to you.

Step 4

Emilia's therapist decided to start with the *my fault* thought. She did not tell Emilia that they would start with this thought, however. So, after reinforcing Emilia for doing a good job with the first three steps, the therapist introduced this idea with a question.

THERAPIST: OK, we have a lot to work with here because you did a good job with Step 3. Sometimes this step is really difficult, but you did really well with it.

EMILIA: Thanks, but look at it all. No wonder I feel like shit.

THERAPIST: These are some pretty rough thoughts. Do you have a thought that you would really like to start with?

EMILIA: I have no idea where to start.

THERAPIST: Well, what about starting up here, with the thought that the rape was all your fault? This thought seems to occur to you quite often, and it seems to be very upsetting.

EMILIA: OK.

THERAPIST: Then let's circle this thought, so we can keep our focus on it. Now let's move to this column. This is where we start to challenge your thought. We are going to gather *evidence for* and *against* your thought. You can think of this in two ways. First, we are going to act like scientists and start finding facts that support and go against your belief. And we are just going to focus on facts. You can also think of this like we are being lawyers, presenting the facts in the case. Now one of the things about facts is that they really can't be argued, unless someone is being unreasonable. For example, it is a generally accepted fact that the world is round. Most people would agree that we can't argue about that. Right?

EMILIA: Right.

THERAPIST: So that is what we are looking for. Facts. We are going to start with the facts, or evidence, that support your belief. My assumption is that you are a smart person, and that you believe what you believe for a good reason. We need to find that reason. So, at the top of this column, write "evidence for," that is *f, o, r. . . .* Now, what evidence supports your belief that the rape was your fault?

EMILIA: Well, if I had done what my parents would have wanted me to do, I would not have gone to the party, and if I had not gone, I wouldn't have been raped that night.

THERAPIST: OK. Now do we know 100% what would have happened if you had stayed home that night? In other words, do we know whether a helicopter might have fallen on the roof? Or whether Daniel might have tried something in your room?

EMILIA: No. I don't know for sure.

THERAPIST: But it does seem reasonable to assume that if you had made a different choice that night, things probably would have gone very differently.

EMILIA: Yes. I would have been with my roommate all night. She wanted us to study together.

THERAPIST: OK. Let's write that down.

[*Commentary: Emilia looks confused. The therapist then models evidence for statement.*]

THERAPIST: So let's write down something like "I could have made a decision that my parents would have liked, and that would have reduced the likelihood of something bad happening, because I would have been with my roommate all night." Does that sound right?

EMILIA: Yes.

THERAPIST: See, it would be difficult to argue that you couldn't have made a different decision, because, theoretically, you could have.

EMILIA: Exactly.

[*Commentary: Although some might argue the logic of this point, the therapist uses this section to highlight that she and Emilia are working together by finding a way to agree on this evidence.*]

THERAPIST: OK, what is other *evidence for*?

EMILIA: I don't know.

THERAPIST: Was this the first time you made a decision for yourself that went against your parents' teachings?

EMILIA: Yes.

THERAPIST: Were you ever raped before?

EMILIA: Of course not!

THERAPIST: So is it fair to say that in the past, when you have followed your parents' teachings, you did not get raped? And when you did go against their teachings and made your own decision, you did get raped?

EMILIA: It's not just fair, it is true.

[*Commentary: It may seem countertherapeutic to point out additional* evidence for. *Cognitive restructuring is more likely to work, however, when patients are able to truly weigh both* evidence for *and* against. *Emilia was unable to articulate this piece of evidence. Thus, her thera-*

pist surmised from Emilia's frequent mention of this point that it played a role in supporting her belief about being at fault. Many patients find it surprising when the therapist helps them with the evidence for *section, because they are waiting for the therapist to side more strongly with the* evidence against *portion of the process. By working as hard to identify* evidence for, *however, you model the balanced approach that is the hallmark of cognitive restructuring.*]

THERAPIST: OK. So write that down. . . . Now, is there other *evidence for* this being your fault?

EMILIA: I once overheard my father saying that a woman had gotten raped because she put herself in that situation. My father doesn't know what happened, but I think he would say it was my fault. For these same reasons I wrote here.

THERAPIST: OK. Let's keep this pretty factual and put down something like "I heard my father blame a woman for getting raped in the past. Therefore, he might blame me if he knew." Because we don't really know for sure what he would say if he knew. Does that seem fair?

EMILIA: Yes.

THERAPIST: So is there any other *evidence for*?

EMILIA: I think that is the main evidence.

THERAPIST: So now let's focus on *evidence against*. Let's leave a little space in case we think of more *evidence for*; write "Evidence Against" here. What is *evidence against* your thought?

EMILIA: I don't know. I think it is my fault.

THERAPIST: Well, let's think about this for a minute. We're you the only one involved in this rape?

EMILIA: I am not sure what you mean.

THERAPIST: Well, were you the only person present during the rape, or were other people involved?

EMILIA: Of course, there were other people involved—you know that.

THERAPIST: Right. You were not the only one involved in this rape. Could you have raped yourself, or did the basketball guys have to be active participants in your rape?

EMILIA: They had to be active participants.

THERAPIST: Did you force them to rape you?

EMILIA: No! Of course not. Besides, I couldn't force them to rape me—that's ridiculous.

THERAPIST: Isn't that *evidence against* the notion that the rape was completely your fault? Imagine being in a car accident where someone ran a red light. Now you could have avoided the accident by deciding to stay home, but you also wouldn't have been in an accident if the other person hadn't run a red light. More than one decision contributed to the accident, and more than one decision contributed to your rape. You decided to go, but those guys made a decision to rape you. And we just agreed that you couldn't make them rape you.

EMILIA: I guess I can't argue that. I still think it is my fault, but they had to rape me for me to get raped. And I didn't make them or ask them to rape me. They could have chosen not to rape me.

THERAPIST: OK, good. We're just gathering evidence at this point, so I'm not surprised your thinking hasn't changed yet.

EMILIA: So what do I write down?

THERAPIST: What do you think?

EMILIA: How about "I couldn't have been raped if they hadn't decided to rape me. I didn't force them to rape me."

[*Commentary: Emilia here demonstrates a common thinking error described by Kubany and Watson (2002) with respect to guilt. In focusing on her role in the rape, Emilia is not recognizing that most events are caused by a several factors.*]

THERAPIST: OK, what else?

EMILIA: Beats me.

THERAPIST: Hmm. When Daniel asked you to the party, what did he tell you about it?

EMILIA: He said that the basketball team was having a small party, and that each of the guys was inviting either a girlfriend or a female student that he liked. He said it would be fun.

THERAPIST: So, Daniel didn't invite you to a party at which you would be the only female, or promise you that you would get raped.

EMILIA: Of course not. I wouldn't have gone if he said that.

THERAPIST: You're sure? If Daniel had told you what was really going to happen, you would have made a different choice?

EMILIA: Absolutely! I never would have gone near that party!

THERAPIST: So the basis for going to this party was that it was going to be a normal party, and that if you had known differently, you would have stayed far away. In fact, Daniel had to seriously lie to you to get you to go, right?

EMILIA: Yes. But I should have known.

THERAPIST: Why?

EMILIA: Because . . .

THERAPIST: Because why? Maybe I'm being stupid, but I'm confused. Given the information you had at the time, why should you have thought that you were being completely lied to and that you were being set up to be gang raped? Actually, let me ask that question a different way. If your friend Amanda had been lied to as a first-year student and ended up getting raped, would you be sitting here telling her that she should have known what was going to happen?

[*Commentary: The therapist starts by "playing dumb." This approach is often referred to as the "Columbo" approach, named after the television detective Columbo, who often acted dumb. This approach is useful in softening questions and facilitating a dialogue regarding patients' thinking, because it forces patients to spell out exactly what they are thinking. One critical factor in using this approach is to ask the questions in a sincere manner that indicates that you really*] *want answers. Although this approach works very well in eliciting* evidence against, *in this case, the therapist changed her mind and tried an alternative approach. Specifically, she asked whether Emilia would treat a friend in the same manner she is treating herself. This is another strategy that can sometimes help patients take a different perspective.*]

EMILIA: No.

THERAPIST: What would you say?

EMILIA: That it is not her . . . fault. I get it. It is that jerk Daniel's fault for lying. I guess that is *evidence against*.

THERAPIST: Let's try to summarize what we just discussed, because I actually think we found two pieces of *evidence against*. First, it sounds like we agree that you chose to go to a nice party, you did not choose to get raped, and that if you had known what was going to happen, you would have made a different decision.

EMILIA: I agree with that. I would have been safer if I had listened to my parents, but I didn't ask to get raped.

THERAPIST: Good. Let's write that down. . . . Now the second piece of evidence is that Daniel purposely lied to you to get you to the party, and that if this had happened to Amanda, you would tell her that it was Daniel's fault.

EMILIA: I really hate him.

THERAPIST: That is understandable. He lied to you and set you up to be raped. So let's add what we just said a minute ago to the *evidence against*.

EMILIA: OK. Daniel lied to me on purpose, which makes this his fault, too.

THERAPIST: Now I think we have sort of addressed this, but I want to make sure that we have fully tackled it. I get the sense—please correct me if I am wrong—that one of the reasons that you think this is all your fault is that you think you should have known what would happen.

EMILIA: That's true—I should have known.

THERAPIST: Now the thought "I should have known" is a separate thought, and we may need to challenge it separately. I want to take just a minute, though, and go down this road a bit, because it may mean we are missing some *evidence for*. Is there some specific reason that you should have known Daniel was setting you up to be gang raped?

[*Commentary: The therapist goes out on a limb here, based on her hypothesis that she might be able to resolve Emilia's belief that she should have known. This would then help Emilia more fully challenge the* my fault *thought. She also goes down this path to determine whether some* missed factual evidence for *is contributing to Emilia's self-blame. The therapist leaves herself a back door, however, by noting that they may have to challenge the* should *thought separately.*]

EMILIA: What do you mean?

THERAPIST: Well, did someone warn you to stay away from him?

EMILIA: No, not before I went to the party. I later heard rumors about him. But not until almost the end of the semester.

THERAPIST: So you didn't have any information *at the time* suggesting that he couldn't be trusted to invite you to a party with other people.

EMILIA: No. He seemed nice. Actually, some of the other girls in class told me they thought he was really good looking and that I was lucky to be invited.

THERAPIST: So is that *evidence against*? In other words, at the time you made the decision, it sounds like you had no evidence or reason not to trust him to take you to a real party. In fact, the other girls were even envious of your invitation.

EMILIA: I guess. I mean, now, looking back, it feels like I should have known. But I guess it would have been pretty hard for me to predict what was going to happen.

THERAPIST: It is actually very common for people to blame themselves for negative events. And one of the reasons we do so is that we sort of assume that we knew more than we really did at the time. We also may take responsibility, because it makes us feel like we have more control over bad things. If we think that we could have prevented something in the past, then we think we can prevent it in the future. But it seems pretty clear to me that if you had known what was going to happen, you would have made a different decision.

EMILIA: OK. So what do I put down?

THERAPIST: How about something like this: "When I made the decision to go to the party, I had no reason not to trust Daniel or to think that something bad would happen. Other girls were even envious, so they don't appear to have predicted anything bad either."

[*Commentary: Kubany and Watson (2002, 2003) have highlighted a number of factors that contribute to guilt in trauma survivors. One such factor is hindsight bias, in which survivors assume that they should have acted in accordance with the amount of information they have in the present, instead of recognizing that they made the best decision they could with the information that was available at that time.*]

THERAPIST: Is there any other *evidence against*?

EMILIA: Well, I guess if Daniel is partly to blame, the other guys also are partly to blame. I mean they raped me too, not just Daniel.

THERAPIST: Absolutely. Let's put that down. (*Emilia writes.*) Anything else?

EMILIA: Not that I can think of.

THERAPIST: Well, you've got down as *evidence against* that Daniel and the other basketball players are partly to blame for what happened. I have a question. If this had happened to Amanda, and she said to you, "OK, Daniel and the other guys are partly to blame" what would you say to her? Would you agree?

EMILIA: Well, it's kind of hard to pretend that this happened to her and not me, but I think I would say that she needs to get real. Basically it is all Daniel's and the other guys' fault. All she did was go to a party. They are really horrible people for doing that to her, and she shouldn't blame herself. She should blame them. She didn't choose to get raped! (*begins to cry*)

THERAPIST: (*softly*) So is that *evidence against*?

EMILIA: I don't know. It seems different when I think about me. I just focus on what I could have done differently, but I didn't ask to have this happen to me. I just wanted to go to a party like other girls do.

THERAPIST: Are you really any different than Amanda?

EMILIA: Not really.

THERAPIST: So can we say that most of the blame should be placed at the feet of the rapists?

EMILIA: Yes. The person who did the bad thing should get the most blame.

THERAPIST: OK, why don't you write that down . . .

This section demonstrates the process of gathering evidence to challenge the belief. Typically, you want to gather as much *evidence for* and *against* as you possibly can. In this scenario, the therapist still had some alternative *evidence against* paths to consider, such as the fact that Emilia fought her rapists, that they were larger than she was, and they outnumbered her. You also may ask patients to brainstorm alternative interpretations of the event by asking them how others might interpret this event. Finally, it can be useful to ask patients to identify the advantages and disadvantages of continuing to hold a belief. This approach is particularly useful when patients are very reluctant to give up a particular belief.

Emilia was able to generate evidence with guidance from her therapist. Some patients can generate *evidence for* easily. They may also offer other thoughts (vs. facts) as *evidence for*. In such situations, it is important to clarify that the patient has confused other thoughts with evidence. One gentle way to do this is to ask the patient whether the statement is truly a fact or whether it is a thought. You might also ask whether someone could argue about the factual status of the statement in a court of law. Usually these two questions help patients to realize that a statement is a thought and not factual evidence. Many patients find this distinction confusing, and you should not gloss over this; if they are struggling to recognize facts, take time to teach this point.

This section also portrays a common occurrence as patients work through guilt. When patients recognize that others played a role in their trauma, they may become increasingly angry. A subsequent task for Emilia is to learn to put aside her anger, at which point she may become sad over what has happened to her. The thoughts contributing to sadness also can be explored with cognitive restructuring, or patients may simply try to accept their loss. At this point, the survivor ideally reaches acceptance. In the words of one rape survivor, "Although I never wanted to be raped and wouldn't want anyone to have to go through what I did, I wouldn't be who I am now if it hadn't happened. So I guess I am no longer wishing it away. It happened, I survived, and I like who I am now—including the parts of me that resulted from the rape."

Steps 5 and 6

It is important not to stop after the challenge column; rather, help your patient formulate a concise and coherent response that summarizes the main persuasive points generated during the challenge step. The response is the take-home message, and you want patients to rehearse it, so that they can respond to unhelpful thoughts if they recur. At times, very successful cognitive restructuring eliminates an entire line of thinking, and your patient may have a revelation during the challenge phase. For example, Charlie, who had been physically abused as a child, had an abusive son. Charlie continued to give his son money, secondary to a belief that it was his duty as a parent to help his children. During cognitive restructuring, Charlie concluded that if he didn't force this son to move out, he would have no emotional or financial resources for his other children. This conclusion produced sweeping changes in Charlie's behavior, thinking, and emotions. In many cases, however, cognitive restructuring involves chipping away at unhelpful thoughts. In such cases, it is important to generate responses that are used actively and repeatedly to replace future unhelpful thoughts.

THERAPIST: Now it is time for us to put this all together.

EMILIA: How do I do that?

THERAPIST: With practice you will probably find different ways of doing this, but early on it is often helpful to work with a bit of a formula. Usually what we do is take the most compelling piece from the *evidence for* list and connect it with some of the most compelling *evidence against*. You could do this a couple of ways. For example, you could say something like "If I had done what my parents would have wanted me to do, I probably would not have been raped, and yet all I did was decide to go to a party. Most of the blame should go to Daniel and the other guys who chose to lie to me and rape me." We prefer to use the terms "and yet" to link the *evidence for* with the *evidence against*, because "but" sort of implies that the *evidence for* isn't as important. Another way to do this is to come up with an "Although . . . in fact . . . " statement. In other words, although the *evidence for* is true, in fact there is also the *evidence against*. The first thing to do is decide which is the most compelling *evidence for* and *against*.

EMILIA: (*looking at sheet for a while*) Well, I definitely think that if I had listened to my parents teachings I likely would have been safer, but—or and yet—I didn't choose to get raped and would have stayed away had I known what was going to happen. Daniel and the other guys went to the party with their eyes open, and they chose to rape me. So they are to blame more than me.

THERAPIST: Excellent. Go ahead and write that down.

EMILIA: OK, what did I just say? . . . never mind, I remember.

[*Commentary: Be prepared to remind your patient of the rational response. Sometimes patients articulate a very clear response, then lose their hold on it as soon as they are done speaking. This also highlights the need to write down the response.*]

THERAPIST: Now, read that out loud. (*Emilia reads it.*) How much do you believe that thought?

EMILIA: I believe it pretty much. Say 95.

THERAPIST: Good. So now let's rerate your emotions. Where is your shame?

EMILIA: Still pretty high. I still feel very dirty because all of those guys had sex with me. Say 85.

THERAPIST: How about your guilt?

EMILIA: That is a lot less. Maybe 30.

THERAPIST: And your anxiety?

EMILIA: Hmm, maybe down a bit. Maybe 40.

THERAPIST: Good. The thought we tackled was very much a guilt thought, and that is what we see here. Your guilt is what came down the most.

EMILIA: You know what, though?

THERAPIST: What?

EMILIA: I'm angrier. I'm angry at them for raping me. It's kind of weird. Until now, I haven't been angry. I was too busy blaming myself. But I am now. They lied to me. They tricked me. And it wasn't fair. At least I'd rather be angry than feel so guilty all of the time.

COMMON PTSD THOUGHTS

Guilt is a common emotional reaction in patients with PTSD and is usually related to self-blame. A variety of other thought patterns also are common in patients with PTSD, and familiarity with common types of thinking makes cognitive restructuring easier (see Figures 8.2 and 8.3 for common PTSD thoughts). For example, many patients report shame-related thinking, which may include thoughts such as "I'm dirty," "I'm bad," and "I'm a monster." In addition to following the standard questions described earlier, ask patients to define the prototypical "dirty" or "bad" person. Then look for features of your patients that do and do not correspond to that definition. Also consider exploring whether there are people who do "bad things" but are not "bad people." Pa-

---

- My anxiety will never go down.
- I feel scared, so it must be dangerous.
- I can't cope with my anxiety.
- If I stay with my anxiety, I might lose control or go crazy.
- If I let myself feel any feelings, I will be completely overwhelmed.
- If I think about what happened, I may get "stuck" there.
- If I think about what happened, I won't be able to turn it off.
- I can't tolerate the discomfort of thinking about what happened.
- Thinking about what happened will be uncomfortable, and it won't help.
- Avoidance is the only way I can stay in control.
- It's dangerous to go out alone.
- I'm never safe in public places.
- All men are dangerous.
- I won't be able to tolerate my anxiety.
- It's too shameful to think about.
- I'm too embarrassed to face what happened.
- If I think about it I'll get so angry I might explode.

FIGURE 8.2. Examples of thoughts that interfere with exposure.

- I'll never get better.
- My PTSD symptoms mean that I am a weak person.
- If I really wanted to, I could have stopped it, so it's all my fault.
- What happened proves that I am a worthless person.
- I thought I could cope with anything, and I was totally wrong. I am a mess.
- There is no safe place in the world.
- Other people do not care about me.
- People can't be trusted.
- I cannot protect my self.
- I'm not safe around people.
- I can't trust myself.
- My uncontrollable feelings and thoughts mean that I'm going crazy.

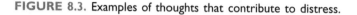

FIGURE 8.3. Examples of thoughts that contribute to distress.

tients with a history of childhood sexual abuse also sometimes report shame based on sexual arousal that occurred during the abuse (e.g., "My sexual reaction means I participated in my abuse"). The goal here is to help patients realize that they cannot control the degree to which their body responds to sexual stimulation. One strategy listed earlier that can be useful is to have the survivor think about how he or she would interpret sexual arousal in a different child of equivalent age. Many survivors far more willingly blame themselves than blame others.

Thoughts related to hopelessness about getting better and "low self-esteem" also frequently occur, particularly among patients with comorbid depression or dysthymia. Many patients are initially excited about starting treatment, but once they start, a variety of factors can bring their mood down. For example, patients may experience an increase in intrusive symptoms as they begin to approach things they have avoided; this sometimes happens after reading the Common Reactions to Traumatic Experiences (Handout 5.1) during psychoeducation. Some patients have unrealistic expectations about the treatment. As they begin to learn more about what is involved, they doubt that they can complete treatment. Alternatively, they may be doing the treatment exercises, but improvement may be slow. At this point, some patients think, "It's hopeless, things aren't going to get better." Be alert for this kind of thinking, because it can rapidly lead to depression and even suicidality in suicide-prone patients. Depression often improves with treatment of PTSD, but severe depression can interrupt treatment, so it is best to intervene with tactics known to be helpful for depression (e.g., activity scheduling; see Chapter 9). Hopeless thoughts also may be modified with cognitive restructuring. For example, Carmen, whose exposure practice was progressing very slowly, felt increasingly discouraged. Figure 8.4 accompanied the following discussion.

THERAPIST: So you found yourself feeling more hopeless after you finished your homework. Can you identify what you were thinking at that time?

CARMEN: It's going so slow. My PTSD is never going to get better.

THERAPIST: OK, let's write that. Anything else?

CARMEN: It should be going faster.

Cognitive Restructuring Worksheet

NAME: Carmen   DATE February 4, 2006

1. Situation	3. Automatic Thoughts	4. Challenge to Automatic Thoughts	5. Response
Describe: • Actual event leading to unpleasant emotion OR • Thoughts or memories leading to unpleasant emotion.	• Write automatic thought(s) that preceded emotion(s). • Ask "What does that mean about me?" to see if an underlying belief is related to the emotion. • Select the thought or belief to challenge and rate how much you believe it is true (0–100%).	• Challenge your automatic thought (for example, list evidence for and against the thought, consider alternative views, and examine the consequences of holding this thought). • Identify your style of thinking.	• Write a response to the automatic thought(s) by summarizing the evidence or alternative views. • If the evidence supports your thought or belief, or you need more information, then make a plan. • Rate how much you believe the response (0–100%).

		% belief		% belief
Doing my exposure homework	~~It's going so slowly.~~ ⟨It's never going to get better.⟩ It should be going faster. I'm a weakling. I'm not going to make it; I may as well just give up now— suicide would be easier.	98	Evidence for: I don't do things I used to do. It's going very slowly. Nothing has happened to make me feel better. Evidence against: I'm coming to therapy. This is a new treatment I haven't tried before. I'm doing the homework. My anxiety is decreasing with exposure. Others benefit from the treatment. Treatment has just begun.	Even though the change is slow in coming, the treatment has just begun and my anxiety is going down. If others benefit from this treatment, so can I.	100

2. Emotions
• Identify the emotion(s) you felt (e.g., sad, anxious, angry, shameful, guilty).
• Rate the intensity of the emotion (0–100).

	SUDS
Hopeless	90
Ashamed	70

6. Emotions
• Rate the intensity of the emotions you identified in Step 2 (0–100).

	SUDS
Sad/Hopeless	50

FIGURE 8.4. Carmen's Cognitive Restructuring Worksheet: hopelessness.

179

THERAPIST: OK, write that too. Anything else? What did it mean to you that its going slowly?

CARMEN: I'm a weakling. I'm not going to make it; I may as well just give up now. Suicide would be easier.

THERAPIST: OK, let's write those thoughts, too.

[*Commentary: As Carmen writes, her therapist notices that the first thought is a fact; Carmen's anxiety has been going down very slowly (see Chapter 7) despite frequent practice.*]

THERAPIST: OK, good. Now we've nailed down some very distressing thoughts. It makes sense that you are feeling hopeless when the treatment is going slowly and you are thinking that it's not going to get better. Actually, it is a fact that it's going slowly, isn't it?

CARMEN: Yeah, I guess so.

THERAPIST: So, let's save that for when we are collecting facts.

CARMEN: (*Crosses it out.*)

THERAPIST: Now, it looks like we have two sorts of thoughts here: that it's not going to get better, and a thought about what that means about you—that you are weak.

CARMEN: I guess so.

THERAPIST: So let's work on the first one on this sheet and save the second for the next sheet.

CARMEN: OK (*circles it*).

THERAPIST: How much do you believe it's true—that your PTSD is never going to get better?

CARMEN: It feels completely true.

Carmen and her therapist proceeded by collecting *evidence for* and *against*. They did not use additional strategies, because time was limited and the therapist could tell that they would be able to generate a believable response using the *evidence for* and *against*.

In the following session they challenged the thought "I'm a weakling," which Carmen had begun challenging at home (see Figure 8.5). They identified important facts that led to this thought (treatment going slowly and having suicidal thoughts) and key *evidence against* (the fact that Carmen showed courage in confronting her trauma memories during exposure, and that she showed courage in filing for divorce and extricating herself from the abusive relationship). Further discussion revealed that rather than a new thought, this was something Carmen had thought repeatedly during her 20 years of abuse. This thought also likely contributed to her staying in the abusive situation. For this reason, the therapist recognized that examining the consequences of this thought could be useful. The final response emphasized Carmen's courage and the counterproductive effect of thinking that she is weak.

Patients with PTSD also often present with thoughts regarding trust ("I can't trust anyone anymore") and safety ("I'll never be safe again," "It is not safe to leave my house," "The world is dangerous"). Many of these thoughts also can be chal-

Cognitive Restructuring Worksheet

NAME: _Carmen_   DATE _March 8, 2006_

1. Situation	3. Automatic Thoughts	4. Challenge to Automatic Thoughts	5. Response
Describe: • Actual event leading to unpleasant emotion OR • Thoughts or memories leading to unpleasant emotion.	• Write automatic thought(s) that preceded emotion(s). • Ask "What does that mean about me?" to see if an underlying belief is related to the emotion. • Select the thought or belief to challenge and rate how much you believe it is true (0–100%).	• Challenge your automatic thought (for example, list evidence for and against the thought, consider alternative views, and examine the consequences of holding this thought). • Identify your style of thinking.	• Write a response to the automatic thought(s) by summarizing the evidence or alternative views. • If the evidence supports your thought or belief, or you need more information, then _make a plan._ • Rate how much you believe the response (0–100%).

1. Situation (cont.)	Automatic Thoughts	% belief	Challenge	Response	% belief
Doing my exposure homework	_I'm a weakling._		_Evidence for:_ _I have thoughts of suicide._ _I have thoughts that I'm not going to make it._ _It's going slowly._ _Evidence against:_ _I'm trying hard and doing all the homework exercises._ _I'm doing very difficult things—it takes courage to face my fear._ _I showed courage by getting a divorce._ _Alternative explanation:_ _The abuse lasted a long time—I have lots of different memories and it had a pervasive effect on my thinking and feeling._ _Living in the house where the abuse took place has slowed my anxiety reduction._ _Consequences:_ _When I tell myself I'm a weakling, things seem hopeless._	_Even though the treatment is going slowly, I have been courageous in doing difficult things and I am facing my fears in therapy. Other things can explain why the treatment is going slowly, like how long the abuse lasted and the fact that I am living in the house where I was abused. Facing my fears takes courage and thinking I'm weak just drags me down._	100

2. Emotions

• Identify the emotion(s) you felt (e.g., sad, anxious, angry, shameful, guilty).
• Rate the intensity of the emotion (0–100).

	SUDS
Hopeless	100
Ashamed	100

6. Emotions

• Rate the intensity of the emotions you identified in Step 2 (0–100).

	SUDS
Sad/Hopeless	40
Shame	40

FIGURE 8.5. Carmen's Cognitive Restructuring Worksheet: shame.

lenged by focusing on *evidence for* and *against*. Asking patients to identify people, including the therapist, whom they trust at all, and helping them realize that trust is not "all or nothing" (i.e., there are shades of gray in trust) can augment standard challenging.

Safety also exists on a continuum. Although we do not consistently teach patients about styles of thinking (Beck et al., 1979; Beck, 1995; Burns, 1980; see Handout 8.6), teaching styles of thinking (e.g., "all-or-nothing thinking") can be very helpful with safety thoughts. Safety thoughts often limit patients' ability to engage in meaningful activities, and an exploration of the specific consequences for a given patient is also helpful. In addition, consider exploring the relative safety of different situations. No situation is 100% safe, and patients must learn to accept certain levels of danger to live their lives. Exploring *evidence for* and *against* the relative safety of situations can help patients gain perspective. Safety thoughts regarding realistically safe situations also can be changed by appropriate *in vivo* exposure assignments/behavioral experiments. Be aware that some patients may not have appropriate thoughts about likely danger in one situation, because they are inappropriately worried about unlikely danger in a related situation (e.g., Jill is willing to run down a dark alley to avoid a chihuahua). Examining relative safety and conducting behavioral experiments to determine how others view the relative safety of a given situation can be useful with these patients.

Finally, many patients with PTSD report thoughts related to control (e.g., "My symptoms mean I am out of control," "Not controlling my emotions means that I am weak"). Defining more precisely what is meant by "out of control" or "weak" can help patients realize that allowing themselves to experience emotions often reflects courage rather than weakness. In addition, efforts to control emotions often have the paradoxical effect of making patients feel more out of control, because the more effort they put toward controlling unwanted thoughts and feelings, the more those feelings and thoughts intrude. Thus, decreasing efforts to control emotions often results in a great sense of control. Challenging thoughts about control can be a critical element of treatment for many patients with PTSD.

COGNITIVE RESTRUCTURING FOR PTSD: POSSIBLE PROBLEMS

It is important to remember that cognitive restructuring may be accompanied by some pitfalls when treating PTSD.

Cognitive Restructuring: A Potentially Invalidating Technique

Validation involves finding the wisdom in our patients' responses (Linehan, 1993a). Recognizing the importance of validation in PTSD treatment, we now openly admit that cognitive restructuring can be an *invalidating* technique for some patients, because cognitive restructuring implicitly suggests that patients' thinking is, to some degree, wrong or incorrect. Although CBT clinicians often skirt this point, this is not the optimal approach for many patients with PTSD. PTSD often is accompanied by a history of invalidation, and many patients with PTSD become distressed and resistant to cognitive restructuring if they believe that their therapist is invalidating their perception of cognitive restructuring.

For example, after being introduced to cognitive restructuring, Kaya became quite upset. She stated that cognitive restructuring indicated that her thinking was *wrong* and that if she thought differently, she would be *better*. Kaya's therapist, who had not used the words "wrong" or "better," initially tried to refocus Kaya on the notion that her thinking could be more helpful or functional. Kaya responded, "You're still saying that my thinking is wrong" and became increasingly distressed. Kaya had a history of dropping out of CBT with another therapist. Thus, Kaya's therapist switched tactics. Instead of trying to convince Kaya that cognitive restructuring did not necessarily indicate that Kaya's thinking was "wrong," the therapist validated Kaya's interpretation. She noted that she understood why Kaya saw cognitive restructuring in this way. The therapist validated Kaya for several minutes, noting that Kaya's response made sense and that cognitive restructuring was not a perfect technique. Kaya began to calm, and the therapist asked her if she believed her thinking helped her at all times. Kaya responded, "Absolutely not. I would feel better if I could think differently." Kaya's response is common. After patients' perspectives are validated, they generate the rationale for cognitive restructuring themselves and can proceed.

Invalidation during Cognitive Restructuring

Patients with PTSD who are prone to self-invalidation also may inadvertently invalidate their own thoughts, emotions, and experiences with cognitive restructuring. We became aware of this problem when a colleague with depression expertise presented a case in which his patient easily generated *evidence against* her own thinking. The patient then noted that the *evidence against* simply proved that she was stupid for having her initial thought. She also became very distressed. The colleague noted, "My depression patients have difficulty generating *evidence against* or don't believe it. They don't usually twist the *evidence against* to say that their own thoughts are just stupid." Yet we have observed that many patients with PTSD, particularly survivors of childhood abuse, call their own thinking "stupid" at some point during the cognitive restructuring process. Three strategies help to reduce invalidation during cognitive restructuring. First, help your patients gather solid *evidence for* their thinking. The *evidence for* section is critical, because it validates why patients hold the beliefs that they do. Validating thinking is a viable strategy for avoiding invalidation and the associated negative affect, which can derail the task at hand.

In contrast to other populations we have treated (i.e., patients with panic, depression, and eating disorders), we are continually struck by how much difficulty some patients with PTSD have identifying *evidence for*. Also, although we teach all patients to identify *evidence for*, some fail to acknowledge the *evidence for*, or generate only superficial evidence. Do not let this slide. Adrienne, a 30-year-old incest survivor, habituated rapidly during exposure, yet she continued to report low self-esteem, shame, and irritability. Her therapist encouraged Adrienne to identify specific situations that triggered low self-esteem and shame. Adrienne stated, "Well, it's all the time. I just always think I'm fat and ugly." Subsequently, the underlying belief "I'm worthless" was identified. In challenging the "I'm worthless" belief (Figure 8.6), Adrienne could not identify any *evidence for*, despite her claim of 100% belief.

Cognitive Restructuring Worksheet

NAME: _Adrienne_   DATE _3/1/06_

1. Situation	3. Automatic Thoughts		4. Challenge to Automatic Thoughts	5. Response	
Describe: • Actual event leading to unpleasant emotion OR • Thoughts or memories leading to unpleasant emotion.	• Write automatic thought(s) that preceded emotion(s). • Ask "What does that mean about me?" to see if an underlying belief is related to the emotion. • Select the thought or belief to challenge and rate how much you believe it is true (0–100%).		• Challenge your automatic thought (for example, list evidence for and against the thought, consider alternative views, and examine the consequences of holding this thought). • Identify your style of thinking.	• Write a response to the automatic thought(s) by summarizing the evidence or alternative views. • If the evidence supports your thought or belief, or you need more information, then _make a plan._ • Rate how much you believe the response (0–100%).	
		% belief	_Evidence for:_ _I am overweight and my father, kids in school,_ _and society generally has taught me that_ _overweight is bad and that overweight people_ _are judged for being overweight._ _My father actually called me worthless._ _I feel worthless._ _Evidence against:_ _My husband loves me._ _I have a good supportive group of friends._ _I make a difference in my work._ _I believe that all people have worth._ _Consequences:_ _When I think I am worthless, I feel hopeless._		% belief
Couldn't fit through a _small space in fence_	~~I couldn't fit through the~~ ~~space in the fence because~~ ~~I'm so big. (This is a fact!)~~ _I'm fat and ugly._ ⟨_I'm worthless._⟩	100		_Although I have always felt_ _worthless and my father called me_ _worthless, in fact I am loved and I_ _make a difference._ ~~If everyone else~~ ~~on the planet has worth then so~~ ~~do I.~~ _When I regard myself as I would_ _others, I feel less hopeless._	20 90

2. Emotions		6. Emotions	
• Identify the emotion(s) you felt (e.g., sad, anxious, angry, shameful, guilty). • Rate the intensity of the emotion (0–100).		• Rate the intensity of the emotions you identified in Step 2 (0–100).	

	SUDS		SUDS
Ashamed	100	_Sad/Hopeless_	0
Hopeless	100	_Shame_	0

FIGURE 8.6. Adrienne's Cognitive Restructuring Worksheet: worthlessness.

THERAPIST: Well, you must have some evidence for this belief, because you believe it 100%.

ADRIENNE: I know, it's just stupid. I'm just stupid. I'm just so stupid, and this proves it.

THERAPIST: Well, if you believe your thought that strongly, I'm guessing you have a good reason for believing it—not just for the heck of it. Earlier, when I asked you how much of your self-esteem you connected to your body weight and shape, you said 90%. I'm wondering then, is the fact that your are overweight somehow evidence to you that you are "worthless"?

ADRIENNE: Yeah, I guess you're right. It's the main thing.

THERAPIST: OK, so why would you believe that being overweight makes you worthless? Where did you learn that?

ADRIENNE: I don't know. Kids in school teased me, and my father used to call me a worthless, fat pig. He used to call me that when he raped me, too.

THERAPIST: There we go. You learned this connection from your father and from kids in school. In fact, what does our larger culture say about being overweight?

ADRIENNE: That it is a bad thing.

THERAPIST: So you also learned it from society. Let's put that down.

ADRIENNE: That I'm fat?

THERAPIST: Well, being overweight doesn't necessarily mean that someone is worthless. Lot's of overweight people don't feel worthless. But you had experiences that taught you to connect these. And those experiences happened; they are facts. Let's write, "I am overweight and my father, kids in school, and even society in general taught me that being overweight is bad, and that overweight people are judged for being overweight. Let's also put down that your father actually called you worthless. Now, has anyone else ever called you worthless?

ADRIENNE: I don't think anyone has actually said it. But I know it is true (*sighs*). My father also said that is why he raped me. He would call me a worthless, fat pig. Then he said that was why he had sex with me. He had to find something useful to do with someone so worthless. Since he had to feed me, I needed a purpose because I was so worthless.

[*Commentary: Weight is highly value laden in our society. Although Adrienne is unable to identify how she learned that her weight is connected to her beliefs about herself, the therapist shows her that her beliefs have some basis in her history and cultural environment. During this exploration, Adrienne also identified other evidence from her rape history that supported her belief about being worthless.*]

Second, watch for too much focus on the *evidence against*, accompanied by an escalation of negative affect. For example, Mike generated a few pieces of *evidence for* his belief that he would never be safe again, then proceeded to produce a flood of *evidence against*. He also became increasingly angry. When his therapist asked him what he was thinking, he responded, "This just proves that I am crazy. I am totally hopeless for thinking such ridiculous things." The therapist responded by validating Mike's invalidating response: "Well, looking at all of the *evidence against* we have generated, I can see why you might think that." He then had Mike revisit the *evidence for* section, and together they generated additional *evidence for*. After this, Mike commented, "I guess there are reasons why I think the way I do."

Finally, many patients benefit from learning about and labeling self-invalidation (Linehan, 1993a). In particular, you can teach patients that (1) invalidation distresses most people, (2) self-invalidation is particularly distressing, and that (3) they are prone to self-invalidation. Once patients understand the concept of self-invalidation, they can often use this as a short cut. For example, Kirsten was prone to self-invalidation. When she started self-invalidating, her therapist simply asked, "What are you doing right now, in the moment." Kirsten reflected for a moment and then gave a short laugh: "I'm doing it again, aren't I? I'm self-invalidating." Her negative affect immediately decreased and Kirsten was able to refocus on cognitive restructuring.

What Do I Say When the Thought Appears to Be True?

If a patient articulates a fact as a thought, explore the meaning of the fact. You also may need to search for underlying beliefs to find an appropriate target for challenging. In an earlier example, the first "thought" Adrienne articulated as contributing to her low self-esteem and shame was "I couldn't fit in between the space in the fence, because I'm too big." Adrienne's therapist recognized this as a fact (Adrienne literally could not pass through the space), and that challenging it would not likely change Adrienne's emotions. So she asked Adrienne, "What did that mean to you?" Adrienne replied, "That I'm fat and ugly; I say this to myself 100 times per day." Her therapist realized that this thought was a judgment and likely related to her distress.

The line between "fat" and "overweight" is tricky in patients who are actually overweight. Adrienne was fairly overweight and out of shape, though not severely obese. Thus, the therapist expected that challenging this thought would be difficult. She imagined what response might result from challenging and came up with "Although I am overweight and couldn't fit in the space, it doesn't mean I am fat and ugly." The therapist did not expect that such a response would be highly believable or markedly affect Adrienne's shame and sadness. She hypothesized that there was a deeper belief underlying the "I'm fat and ugly" thought that might reduce shame and sadness, if successfully challenged. She also hypothesized that the underlying belief would be more global and more amenable to challenging.

THERAPIST: Adrienne, I might be going out on a limb here, but some people who have told me that they think of themselves as "fat and ugly" have said that, as a result, they feel they are worthless. Is that what you believe about yourself?

ADRIENNE: *(crying)* Definitely. All the time. I know I'm worthless. And you know, I think I even believed that back when I lost all that weight and only weighed 100 pounds.

[*Commentary: The more extreme the statement, the less likely it is true. It is easier to challenge a statement containing extreme words such as "always," "all," or "complete," or "never."*]

Adrienne's therapist began by challenging this pervasive underlying belief rather than the more superficial "I'm fat and ugly." The therapist also realized that she might still have to address Adrienne's linking of fat and ugly, and self-esteem at some point.

In other words, Adrienne would ultimately benefit from realizing that she could be attractive and overweight at the same time. Although Adrienne's thoughts may seem to have strayed from the topic of PTSD, patients often present with a wide array of thoughts contributing to their distress. This is particularly true of patients with histories of child abuse. You often need to address these thoughts to fully resolve emotions such as shame and sadness. Also, as with Adrienne, such thoughts sometimes have a basis in patients' trauma histories.

What If the Patient Does Not Believe the Response?

Some patients may not believe the response generated by linking together the facts. When this happens, you need to dissect the response to determine which part is not believable. Doing this might simply reiterate for your patient that all the component facts are true and result in stronger belief in the response. Other times, you identify the weak link in the response, which you alter to make the response believable. Often, a subtle change in the response can make the difference. Adrienne's challenge to the belief "I'm worthless" brought up several points of *evidence for* and *against it*. Her therapist also asked her to define a "worthwhile" human being. This strategy can be helpful when challenging thoughts involving inherent judgment. When asked the "worthwhile" human being question, most patients offer one of two answers. Some say that they all humans have worth/value. Others respond that all humans have worth except those who hurt others, such as murders, rapists, and child molesters. Adrienne subscribed to the first definition, so her therapist gently pointed out the inconsistency.

THERAPIST: So, are you saying that you are the only person on the planet who doesn't have worth?

ADRIENNE: *(tearfully)* It feels that way!

Subsequently in constructing the response, Adrienne wrote, "Although I have always felt worthless and my father called me worthless, in fact I am loved and I make a difference."

THERAPIST: It might be useful to include something of our discussion about your worth relative to everyone else's. How about "If everyone else on the planet has worth, so do I." (*Adrienne writes this down.*) OK, lets read the response out loud. (*Adrienne reads it.*) How much do you believe this is true?

ADRIENNE: About 20%.

THERAPIST: OK, so it's not working for you. Let's look at it more closely. The first part is "I have always felt worthless." How much do you believe that?

ADRIENNE: It's just a fact—100%!

THERAPIST: The next part is "My father called me worthless." How much do you believe that?

ADRIENNE: Also fact, it happened—100%.

THERAPIST: The next part is "In fact, I am loved and I make a difference." How much do you believe that?

ADRIENNE: Definitely 100%.

THERAPIST: OK, so the last part is not working. "If everyone else on the planet has worth, so do I." Let's see if we can tweak this a bit to make it work for you. It seems like it's hard to think of yourself in the same way that you think of others. Yet thinking of yourself as the only worthless person seems to result in feeling extremely hopeless. What happens when you think of yourself as being like other people?

ADRIENNE: Well, less hopeless.

THERAPIST: Would it work to say, "When I think of myself as I do of others, I feel less hopeless"?

ADRIENNE: Maybe. (*Writes it down.*)

THERAPIST: Now, read the response again. (*Adrienne reads it.*) How much do you believe that?

ADRIENNE: About 90%.

THERAPIST: OK. When you think that way, how strong is the hopelessness and shame?

ADRIENNE: Well, hopeless is 40, and shame is 40, too.

What If the Patient Seems Not to Retain Cognitive Changes across Sessions

Some patients appear to challenge a thought successfully in one session, then return, appearing to have lost ground. Two issues are important in producing lasting changes in your patients' thinking. First, patients need to recall what you did in the session. Second, they need to rechallenge the thought, if the same thought is triggered again.

Retaining cognitive changes can be a bigger challenge in treating PTSD than in many other disorders. The reasons for this are the same as those we discussed relative to psychoeducation, namely, that highly aroused patients may have difficulty concentrating and retaining information. Patients who are prone to dissociating also may have difficulty, particularly if trauma discussion triggers intermittent dissociation. As with psychoeducation, audiotaping cognitive restructuring sessions to supplement the use of handouts and worksheets can be very useful for these patients. One highly aroused patient liked to listen to her most recent tape repeatedly between sessions. She noted that listening to the tapes "really help what I learn and figure out to sink in."

Patients without these difficulties also may struggle to translate in-session changes into their daily lives. Adrienne noted that the thought "I'm fat and ugly" and the underlying belief "I'm worthless" came into her mind so frequently that it felt like she thought it "constantly." Challenging this thought once in session may not result in a change in her daily thinking. Validate the challenge of learning to think differently for such patients, and let them know that some thoughts are so habitual that changing them takes a lot of practice.

ADRIENNE: I believe this thought right now, but I have a feeling that when I am back at home and look in the mirror or something like that, I am going to think the old way again. I'm not sure how to remember this.

THERAPIST: You've been thinking this thought hundreds of times every day for 30 years.

We can't know for sure what got you started thinking this way, but it's a habit you've practiced for a long time. Changing a habit you've had for this long isn't going to happen overnight, but now that you know how to challenge this thought, you can begin to practice noticing it and rehearse the alternative we came up with today.

[*Commentary: Although sometimes you emphasize practicing the entire challenging process, when a thought is this frequent and habitual, just rehearing the response is a shortcut that works if patients really believe the response. They can also carry around the written response on a card to read.*]

CONCLUSION

Cognitive restructuring is an important additional technique for reducing negative emotions that do not respond to exposure. It also may be used to challenge thoughts that impair patients' ability to participate in exposure, and as an alternative in patients for whom exposure is not appropriate. There are, however, a number of ways that patients with PTSD can go off course with cognitive restructuring for PTSD. We have reviewed and offered suggestions for handling some of these issues; you may develop strategies of your own as you become more familiar with implementing cognitive restructuring in this population.

Cognitive restructuring enables you to have better control over your feelings. The premise of cognitive restructuring is that you can learn to control the intensity of your emotional reactions by modifying the way you think about things that happen in your life. At first glance, you may feel uncomfortable with the notion that the way you think about things may contribute to your distress. Remember, though, that your way of thinking has been influenced by your traumatic experiences.

That is:

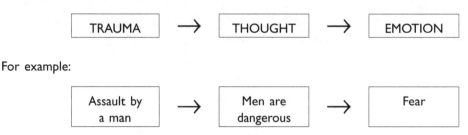

For example:

From this, you may recognize that to free yourself of the effects of trauma, you must take control of your own thoughts rather than allowing them to be dominated by fear or other negative emotions.

Emotional reactions are often related to thoughts. Survivors of trauma often experience strong emotional reactions to current situations. Such intense reactions are a common effect of traumatic events. For example, because of your past trauma, you may suddenly become very intensely frightened, sad, guilty, or angry in some situations, often without knowing why. You may feel that your emotions are out of your control. Although it is true that events affect us in important ways, it is also true that we can learn to have more control over our emotional reactions to events by taking control of the thoughts related to them.

How you think affects how you feel and act. Almost every minute of your life you are engaging in self-talk. This is like a conversation with yourself. This internal self-talk is how you interpret and make sense of the world. Your self-talk can affect the way you feel and behave. If your self-talk is unrealistic or unhelpful, your emotions may be overwhelming.

A traumatic experience can affect your thoughts about yourself and the world. Your traumatic experiences may have convinced you that the world is a dangerous place. Fear and anxiety related to the trauma may have shaped the way you think. As a result you may, understandably, think that many situations are more dangerous than they really are. As described in the "Safety–Danger Continuum" (below), even though a bathtub may feel very scary to the person who survived shark-infested waters, realistically, it is safe. Therefore, avoiding bathtubs is not likely to make the shark survivor realistically any safer, even though he or she may temporarily feel less anxiety.

The traumatic experience may also influence your thinking in other ways. For example, it may lead you to think you are not in control, or that you are unworthy or unable to cope with stress. Beliefs that the world is dangerous and that you are unable to cope were shaped by your experiences and have helped you to survive the trauma. However, they may not necessarily be true for all the situations you encounter in your daily life.

(continued)

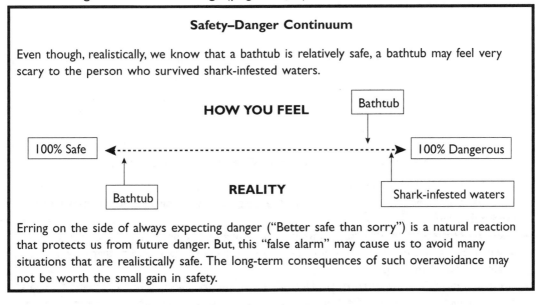

Safety–Danger Continuum

Even though, realistically, we know that a bathtub is relatively safe, a bathtub may feel very scary to the person who survived shark-infested waters.

Erring on the side of always expecting danger ("Better safe than sorry") is a natural reaction that protects us from future danger. But, this "false alarm" may cause us to avoid many situations that are realistically safe. The long-term consequences of such overavoidance may not be worth the small gain in safety.

Typically, we are not aware of our self-talk. Our self-talk is usually *automatic*. Self-talk, in the form of "automatic thoughts," comes into our minds so quickly that we may not be aware of it, so the feelings it produces seem out of our control.

Automatic thoughts contribute to distress. Automatic thoughts can contribute to feelings of anxiety, sadness, anger, and guilt. They can lead you to feel out of control and overwhelmed, because automatic thoughts often follow a pattern or style of thinking that is not helpful.

You may prefer to avoid focusing on automatic thoughts. You may feel that the only way to cope with these distressing thoughts is to avoid thinking about them. This may help you feel better for a little while, but troublesome thoughts about your traumatic experiences play a major role in the distress you experience. Avoiding them does not help to reduce their intensity or help you to feel better in the long run. Although it may be difficult at times, paying attention to unhelpful automatic thoughts will enable you to have more control over your emotional reactions to situations. This in turn will result in lasting change in the distress you experience.

Believing a thought is true does not automatically mean it is. Because automatic thoughts are knee-jerk reactions, they are usually based on feelings rather than fact. Although it may *feel* like it is true, just having a thought does not *make* it true! You will learn ways to challenge those thoughts, so that we can make a more objective decision as to how closely they reflect reality.

By paying attention to your thoughts, you can learn to detect problems in your thinking and replace unhelpful thoughts with more balanced ones. Cognitive restructuring follows a series of steps to help you learn to notice your thoughts, examine them carefully, and bring together all the information about the situation to create a balanced and helpful response.

LEARN TO OBJECTIVELY EXAMINE YOUR THOUGHTS

Cognitive restructuring is a coping skill that involves learning to examine how realistic your thoughts are. This skill will help you to have more control over how you think, feel, and behave in stressful situations. Research has shown that cognitive restructuring is very effective at reducing and controlling feelings of depression and anxiety. It can help you manage your distressing emotional reactions to trauma-related situations.

Six Main Steps to Learning Cognitive Restructuring

- **Step 1—Notice the situation.** Involves identifying the situation or events that triggered your distress. When you become aware of the triggers of your distress, it becomes more predictable and easier to control.
- **Step 2—Notice your emotions.** Involves identifying your emotions and rating their intensity. Being aware of your emotions helps you to identify the thoughts that may be related to your emotions.
- **Step 3—Identify your automatic thoughts.** Involves recognizing the automatic thoughts that contribute to your distress. Becoming more aware of your automatic thoughts opens the door to modifying them.
- **Step 4—Challenge your automatic thoughts.** Involves evaluating your thoughts and recognizing styles of thinking that may lead to negative emotions. You will learn techniques to help you to interpret events realistically and in helpful ways.
- **Step 5—Respond to unhelpful thoughts.** Involves replacing unhelpful automatic thoughts with more helpful ways of thinking. Developing alternative ways of thinking can help you feel a greater sense of control and personal effectiveness.
- **Step 6—Noticing your emotions.** Involves rerating the intensity of your emotions. This enables you to see whether your cognitive restructuring work was effective in reducing the intensity of your emotions.

USING THE AUTOMATIC THOUGHTS LOG

Let's start with Steps 1, 2, and 3—noticing the situation, your emotion, and your automatic thoughts. Use the Automatic Thoughts Log (Handout 8.3) as a tool to help you learn to be aware of your trigger situations, emotions, and automatic thoughts. The example of a completed Automatic Thoughts Log in Handout 8.3 shows how it works.

(continued)

Step 1—Notice the Situation

If you are like many people who have PTSD, it may seem that your distress is like a wave out of the blue that sweeps over you. You may not be aware of what triggered your distress or where it is coming from. Very often, by the time you are aware of your distress, you are out of the situation that triggered it. When you become aware of the triggers of your distress, it becomes more predictable and easier to control. Knowing what situations are likely to trigger certain feelings helps you to be prepared with a helpful response.

- In the first column of the Automatic Thoughts Log, describe the situation you were in or the events going on when you felt distressed. (*Hint*: Sometimes the trigger event might not be around you; instead, it could be a thought or a memory of something from the past.)

Step 2—Notice Your Emotions

This may be hard at first, because, if you are like many people with PTSD, you have put a lot of effort into *not noticing* your emotions. You might be used to thinking of your emotions as bad. If you think of your emotions as entirely negative experiences, it makes sense that you try to get to get rid of them. In fact, you may be so skillful at ignoring your emotions that you may find it hard to recognize and label them. Yet paying attention to your emotions is critical to change. Being mindful of your emotions is easier when you accept them as a valuable human experience. Emotions are valuable because they have a purpose in our lives. Emotions serve as signals of certain kinds of situations and prompt us to act in particular ways. Learning to identify and observe these signals is an important step toward acceptance of your emotions. (*Hint.* You can sometimes identify your emotions by the urge you feel when you are distressed.) Knowing the purpose of your emotions makes it easier for you to accept them as part of normal human experience. Knowing what your emotions signal enables you to respond effectively. Below is a list of common urges that people feel with each emotion, and its purpose.

UNDERSTANDING YOUR EMOTIONS		
Emotion	**Urge**	**Purpose**
Fear	To escape	Signals danger and prompts you to protect
Anger	To attack	Signals injustice and prompts you to correct the unfair situation
Guilt	To repair	Signals that you did something wrong and prompts you to repair the transgression
Shame	To hide	Signals that thoughts, feelings, or behaviors are socially unacceptable and prompts you to refrain from acting on them
Sadness	To quit	Signals loss and prompts you to promote grieving

- In the second column of the Automatic Thoughts Log, list all the emotions you notice. Then, rate their intensity using the 0–100 SUDS scale.

(continued)

Step 3—Identify Your Automatic Thoughts

Now that you have identified the triggering event and the emotions that you are feeling, the next step is to become aware of your automatic thoughts. This is not easy. You kind of have to step outside your thoughts to notice them—as if you were listening to a tape recording of them. Very often, we confuse our thoughts with reality. But if you think about it, our thoughts may accurately reflect reality, or they may *not*. I can think anything I want, but that doesn't make it true. I can think that a pink elephant is in the room as hard as I like, but it's not going to be true. So, you see, our thoughts exist apart from reality, although sometimes they may reflect reality, and sometimes they may not. Once we accept this, it becomes easier to step outside our thoughts to observe them.

- Write down the first automatic thought that came to mind in the situation. Write it down exactly as it went through your head, in the first person ("I") and using *your own* words. Then, from 0% to 100% rate how much you believe that thought.

Your Emotions Can Help You Identify Your Automatic Thoughts

If you find it difficult to identify your automatic thoughts in a given situation, you may find it helpful to use your emotions as a cue to your thoughts. The Guide to Emotions and Related Thoughts (Handout 8.5) shows the link between emotions and particular kinds of thoughts. For example, feelings of *sadness* are often related to *thoughts of loss*. The loss can take many forms. Some common forms of loss include the loss of a person, hope, innocence, or self-worth. If you have trouble recognizing your automatic thoughts, try this approach:

- Notice your emotion. (*Hint*. You can recognize your emotion by paying attention to an urge you feel. For example, sadness is typically related to an urge to quit.)
- Ask yourself the question that corresponds to that emotion (e.g., for sadness, "What have I lost?")

Using the Cognitive Restructuring Worksheet

Once you have identified your unhelpful automatic thoughts, you are ready for Steps 4, 5, and 6. Here, you take control of your unhelpful automatic thoughts by challenging them, forming new thoughts to replace the unhelpful ones, then rerating the intensity of your emotions. The Cognitive Restructuring Worksheet (Handout 8.4) helps you observe your reactions to stressful situations and challenge unhelpful thoughts. The more you practice filling out Handout 8.4 for stressful situations, the more you will improve your skills and gain control of unhelpful thoughts. So try to fill it out at least once each day. You may find this difficult at first. Your therapist will help when you have trouble challenging a thought.

(continued)

Step 4—Challenge your Automatic Thoughts

This step involves evaluating your thoughts and recognizing styles of thinking that may lead to negative emotions. Some techniques that may help you to interpret events realistically and in helpful ways are listed below.

- Challenge the thought by answering the following questions in the space provided:
  - What evidence do I have for this thought?
  - Is there an alternative way of looking at the situation—an alternative explanation?
  - What are the consequences (advantages–disadvantages) of thinking this way?
- *Hint.* When weighing the evidence for and against the thought, remember to use facts, not feelings. The "evidence" should be able to stand up in court as fact.

Step 5—Respond to Unhelpful Thoughts

This step involves replacing unhelpful automatic thoughts with more helpful ways of thinking. Developing alternative ways of thinking can help you feel a greater sense of control and personal effectiveness.

- Create a response to your thought that combines the *evidence for* and *against* he thought, and the consequences for continuing the thought into a whole statement. Use your this response to help you cope if you have this thought again in the future. (*Hint.* If you are having trouble blending the evidence, use the format, *Although ... in fact ...*).
- Rate how much you believe this response (0–100%).
- *Note.* Sometimes you may find that the evidence supports your automatic thought. If so, then it may instead be helpful to develop a plan of action to respond to the situation.

Step 6—Notice Your Emotions

This step involves rerating the intensity of your emotions. This enables you to see whether your cognitive restructuring was effective in reducing the intensity of your emotions.

- Rate the intensity of the emotions you feel when thinking the new thought using the SUDS scale.

HANDOUT 8.3. Automatic Thoughts Log (page 1 of 2)

Use this log to help you become aware of your automatic thoughts when you are feeling distressed.

Name: _Example_   Date: _____

1. Situation Describe: • Actual event leading to unpleasant emotion OR • Thoughts or memories leading to unpleasant emotion	2. Emotions • Identify the emotion(s) you felt (sad, anxious, angry, guilty, ashamed) • Rate intensity of the emotion(s) (0–100 SUDS)		3. Automatic Thoughts • Write automatic thought(s) that preceded your emotion(s) • Rate how much you believe the thought is true (0–100%)	% Belief
In Walmart	Anxious	95	I'm not safe. That man might attack me.	80%
Driving in car	Anxious	80	If I have another accident, I could be paralyzed.	90%
Watching TV—a car crashed and I got upset	Sadness	100	Getting upset means I'm weak.	100%
Newspaper story about a rape	Guilty Ashamed	85 75	It was all my fault—I never should have gone there. I'm dirty.	80%
Attending therapy session	Sadness	95	I'll never get any better.	100%
Getting ready to leave the house.	Anxious	60	I'm not safe unless I stay in my house.	100%
I trusted my coworker, and she didn't support me.	Sadness	100	I can't trust anybody.	100%
Thinking about the rapist	Angry	80	It's not fair that he's not suffering.	95%

196

- Bring awareness to listening and talking. Can you listen attentively without agreeing or disagreeing, giving advice or planning what you will say when it is your turn? When talking, can you just say what you need to say without the usual labels and judgments, and without overstating or understating things? Can you notice how your mind and body feel?

- Whenever you wait in a line or at a red light, use this time to notice standing/sitting and breathing. Feel the contact of your feet on the floor or the seat underneath you, and how your body feels. Bring attention to the expansion and contraction of your abdomen.

- Be aware of any points of tightness in your body throughout the day. See if you can breathe into them and, as you exhale, let go of excess tension. Is there tension stored anywhere in your body? For example, your neck, shoulders, stomach, jaw, or lower back? If possible, stretch or do yoga once a day.

- Focus attention on your daily activities such as brushing your teeth, washing the dishes, brushing your hair, putting on your shoes, doing your job. Bring curiosity and awareness to each activity.

- As you go to sleep at night, bring your attention to your body and your breathing. Let go of tension in the body and feel the warmth and softness of your bed.

As you do this experiment, notice the effect it has on your day (and night). Talking point within the group, consider sharing with other learners five things that you would normally do on automatic pilot. They can be from the suggestions provided or something else you think of. Commitment to engagement Over the next week, please select at least one activity or task (feel free to do this with as many as you like) and then make a commitment to engage fully with it, just to be mindful of the effect this has. You will have an opportunity to share what you discover next week.

Remember share only what you are comfortable sharing, there is no obligation to share.

Mindfulness of everyday activities – the informal practice of mindfulness

Our lives are comprised of moments, one after another. For instance, today you may have woken up, turned off your alarm, got up, showered, dried yourself, had breakfast, travelled to work or school/university, etc. We can engage in each of these moments/activities with a sense of curiosity and engagement, or on automatic pilot.

We can intentionally bring this attitude to whatever we are doing to help us become more present and awake in every moment of our lives. We can be especially mindful to everyday activities like breathing, travelling and communicating - which we normally tend to on automatic pilot. The more we make effort to bring mindfulness to our experiences, the more we will find ourselves spontaneously just "dropping into the moment" without even trying during the day.

Bringing mindfulness to everyday activity

For the next week, pick some everyday activities and try doing them mindfully. Simply bring curiosity to them and engage with them fully. You may like to experiment with a few of them, or you may prefer to pick one each day. Here are some suggestions. Feel free to use these or create your own.

- When you first wake up in the morning, before you get out of bed, feel your body. Stretch like you did when you were a kid, just whatever feels right. Take a few mindful breaths. Connect with your intention for the day ahead. Notice which foot first touches the floor.

- Find some touchpoints in your body, for example, feeling your feet on the floor, your breath coming and going, the sensations around your heart. Reconnect with these as much as possible throughout the day.

- Throughout the day, take a few moments to bring your attention to your breathing. Set a timer to remind you to be present.

- Notice the sounds around you throughout the day. Really tune into the sound of the wind, rain, traffic, and birdsong etc. Listen to the background hum of conversation.

- Whenever you eat or drink something, take a moment to really connect with it. Pause and notice how your body feels, whether you are hungry and what kind of food your body feels like it needs. Reflect on where the food has come from, the fact that it grew somewhere or was made by someone, perhaps wondering who was involved in its creation and transport. Connect with the sensory experience of eating – with the taste, the smell, the texture. Notice the chewing, the urge to swallow, the actual swallowing. Tune in to the effect of eating certain foods on your body.

- Notice your body while you walk or stand. Take a moment to notice your posture. Pay attention to the contact of the ground under your feet. Feel the air on your face, arms, and legs as you walk. Are you rushing? Is your mind already where you are going? Come back to each step.

Automatic Thoughts Log (page 2 of 2)

Use this log to help you become aware of your automatic thoughts when you are feeling distressed.

NAME: _____   DATE: _____

1. Situation	2. Emotions	3. Automatic Thoughts	
Describe: • Actual event leading to unpleasant emotion OR • Thoughts or memories leading to unpleasant emotion	• Identify the emotion(s) you felt (sad, anxious, angry, guilty, ashamed) • Rate intensity of the emotion(s) (0–100 SUDS)	• Write automatic thought(s) that preceded your emotion(s) • Rate how much you believe the thought is true (0–100%)	
			% Belief

HANDOUT 8.4. Cognitive Restructuring Worksheet

NAME: _____   DATE _____

1. Situation	3. Automatic Thoughts	4. Challenge to Automatic Thoughts	5. Response
Describe: • Actual event leading to unpleasant emotion OR • Thoughts or memories leading to unpleasant emotion.	• Write automatic thought(s) that preceded emotion(s). • Ask "What does that mean about me?" to see if an underlying belief is related to the emotion. • Select the thought or belief to challenge and rate how much you believe it is true (0–100%).	• Challenge your automatic thought (for example, list evidence *for* and *against* the thought, consider alternative views, and examine the consequences of holding this thought). • Identify your style of thinking.	• Write a response to the automatic thought(s) by summarizing the evidence or alternative views. • If the evidence supports your thought or belief, or you need more information, then *make a plan.* • Rate how much you believe the response (0–100%).
	% belief		% belief

2. Emotions

• Identify the emotion(s) you felt (e.g., sad, anxious, angry, shameful, guilty).

• Rate the intensity of the emotion (0–100).

SUDS

6. Emotions

• Rate the intensity of the emotions you identified in Step 2 (0–100).

SUDS

HANDOUT 8.5. Guide to Emotions and Related Thoughts

Emotions	Related Thoughts	Ask Yourself:
Fear or anxiety (urge to escape or avoid)	Thoughts that something bad will happen: • Harm to yourself or someone else • Being punished • Being embarrassed • Being unloved • Being abandoned	What bad thing do I expect to happen?
Sadness (urge to quit)	Thoughts of loss: • Loss of self-worth • Loss of innocence • Loss of a connection with another person • Loss of hope	What have I lost?
Guilt or shame (urge to repair/hide)	Thoughts of having done something wrong: • Being humiliated or ridiculed • Being bad or evil • Having bad thoughts or desires • Being responsible for bad things happening	What bad thing have I done?
Anger (urge to attack)	Thoughts of being treated unfairly: • An injustice or harm done to you • Being taken advantage of • Things not going as you want them to	What is unfair about this situation?

From Zayfert, Becker, and Gillock (2002). Copyright 2002 by Professional Resource Exchange, Inc. Reprinted with permission in *Cognitive-Behavioral Therapy for PTSD* by Claudia Zayfert and Carolyn Black Becker. Permission to photocopy this handout is granted to purchasers of this book for personal use only (see copyright page for details).

It can be helpful to recognize patterns in thinking that are problematic. The list below describes common types of automatic thoughts. Sometimes thinking in these ways can be unhelpful and may contribute to your distress. For example, when you think in "all-or-nothing" ways, you may be overlooking important information about a situation. When you "overgeneralize," you may be applying a belief about one person to someone else, when there is no evidence that it is true for that person. When you engage in emotional reasoning, you may respond too quickly to notice the facts in the situation. These styles of thinking are important, because they can affect a large number of thoughts. Learning to recognize these patterns in your thinking can help you to challenge your automatic thoughts and develop more realistic alternatives.

ALL-OR-NOTHING THINKING

When a person is thinking this way, he or she sees everything in black-or-white terms. For example, someone might label all people as either "good" or "bad," without thinking about any middle ground. If you cannot see any "shades of gray" in between, you may be engaging in "all-or-nothing thinking." An example of all-or-nothing thinking is falling just short of meeting your goals and, regardless of how close you came, thinking:

- "I am a complete failure."

    People who have experienced traumatic events often see personal safety in an all-or-nothing manner: if a situation is not completely safe, then it is completely dangerous. There is no middle ground. Another example of all-or-nothing thinking is when a person takes complete responsibility for something that happened even if the situation may not have been fully within their control. For example, someone who was assaulted on a date might think:

- "It's all my fault because I agreed to kiss him."

OVERGENERALIZATION

Overgeneralizing is when you draw a conclusion from one incident and apply it to all incidents. When you assume that the negative results of one event will happen all the time, you are overgeneralizing. Examples of this type of thinking follow:

- "I had no control during the earthquake; I have no control over anything."
- "I went on a date with a man who assaulted me. Anytime I go on a date with a man, I will get assaulted."

(continued)

EMOTIONAL REASONING

Most of the time, your experience determines your expectations about the future. If you are engaged in emotional reasoning, your emotions determine your expectations. Most of us assume that our feelings are an accurate reflection of how things really are. This is a reasonable thing to assume in many situations. At times, however, our emotions may not completely match the reality of the situation. A person using emotional reasoning might think:

- "I feel scared when I get into a car, so riding in a car is dangerous."
- "I get nervous whenever I go to the grocery store, so there must be something in the grocery store that can hurt me."

"SHOULD" STATEMENTS

These are unwritten rules you have for yourself or others that are based on wishful thinking rather than fact. "Should" statements create expectations that are unrealistic and can produce guilt, shame, frustration, and anger. "Should" statements also might include words like "must," "ought," or "have to." Examples of this type of thinking follow:

- "I should be over this by now."
- "My mother should have protected me."
- "I should have stopped the abuse."

PERSONALIZATION

This occurs when you hold yourself personally responsible for bad things that happened, even if you did not have complete control of them. When you engage in this form of thinking, you may be ignoring evidence that other people shared responsibility for events. Examples:

- "It was all my fault."
- "I let it happen."

NINE

Supplemental Tools

This chapter provides an overview of useful, supplemental CBT tools for treating complicated cases of PTSD. Supplemental tools are drawn from empirically supported or promising therapies developed for other disorders or problems that commonly co-occur with PTSD. Developing familiarity with some of these interventions expands your ability to address the full clinical picture of PTSD using the case formulation approach. For example, familiarity with panic control treatment (Barlow & Craske, 2000), the treatment for panic disorder that has the most empirical support, helps you to tailor treatment for patients with co-occurring PTSD and panic disorder.

Some patients only need PTSD treatment, because no additional problems are present. Comorbid problems also often resolved along with PTSD, and some patients do not wish to address comorbidity. Yet comorbid problems often warrant intervention. Thus, in addition to using a systematic approach to develop an appropriate treatment, you may find it useful to have a "toolbox" that includes interventions for common comorbid problems.

For some problems, the toolbox may simply contain appropriate referral sources. For example, you may not wish to become expert in treatment of eating disorders. If so, you can monitor patients' eating disorder symptoms and refer them to an expert in eating disorders after completion of PTSD treatment or, if necessary for safety, prior to or during PTSD treatment. Similarly, you might choose to refer patients to a formal pain management program rather than implementing pain management interventions along with or subsequent to PTSD treatment. We also typically refer patients with substance abuse dependence problems to substance abuse experts for either staged or concurrent treatment. The extent to which you supplement your toolbox with intervention skills in adjunctive areas depends, in part, on the availability of specialists in these other issues in your area.

Some skills, however, are invaluable regardless of referral source availability. For example, formal dialectical behavior therapy (DBT) programs may be available to accept referrals of individuals with borderline personality disorder (BPD) who have marked suicidality and emotion dysregulation. Yet many individuals with PTSD and milder forms of BPD do not qualify for such programs. Borderline symptoms also may be severe enough to disrupt treatment but not severe enough to warrant derailing PTSD treatment in favor of admission to a DBT program. Thus, we recommend that you develop some familiarity with DBT.

In addition, often there are distinct advantages to addressing comorbid problems. For example, should you decide to treat residual sleep problems behaviorally in a patient who responded to CBT for PTSD, you would have a running start, because you already have a working alliance with the patient. You also would be familiar with the patient's knowledge base and skills, as well as his or her strengths and areas of difficulty. Moreover, the patient would likely have significant trust in you if treatment had thus far produced improvement. In contrast, if a patient experienced sleep disruption following CBT for PTSD and you referred that patient to a sleep clinic, a new rapport and confidence in the therapist and therapy would have to be established.

DIALECTICAL BEHAVIOR THERAPY

As noted throughout this book, we find many facets of DBT (Linehan, 1993a) helpful in treating trauma survivors. DBT is a complex treatment, and it is beyond the scope of this book or chapter to detail fully the many ways we find DBT useful in treating trauma. Interested readers should see Becker and Zayfert (2001) for additional discussion of the application of DBT to CBT for PTSD. Training in DBT also is available throughout the United States by Behavioral Tech (see www.behavioraltech.com), which offers both online training and a database of trained DBT providers at their website.

Many DBT concepts are very useful in treating trauma. In particular, however, we rely most heavily on the biosocial theory that underpins DBT, the dialectic of acceptance and change (Linehan, 1993a), and a variety of DBT skills. The biosocial theory argues that BPD (or profound problems in emotion dysregulation) is produced when an inborn temperamental vulnerability to emotion dysregulation is combined with an invalidating environment (Linehan, 1993b). Developing a good grasp of the biosocial theory and the concept of invalidation (including self-invalidation) helps you develop comprehensive case formulations for many patients. In addition, patients often seem to benefit from having their emotion dysregulation difficulties explained via the biosocial theory.

The dialectic of acceptance and change (Linehan, 1993b) explicitly acknowledges the need for a balance between acceptance and change throughout therapy. This dialectic operates both in your patients (i.e., some things they can change and others that they must simply accept) and in you (i.e., the need to balance your use of acceptance and change strategies; Becker & Zayfert, 2001). Becoming thoroughly acquainted with the dialectic of acceptance and change helps you better conceptualize the tasks a given patient faces. It also helps you appropriately interweave acceptance and change strategies. CBT rests heavily on a technology of change. Even acceptance typically is produced with the use of change techniques. For example, patients need to accept their trauma. We teach them to accept their trauma during exposure by changing their primary coping strategy of avoidance. We also use cognitive restructuring to change their thinking. At times, however, skillful introduction of specific acceptance-based strategies facilitates the progression of treatment. For example, the notion of adopting a mindful, accepting stance toward anxiety (and emotions in general) is helpful for many patients (see Handout 9.1). The therapist example below demonstrates how you can utilize acceptance strategies to facilitate engagement in exposure.

> "I've noticed that you have expressed quite a bit of reluctance to feel anxiety, which is understandable, because the intense anxiety that you sometimes feel can be overwhelming and quite unpleasant. As we've discussed, anxiety is a useful human emotion. It serves a very important function in protecting us when we are faced with danger. It becomes a problem for you, however, when you feel it in situations that present minimal danger. The goal of this treatment is to learn that your anxiety is unnecessary in certain situations. Yet in order to learn this, you need to feel the anxiety. In other words, your success in doing this therapy may depend on your willingness to accept anxiety. We can also think of this as the mind-set that you bring to the therapy tasks. If you tend to believe that all anxiety is bad and that you should work hard to "get rid of" your anxiety, you may approach the therapy tasks as something that you must *endure* to be rid of anxiety for good. We sometimes call this 'white knuckling it.' You sort of grip your fists and grit your teeth, and wait for it to be over. This kind of mind-set tends to make it harder to stay with the therapy tasks and the program. Another way of approaching the therapy tasks is to acknowledge and accept that although anxiety may be uncomfortable, it helps us to survive. In addition, some people find it helpful to practice radically accepting anxiety as a valuable life experience. Adopting an accepting stance toward your anxiety can enhance your likelihood of success."

Many patients find it easier to adopt an accepting stance toward anxiety and other emotions after being taught specific DBT acceptance skills. For example, in the preceding example, the therapist talks about the DBT skill of radical acceptance, which involves an extreme acceptance of things formerly rejected. Mindfulness skills, which are based on Buddhist mediation, teach patients to accept the present with out judgment. Mindfulness, which is incorporated into Handout 9.1, is further addressed in Handout 9.2. Mindfulness skills can be very helpful for patients who dissociate, numb out, or have difficulty distinguishing and experiencing their emotions.

We also utilize the DBT concept of "states of mind," which is introduced early in formal DBT mindfulness training. The therapist presents the notion that patients can be in one of three states of mind: reasonable (or rational) mind, emotion mind, or wise mind. The reasonable mind is analytic and rational, whereas in emotion mind, emotions dominate. It is unfortunate that Western culture often rewards us for being in reasonable mind because we are most effective when we combine emotion with reason, a state labeled "wise mind." Patients most often see the utility of this when asked to identify a time when they "truly knew something deep down in their gut." When we are in our wise mind state, we know things in a truly meaningful way. One example of wise mind that resonates with the vast majority of patients with PTSD is the decision to seek treatment for PTSD. For example, when Amira was asked about her decision to seek treatment, she responded, "I was terrified and I didn't want to do it. But I *knew* I needed to, even though I was scared, because it was the only way that I could heal." In this response, Amira demonstrates wise mind thinking. She incorporates both rational thought (i.e., "Treatment was the only way I could heal") and emotions (i.e., "I was terrified") without invalidating either (e.g., she does not say that her fear is unfounded).

Amira also "knows" that she needs to seek treatment. Handout 9.3 summarizes the different states of mind. In the course of this discussion we frequently also draw for our patients Linehan's (1993b) intersecting circles, which illustrate wise mind as the integration of emotion mind and reasonable mind.

For many patients it can be helpful to discuss the effects of traumatic experiences on state of mind. We find that the metaphor "The Seesaw of Emotion and Reason" (see Handout 9.3) is a useful tool for normalizing reactions to trauma and conveying the effects of trauma on the ability to remain balanced in the wise mind state (Zayfert, Becker, & Gillock, 2002). Using this metaphor, we emphasize that all human beings live on this seesaw and must try to balance emotion and reason. Those who have not experienced trauma are perched in the center of the seesaw, and their movements are contained within a short distance of the fulcrum, making the task of remaining balanced relatively easy. A traumatic event, however, typically thrusts a person rapidly into emotion mind, which often is perceived as being out of control, and it is common to attempt to escape quickly from this state. Rapid retreat to the opposite end results in a reasonable (often numbed-out) state. This sets the stage for flip-flopping between emotion mind and reasonable mind. Once the seesaw is in motion, it can be harder for people to regain the balance they had when perched at the center. The seesaw metaphor helps patients conceptualize their own tendency to ricochet back and forth between emotion and reason mind as an understandable consequence of traumatic experiences.

Another tool we employ to help patients regain this balance is the worksheet for recognizing states of mind (Handout 9.3). Our goal in this worksheet is to help patients identify cues that indicate they are in reasonable or emotion mind, and steps they can take to help reestablish balance between the states of mind.

We find that many patients benefit from short, or sometimes longer, courses of mindfulness training. Thus, we encourage you to develop a background in mindfulness training. You also may find it helpful to learn about mindfulness from other sources (e.g., Kabat-Zinn, 1994) and to compile a list of resources for mindfulness (or meditation) practice in your local area.

As we noted earlier in this book, other skills also can facilitate the delivery of CBT for PTSD. For example, self-soothing strategies and distraction skills drawn from DBT can help patients modulate their emotional response during treatment. In summary, DBT has much to offer trauma therapists, including those who never intend to implement full-blown DBT.

ACTIVITY SCHEDULING

Activity scheduling (also referred to as "behavioral activation" and "pleasant activities scheduling") is one of the core components of CBT for depression (Beck et al., 1979). Dismantling research suggests that activity scheduling alone may produce similar reductions in depression compared to activity scheduling plus other CBT elements, such as cognitive restructuring (Jacobson et al., 1996). Thus, activity scheduling can be very useful in managing depressed mood in PTSD patients.

On the surface, activity scheduling is quite simple: You and your patient schedule activities. We often focus on pleasant activities during activity scheduling, because many trauma survivors have ceased all engagement in pleasant activities, and many others never learned how to use pleasant events to modulate affect. Other patients, however, stop most of their activities altogether, and need help in resuming basic activities of daily living. Despite the apparent simplicity of activity scheduling, the nuances of this technique are important, if you want it to be effective. Thus, we recommend that you become familiar with these nuances. Interested readers are referred to Beck et al. (1979) and to Persons et al. (2001) for a more detailed discussion of activity scheduling. Understanding the nomothetic formulation that underlies CBT for depression also is useful in developing your case formulations with depressed patients with PTSD. Information on the nomothetic formulation for depression is available in the same references.

ASSERTIVE COMMUNICATION SKILLS

Patients with PTSD frequently present with deficits in assertive communication skills, which can generate significant life problems that derail treatment. For example, Adele came to session reporting that she was about to be thrown out of her apartment for not paying her rent. Adele made sufficient money at her job to pay her rent and basic expenses, but her former husband, who had left her for another woman, continued to ask for money. Adele reported that she could not imagine refusing his request for money, or any other request for that matter. A quick review of Adele's history revealed a long-standing pattern of lack of appropriate assertiveness.

Adele's lack of assertiveness created a logistical problem that threatened to derail treatment. Thus, her therapist briefly integrated assertiveness training into treatment, then continued with CBT for PTSD. You likely will encounter plenty of patients like Adele. Many other patients, however, will benefit from more comprehensive assertiveness training before or after the completion of CBT for PTSD. Such training should precede CBT for PTSD when, for example, patients are in relationships or living situations that involve active emotional, physical, or sexual abuse, or if they experience repeated assaultive violence in other areas of their lives. There are a variety of good references for learning about assertive communication skills, and much of this literature has been translated into easy-to-read self-help books (e.g., see Jakubowski & Lange, 1978; Alberti & Emmons, 1986). For the most part, we find it insufficient just to give these books to patients, because many patients with PTSD need more intensive instruction and assistance with practicing assertive communication skills. These references will help you develop a stronger background in assertiveness, however, so that you can interweave in-session assertiveness training with bibliotherapy.

PROBLEM-SOLVING SKILLS

Many CBT interventions include problem-solving steps (e.g., CBT for bulimia nervosa; Fairburn et al., 1993) and/or are based on problem solving for depression (Nezu, 1986). Patients with PTSD frequently come to treatment with problems that impair the quality of their lives and/or their ability to proceed through treatment. Thus, it often is helpful to teach them the seven simple steps of problem solving.

Problem solving can be done both formally and informally. Formal problem solving involves explicitly teaching the seven steps. Informal problem solving may consist of taking the patient through the seven steps, without being as explicit in the teaching process. The latter option sometimes works better for patients who are extremely distressed about a problem and cognitively overwhelmed. The main goal in informal problem solving is to solve the problem as quickly as possible using the seven steps, not to teach problem solving.

Step 1 of problem solving consists of identifying the problem in language that is as specific as possible (see Handout 9.4). If patients lump multiple problems together, these should be separated and addressed independently. Step 2 involves brainstorming as many ways to address the problem as possible. Encourage patients to move beyond the easy answers and really try to explore all solutions without judgment. Even absurd answers should be written down at this point to highlight the expansive nature of this type of brainstorming. The rationale behind this stage is that a good solution is more likely to emerge if many solutions are generated. For example, in brainstorming solutions to a lack of transportation problem, Jeremy jokingly said, "I could get on my pet donkey, ride him here, and tie him up outside the hospital." He did not want to write that answer down, however, because it was "ridiculous." His therapist had him write it down, at which point Jeremy laughed and said, "You really are looking for *all* solutions, aren't you?"

For the Step 3, you and your patient evaluate the feasibility and likely success of each solution. After this, the patient chooses a solution (Step 4), which may consist of a combination of solutions. Step 5 involves describing what the patient needs to do to carry out the solution. Steps 6 and 7 consist of implementing the solution, then evaluating how things turned out.

EXPOSURE FOR COMORBID ANXIETY DISORDERS

PTSD often is accompanied by other anxiety disorders. For example, we found in a recent clinical practice study that 74% of patients with a principal diagnosis of PTSD met criteria for at least one other anxiety disorder (Zayfert, Becker, Unger, & Shearer, 2002). Thus, clinicians who treat PTSD need to be prepared to manage co-occurring anxiety disorders.

Other anxiety problems may develop together with PTSD, predate the onset of PTSD, or emerge later in the course of PTSD. Regardless, it is important in most cases to *consider* potential interactions between PTSD and other anxiety problems when developing the case formulation, so that you are prepared to manage such problems. Management of a comorbid anxiety disorder may simply include monitoring the ongoing symptoms associated with the anxiety disorder, or it may involve treatment (i.e., active intervention).

In some cases, there is good reason to hypothesize that comorbid anxiety disorders will diminish with PTSD treatment. For example, Marsha, who survived extensive childhood physical and sexual abuse, met criteria for both PTSD and obsessive–compulsive disorder (OCD). Marsha's behaviors included spending 3–4 hours per day cleaning her house, and frequently counting objects in her environment. Marsha was unable to control her cleaning and reported that it often interfered with her life. The counting, which started in childhood, was disturbing, but it did not interfere significantly with daily functioning. Marsha's OCD behaviors appeared to be functionally related to her PTSD, in that they increased when she encountered anxiety-provoking, trauma-related stimuli. Thus, the therapist hypothesized that counting was a distraction technique that Marsha had first used during the abuse, then later employed in many types of uncomfortable situations, or when reminded of the abuse. Marsha was participating in several hours per day of exposure, cognitive restructuring, and activity scheduling. Instead of devising additional exposure and response prevention tasks (drawn from the nomothetic model of OCD) to address the cleaning and counting directly, the therapist suggested that treatment initially target PTSD and depression. She also suggested that they monitor the severity of OCD symptoms during treatment and reassess them at the end of PTSD treatment to determine whether the OCD symptoms persisted and required additional, focused intervention.

In some cases, the comorbid anxiety problem may take on "a life of its own" and be so distinct from the PTSD that interventions for PTSD do not generalize to the distinct anxiety problem. For example, social phobia is one of the most common comorbid anxiety problems among individuals seeking treatment for PTSD (Zayfert, Becker, Unger, et al., 2002). Although evidenced-based treatment for social phobia includes exposure and cognitive restructuring, the target of these methods may be so different than that for PTSD that the PTSD treatment effects do not generalize to social phobia. Julian reported a long-standing history of social phobia, in addition to PTSD related to childhood physical abuse. Julian reported always being "shy and quiet," and noted that this did not fit well with his father's desire for a son who was a "man's man" and a popular athlete. Julian completed exposure to memories of being beaten by his father and successfully used cognitive restructuring to challenge beliefs that the abuse was his own fault, because he did not live up to his father's expectations. At the end of treatment, however, he still experienced significant anxiety about dating, talking with women, and speaking in public. Thus, Julian's therapist had him participate in a group social phobia treatment, which consisted of exposure to social situations, social skills training, and cognitive restructuring.

Sometimes you may not be able to address disorders sequentially, and will instead address problems simultaneously. For example, Lois met criteria for both PTSD and OCD. One of her traumatic events involved seeing her father's remains after he shot himself. Lois reported that there was blood everywhere, and that her father had soiled himself. She avoided blood, urine, feces, and stains that reminded her of blood, feces, or urine, because they triggered both OCD-related fears of contamination and trauma-related fear and memories. Lois's therapist implemented integrated treatment of both disorders, which involved having Lois focus on either PTSD- or OCD-related fear during the first exposure to a given stimulus. Once she had habituated to the first fear associated with the stimulus, Lois completed exposure to her second fear of the same stimulus (for a detailed discussion of another case involving integrated OCD and PTSD treatment, see Becker, 2002).

Sometimes we also find it useful to integrate panic and PTSD treatment. For example, Erica, who met criteria for both panic disorder and PTSD, reported unexpected panic attacks and cued panic attacks. The latter typically were in response to traumatic stimuli. Erica was extremely frightened by her panic symptoms and reported believing that she was going to have a heart attack or stroke during her panic attacks. Given her fears about her panic attacks, Erica's therapist hypothesized that she might have trouble with trouble with PTSD exposure, which was likely to elicit fears of both panic and of traumatic stimuli and memories. Thus, Erica's therapist blended some panic psychoeducation into PTSD psychoeducation. She also started Erica on breathing retraining and interoceptive exposure for panic attacks (Barlow & Craske, 2000) prior to starting *in vivo* trauma exposure. The goal was to have Erica learn to not fear the sensations associated with acute anxiety prior to starting trauma exposure.

A recent survey indicates that many therapists trained in CBT for PTSD *have not* been trained in CBT for other anxiety disorders (Becker et al., 2004). This is not an optimal situation in our opinion. Thus, we encourage you to gain some background in CBT/exposure for other anxiety disorders. You can obtain training at the annual convention of the Association for Behavioral and Cognitive Therapies (ABCT; www.abct.org). Treatment manuals for other anxiety disorders (e.g., panic, generalized anxiety disorder, etc.) can be obtained from Oxford University Press.

DECISION ANALYSIS

A commonly used CBT technique, decision analysis (Janis & Mann, 1977), can be very useful in resolving patients' ambivalence regarding therapy in general, and exposure in particular. Decision analysis is a relatively simple technique that involves having patients identify the pros and cons of maintaining their behavior and of changing that same behavior. In PTSD treatment, the behavior is usually some form of an avoidance behavior. It is usually best to do this on paper (see Handout 9.5, which includes a completed worksheet as an example). Quite often the difficulty in decision making relates to difficulty retaining and organizing all the information in one's head.

Decision analysis is a nonthreatening way to explore patients' ambivalence about giving up avoidance. In addition, when patients examine the pros and cons of their avoidance behaviors, they more easily recognize that short-term reductions in anxiety are associated with profound long-term costs. For example, Roberta came to treatment at the urging of her former therapist and was very reluctant to start PTSD treatment. Rather than trying to convince Roberta that PTSD treatment would be a good idea, the therapist said, "Tell you what, why don't we examine the benefits and costs of facing your trauma memories and the benefits and costs of continuing to keep those memories boxed away." As Roberta filled in the Decision Analysis Worksheet (Handout 9.5), she noted "There are a lot of reasons in the short term for me to stay with what I am doing. But look at the long term. I never realized all of the long-terms costs. I just never thought about it."

You also can use decision analysis to directly address patient ambivalence regarding exposure. For example, after completing psychoeducation, Ron reported, "This all makes a lot of sense and I actually feel somewhat better. I'm having a hard time, though, with the idea that I am going to have to think about what happened. I just can't see going through that. It is going to be too awful." The therapist realized that he had several options, including using cognitive restructuring to address Ron's thinking, and trying to verbally persuade Ron to give exposure a chance. Instead, the therapist decided to see whether Ron could persuade himself through the use of decision analysis.

As Ron completed decision analysis, he realized that the consequences strongly favored proceeding with exposure. By the end of the session, Ron was explaining to the therapist why he needed to do exposure.

Two major considerations are important in the use of decision analysis (readers interested in further discussion of the use of decision analysis in PTSD treatment should see Zayfert, Becker, & Gillock, 2002). First, decision analysis typically is easier when you target a very specific avoidance behavior. In other words, patients find it more difficult to identify specific consequences (positive and negative) if the stated behavior is just "avoidance." In contrast, they find it easier to generate consequences if the stated behavior is "avoiding trauma treatment" or, even better, "avoiding thinking about being raped by my neighbor," or "avoiding the grocery store."

Second, we typically start decision analysis by asking patients to identify the short-term benefits of maintaining their avoidance behavior. Short-term benefits of continuing avoidance are usually very easy for patients to identify. In addition, by starting here, you step out of the role of persuading patients to do something frightening. Instead, you validate the reasons for their current behavior, which helps build rapport.

TREATMENT FOR INSOMNIA

Difficulty falling or staying asleep, the most commonly reported symptom among various types of patients with PTSD (Green, 1993), is endorsed by as many as 70% of those meeting diagnostic criteria for PTSD (Ohayon & Shapiro, 2000). Although sleep problems initially may be precipitated by nightmares and hypervigilance, insomnia associated with PTSD often persists after otherwise successful treatment of PTSD (Zayfert & DeViva, 2004), suggesting that additional factors may maintain PTSD-related insomnia. For example, some patients with PTSD may develop a fear of sleep secondary to nightmares, fear of the bedroom, and/or fear of letting their guard down during sleep. Such fears and maladaptive, sleep-related behaviors sometimes persist after the nightmares and other PTSD symptoms have diminished. In addition, like general insomnia patients, patients with PTSD may develop anxiety and maladaptive beliefs about not sleeping, along with poor sleep hygiene.

If patients continue to struggle with insomnia after successful treatment of PTSD, it may be helpful to address perpetuating factors that maintain insomnia. CBT for insomnia is a brief, highly effective intervention that may help residual sleep problems (DeViva, Zayfert, Pigeon, & Mellman, 2005). At this point, it is unclear whether it is advisable to administer this approach in tandem with PTSD treatment. Given that approximately half of patients with PTSD experience remission of their insomnia as a result of PTSD treatment alone, however, we recommend administering CBT for insomnia after PTSD treatment.

Morin (1993) outlines CBT for general insomnia in detail. CBT for PTSD-related insomnia, however, usually can be abbreviated due to the overlap in skills with CBT for PTSD (DeViva et al., 2005; Figure 9.1). An abbreviated insomnia intervention typically includes the usual components of CBT for insomnia (e.g., stimulus control strategies and sleep restriction, see Morin, 1993), with a focus on targeting residual nighttime vigilance and avoidance of sleep. For example, despite having learned to determine more accurately what constitutes safety during the day, some patients continue to perceive

Session	Contents
1	Insomnia evaluation
2	Sleep restriction and stimulus control
3	Review sleep restriction and stimulus control homework; begin cognitive restructuring
4	Review cognitive restructuring homework; sleep hygiene and progressive muscle relaxation training
5	Review/integrate components; relapse prevention

FIGURE 9.1. Outline of CBT for PTSD-related insomnia.

the bedroom as dangerous, or to engage in habitual vigilance and checking before bedtime. They also may continue the habit of leaving the television or radio on, donning heavy blankets, or sleeping with a light on to feel safe. In addition, they may continue to believe that letting their guard down during sleep is dangerous. Such beliefs may then lead to sleep-interfering behaviors, such as avoidance of the bed, bedroom, darkness, or quiet.

In some cases, once identified, the particular behaviors themselves can be modified to induce sleep, such as turning off the television, radio, or lights. In other cases, however, behavior change alone will not improve sleep without successfully challenging the faulty cognitions about danger that underlie the nighttime vigilance. For example, Jessica reported that if she awoke in the night, she would remain very still out of fear that her husband would be awakened and insist on having sexual relations. Remaining still and uncomfortable often prevented Jessica from falling back to sleep. Using cognitive restructuring, Jessica concluded that although her brother had forced intercourse on her in the middle of the night, her husband had never coerced her to have sex, nor had he ever initiated intimacy late at night. Therefore, he was unlikely to coerce her. As a result, she was able to shift positions comfortably and fall back asleep. Insomnia treatment is not overly complex. Thus, we encourage to you see Morin (1993) and DeViva et al. (2005) for further details regarding insomnia treatment and the abbreviated treatment for patients who have completed CBT for PTSD.

TREATMENT FOR EATING DISORDERS

Research indicates that traumatic experiences are a nonspecific risk factor for development of eating disorders (Dansky, Brewerton, Kilpatrick, & O'Neil, 1997; Fairburn, Cooper, Doll, & Welch, 1999). As noted by Brewerton (2005), however, "nonspecific" does not mean unimportant. In addition, in our exploratory study of eating disorder prevalence among clinical practice patients with anxiety, one out of every six female patients with PTSD likely had an eating disorder (Becker et al., 2004).

In some cases, eating disorders develop shortly after a critical traumatic event, and it is easy to hypothesize a functional relationship between the eating disorder and the trauma history. For example, Karen's eating disorder developed at age 35, after the traumatic miscarriage in her first pregnancy. After her miscarriage, Karen reported clearly thinking that if she could not be a mother, then she wanted to be thin. In cases in which the eating disorder predates the traumatic event or develops many years later, hypotheses about a causal or maintaining relationship typically are substantially more tentative.

Even in cases in which there is no causal relationship, eating disorders may present a challenge to trauma treatment, because patients may use their eating disorders to avoid thinking about their trauma. For example, Karen noted that she believed she used her eating disorder to avoid thinking about her miscarriage. Patients also may experience an increase in eating disorder symptoms secondary to increases in negative affect. For example, patients who use binge eating and/or purging to modulate negative affect often engage in these behaviors to a greater extent when they experience temporary increases in negative affect associated with CBT for PTSD. Jane reported a worsening of her eating disorder symptoms (i.e., increased dietary restriction and purging) whenever she started exposure to a new trauma memory. Although there was no evidence that her eating disorder had been caused by her trauma, the therapist hypothesized that the eating disorder was worsening because Jane used the eating disorder behaviors to modulate her anxiety.

Therapists who treat patients with PTSD and a comorbid eating disorder need to consider the risk of colluding with their patients who may wish to avoid trauma-focused work. In the previous case, Jane's previous therapists had terminated trauma-focused treatment whenever her eating disorder symptoms worsened, which potentially negatively reinforced the eating disorder symptoms. Worsening of eating disorder symptoms, however, can present a genuine physical danger for some patients. We advocate proceeding with trauma treatment whenever possible, because of the likelihood that exposure will rapidly reduce negative affect, which often makes treatment of the eating disorder easier. This clinical decision, however, must be made on a case-by-case basis.

Given that eating disorders may be associated with significant medical complications, we suggest that clinicians who treat female patients with PTSD (1) assess such patients for the presence of an eating disorder, and (2) have enough knowledge about eating disorders to refer appropriately, treat, and/or monitor these conditions. Monitoring may consist of tracking purging and binge eating episodes, weight, or dietary restriction. Patients who purge should be referred to a physician for assessment of physical indicators, such as low blood levels of potassium, which can place them at risk for cardiac arrhythmias. If you do not have eating disorders expertise and you encounter a patient who purges to the point of disrupting potassium levels, then she should be referred to an eating disorders specialist for concurrent monitoring and/or treatment of her eating disorder. Treatment of eating disorders typically is viewed as a clinical specialty, and we are not suggesting that all PTSD therapists need to be able to treat the full spectrum of eating disorders effectively. Yet a certain minimal background in the treatment of eating disorders is likely to be useful.

CBT for bulimia nervosa (Fairburn et al., 1993) is the most well-studied form of treatment for any eating disorder, and a significant amount of research supports the efficacy of this treatment. Clinicians who are interested in learning more about CBT for bulimia nervosa should see the manual by Fairburn et al. Additional training can be obtained either from the ABCT, or the Academy for Eating Disorders (www.aedweb.org). Recently, Fairburn and colleagues (1993) developed a more flexible version of this treatment, aimed at the full spectrum of eating disorders. Fairburn, Cooper, and Shafran (2003) described the model underlying this treatment. You may find the model helpful in developing case formulations with your patients. Treatment recommendations are also provided in that article.

SUBSTANCE ABUSE AND DEPENDENCE

As noted earlier in this book, we do not typically treat patients who have significant problems with substance dependence and/or abuse. Instead, we refer them to substance abuse experts either for concurrent treatment or for detoxification, or other treatment prior to starting PTSD therapy. Some substance abusers, however, can complete PTSD treatment if therapists are careful to monitor the substance use during treatment and make a plan for how to manage increases in substance use. You also may find it helpful to use decision analysis (discussed earlier) as a tool to explore patients' substance abuse behavior. Finally, in some cases, it is effective simply to be able to instruct patients to limit their substance use during PTSD treatment. For example, after beginning exposure, Leigh reported that he resumed drinking three to five drinks on weeknights. After exploring the pros and cons of Leigh's drinking behavior and the ways it might interfere with PTSD treatment, his therapist suggested that Leigh stop drinking on weeknights and limit his weekend consumption to three beers at night. They made a plan for other activities to help Leigh cope with his low mood. Leigh was amenable to this "homework assignment" and successfully reduced his drinking with little trouble.

CONCLUSION

The supplemental tools in this chapter are the methods on which we routinely rely when conducting treatment for PTSD. We recognize that not all clinicians will want to develop expertise in each of these areas. Yet we strongly encourage you to consider developing some expertise in DBT and exposure for other anxiety disorders. Activity scheduling, decision analysis, problem solving, and insomnia treatment, which are not particularly difficult to learn, are clinical skills that you may find helpful with a wide range of patients. Of the areas discussed in this chapter, we expect that eating disorders expertise will be the one pursued by the least number of readers. Nonetheless, given the medical consequences of many eating disorders, we encourage you to develop an awareness of this comorbid condition, so that you can appropriately refer and monitor patients.

A MINDFUL APPROACH FOR MANAGING ANXIETY

Your success in doing this therapy may also depend on the mind-set that you bring to the therapy tasks. If you tend to believe that all anxiety is bad and that you should work hard to "get rid of" your anxiety, you may approach the therapy tasks as something that you must *endure* to be rid of anxiety for good. This kind of mind-set tends to make it harder to stick with the therapy tasks and the program. Another way of approaching the therapy tasks is to acknowledge that, although anxiety may be uncomfortable, it helps us to survive. (In other words, a life without anxiety would be a short one.) Practice cultivating a mind-set that accepts anxiety as a valuable life experience. Adopting an accepting stance toward your anxiety will enhance the likelihood of success.

A.W.A.R.E.

- **Accept** your anxiety. Welcome it. Expect and allow your fear to arise. Decide to be present with the experience. When fear appears, wait and let it be.
- **Watch** your anxiety. Rate your fear on a scale from 0–100 and watch it go up and down.
- **Act** with the anxiety; normalize the situation by acting as if you are not anxious. Focus on and perform manageable activities in the present and in natural environments.
- **Repeat** acceptance. Float with your anxiety. Let time pass. Observe and act with the anxiety until it diminishes.
- **Expect** and allow fear to reappear. Expect and accept future anxiety by giving up the hope that the anxiety will never recur, and replace that with trust in your ability to handle your anxiety.

WHAT ARE "MINDFULNESS" SKILLS?

Being with the Moment

Mindfulness is about being present in the moment. Being mindful means being present with and accepting what is actually happening right in this moment.

WHY IS MINDFULNESS IMPORTANT?

Trauma Takes You Out of the Present

If you are like many people who have lived through traumatic experiences, you may tend to have difficulty being in the present. You may feel as though you are stuck between the things that remind you of the past and the fears you have about the future. Trauma survivors tend to be preoccupied with the past and worried about the future. As a result, the present goes by, and you do not participate in it.

Be Present in the Here and Now

The best way to deal with what is happening in your life is to be where you are right now and address what you have to deal with right here. Learning to live life in the moment puts you in the best position to solve your problems, manage your emotions, and cope with life, even when it is throwing you its worst. At such times, it is most helpful to be able to stay where you are, so you can deal with what is happening. For example, when you are feeling strong negative emotions, you may focus on worries about what is going to happen in the future. When you focus on the future, you are less attentive to things happening right now and tend to respond less effectively to them. Mindfulness teaches you how to stay in the moment, so you can effectively respond to what is happening in your life now.

Getting to Your Wise Mind

Mindfulness skills help you get to your wise mind. Wise mind is a state of mind that enables you to be most effective in dealing with what is happening in your life. When you are in wise mind, you are able to make decisions and choices that help you get what you want in life. To get into wise mind from emotion mind or reasonable mind, you need to be present with and aware of your emotions and your thoughts. (Remember, if you are blocking out or numbing your emotions, you are in reasonable mind. If you are ignoring reason or logic, you are in emotion mind.) When you participate in all of your experiences, both emotional and logical, you will be able to make the best choices to reach your goals.

(continued)

HOW DO I PRACTICE MINDFULNESS?

Focus on What Is Going On Right Now

When you are focusing on what happened in the past or what might happen in the future, you are not in the present moment. Instead, try to observe and describe your experience objectively. Be fully present in the moment and participate in all that is happening. Participating has to do with staying present with what you are doing right now. Attend to and experience what is happening right now. This may be easiest to practice using your five senses. Notice sensations of sight, sound, touch, taste, and smell. Participate in this moment by fully attending to the sensations.

Accept Your Experience without Judging

Control your attention but not what you see. Accept whatever is happening without judging it. Accept reality as it is. Let go of trying to change reality. Accepting is not the same as liking what is going on; it is simply letting go of fighting reality.

Psychologist Marsha Linehan (1993a, 1993b) has highlighted the importance of becoming aware of your state of mind. When we integrate emotion and reason, we can achieve a state she calls "wise mind." Wise mind is a state of balance that neither ignores rational thinking nor "numbs out" emotions. In other words, when you are in wise mind, both your brain and your heart are guiding you. The decisions you make from wise mind, will "feel right" and are the most effective decisions for you.

Emotion Mind

- Your behaviors and thoughts are dominated by emotion
- Emotions run the show; you are ruled by your feelings
- Hard to think clearly
- Emotions tend to be intense (either positive or negative) and overwhelming
- Society often says that this is bad

Reasonable Mind

- Your behaviors and thoughts are dominated by reason
- You ignore your emotions; feelings are not considered in your decisions
- Calm, rational, logical
- "Numbed out"—you clamp down on emotions and use rationalization to cope
- Society often says this is good

Wise Mind

- Combines the two sides—emotion and reason
- Not ignoring, running away from, or numbing out emotions
- Having emotions, validating them, but still being able to think clearly
- Often feel "at peace" or centered when in wise mind

THE SEESAW OF EMOTION AND REASON

Traumatic experiences thrust you into emotion mind. Naturally, you try to escape the intense and unpleasant emotions by moving quickly to a reasonable state. However this starts you seesawing between emotion and reason, making it harder and harder to stay balanced. Healing from trauma involves learning to stay balanced in the center of the seesaw, the place we call "wise mind."

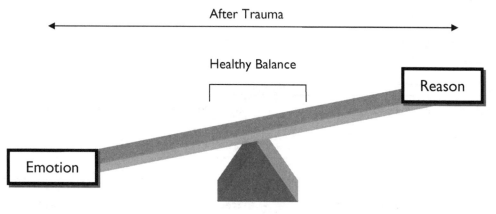

After Trauma

Healthy Balance

Reason

Emotion

(continued)

RECOGNIZING STATES OF MIND

You may find it helpful to recognize signals that indicate your state of mind. A signal might be a physical sensation, an urge, a thought, an image, or a behavior. In the next week, pay attention to such signals and make note of several signals that may serve as easily recognizable cues as to your state of mind. Also, brainstorm steps you can take to bring yourself into *wise mind*. These may be different if you are in reasonable mind or emotion mind. Below is an example of signals and steps to take to move into *wise mind*. Note yours on the blank worksheet that follows.

Signals that I am in **wise mind**:	
1. I can think clearly and focused even while feeling upset	
2. When I make a decision, it feels right	
3. I do what I know I ought to do, even while feeling anxious	
Signals that I am in **emotion** mind:	Steps to take to move to **wise mind**:
1. feeling suicidal	1. take a warm bath with candles
2. wanting to run away from everything	2. take a walk
3. yelling at my husband	3. talk it over with someone
Signals that I am in **reasonable** mind:	Steps to take to move to **wise mind**:
1. pretending everything is all right	1. practice mindfulness of emotions
2. feeling numbed out	2. call my support person
3. rationalizing	3. play with my dog

STATES OF MIND WORKSHEET

Signals that I am in **wise mind**:	
1. _____	
2. _____	
3. _____	
Signals that I am in **emotion** mind:	Steps to take to move to **wise mind**:
1. _____	1. _____
2. _____	2. _____
3. _____	3. _____
Signals that I am in **reasonable** mind:	Steps to take to move to **wise mind**:
1. _____	1. _____
2. _____	2. _____
3. _____	3. _____

1. **Identify the problem.**

2. **Identify an achievable goal.** (What do you want to accomplish?)

3. **Brainstorm.** (Generate possible solutions.)

4. **Evaluate solutions.** (What are the positive and negative consequences of each possible solution?)

Solutions	Pros	Cons
a)		
b)		
c)		
d)		
e)		
f)		

(continued)

5. **Make a decision.** (Choose a solution.)

6. **List steps to implement a solution:**

a)

b)

c)

d)

e)

7. **Evaluate.** (Did you meet your goal?)

HANDOUT 9.5. Decision Analysis Worksheet (page 1 of 2)

Decision Analysis: The Consequences of Avoiding _people_

Name: _Example_   Date: _____

	Immediate (short-term) consequences		Delayed (long-term) consequences	
	Positive	Negative	Positive	Negative
If I continue to avoid: _people_	Less anxiety Can't get hurt Feels safe No expectations More relaxed	Missing out on potential friendships and positive interactions	Can feel OK	Missing out on friendships Isolation Loneliness Remain fearful of people
If I stop avoiding: _people_	Opportunities to interact Confidence increases	Feel afraid Physical discomfort Could get hurt	Opportunity for a better life Anxiety goes down Less isolated World gets bigger Increased social support, trust, confidence, and intimacy	Might lose friends and relationships

(continued)

Decision Analysis Worksheet (page 2 of 2)

Decision Analysis: The Consequences of Avoiding _____

Name: _____   Date: _____

	Immediate (short-term) consequences		Delayed (long-term) consequences	
	Positive	Negative	Positive	Negative
If I continue to avoid:				
If I stop avoiding:				

TEN

Putting It Together

At this point, we hope you understand the principals and goals of CBT for PTSD and have a sense of supplemental tools that will help you meet the multiple needs of your patients with PTSD. In this chapter we offer guidance in handling treatment stumbling blocks, including decision making when treatment does not proceed as expected. We also discuss transitioning between treatment phases aimed at different problems and treatment termination.

COMMON STUMBLING BLOCKS

Poor Adherence

Poor adherence is not uncommon in CBT for PTSD, because the treatment is inherently challenging and anxiety provoking. As one CBT colleague noted with respect to both patients and therapists, "I know exactly why people don't want to do this treatment. It is seriously anxiety provoking and forces you to examine truly awful events. I wouldn't *want* to do it. Doesn't mean I wouldn't do it, I just understand why people have trouble." Given that you are asking your patients to face their worst fears, it is important to validate the difficulties they face, whether with psychoeducation, cognitive restructuring, or exposure. Then, explore any obstacles they encounter in completing assignments. Did she not understand the assignment or have trouble fitting it in her day? Did he grit his teeth to just get through it, versus accepting his anxiety, or race too quickly on to the next assignment without fully completing the first one? Is the patient incapable or unwilling at this point to complete home practice? Clarifying the assignment, scheduling time to do it, and problem-solving obstacles can go a long way to improve adherence in many cases. If your patient is simply not ready to do it on his or her own, complete the assignment, or a modification of it, in session. Nothing sends a clearer message about the importance of the tasks than simply stating, "OK, you ran into trouble, and that is understandable. Let's just do the exercise right now, here in session." Below, we provide two examples of patients who returned without fully completing an assignment.

Sample Dialogue: Patient Returns without Completing Exposure Records

After her first *in vivo* exposure assignment, Jill reported that she did the assignment but did not keep records. The following dialogue illustrates how the therapist responded to Jill's difficulty with record keeping during exposure, which is critically important. Homework records provide the ongoing assessment data that enable you to determine whether exposure is proceeding as expected. Failure to maintain records also may indicate that the patient did not complete other aspects of home practice, although this is not the case in the sample dialogue.

THERAPIST: So you were going to spend 30–45 minutes each day with your sister's golden retriever Toby and keep track of your anxiety levels on the form I gave you. How did it go?

JILL: Well, I did it a few times, but I didn't write it down.

THERAPIST: OK, that's understandable. You may not be used to keeping track of things as carefully as I'm asking you to. I'm glad you got started with the golden retriever. Some people find it hard just to get going. (*Pulls out a blank form.*) Tell me more about what you did. When was the first time you went to your sister's house to work on exposure to Toby?

[*Commentary: The therapist validates Jill's difficulty, reinforces her efforts, then behaviorally communicates that they are going to complete the record keeping task together in session. The therapist also communicates that record keeping is an important task, and models record keeping behaviors for Jill. If Jill persists in not completing her records, then the therapist may need to explore Jill's reasons for not doing so.*]

JILL: Last Monday.

THERAPIST: OK. What was your anxiety level before you saw Toby?

JILL: You mean at her house or before I left mine?

THERAPIST: Was it different?

JILL: Yeah. My anxiety was 40 when I left my house, but by the time I got to her house, it was already up to 60.

THERAPIST: It's common to feel a lot of anticipatory anxiety. Let's use your anxiety rating at her house before you saw Toby. That way we'll track your anticipatory anxiety as well. Most people find that the anticipatory anxiety reduces after a few trials. Let's see if that happened to you. (*Writes 60 in space for preexposure anxiety on the form.*) OK, what happened next?

JILL: Sarah kept Toby on the lead in the living room while I stood by the door, just as you and I had discussed.

THERAPIST: Sounds good. Then what happened?

JILL: I started to feel my heart pounding and I was shaking. I wanted to get out of there. I was really scared.

THERAPIST: But you stayed?

JILL: Yes. I reminded myself that it was just Toby, and he's never hurt anyone.

THERAPIST: Good. How high did your anxiety get?

JILL: Pretty high. I wasn't quite as anxious as when I last saw a bull mastiff, but it was up there. I'd say maybe 85.

THERAPIST: OK, let's enter that here (*writes down 85*). How long did you stay?

JILL: About 20 minutes.

THERAPIST: OK (*writes 20 minutes on the form*). And, what was your anxiety level at the end, when you left?

JILL: Well, like you told me to, I stayed until my anxiety went down by half, so I finally went into the kitchen when it was about 40.

THERAPIST: Good! OK . . . when was the next time you did exposure with Toby?

[*Commentary: Continued recording and analysis of homework data also demonstrate to Jill how they use the data to guide treatment decisions.*]

Sample Dialogue: Patient Returns without Completing Exposure

Elena returned to session without having completed home practice of imaginal exposure to the memory of her rape. She had habituated in session, but reported being unable to pick up the tape to practice at home.

ELENA: I looked at the tape a lot. But I couldn't bring myself to do it.

THERAPIST: That is understandable. Tell you what. Let's do the exposure here in session again. Then, when we're done we can look at the home practice and see whether we can't find some ways to make it work for you. I want to make sure, though, that we have enough time in session to do the exposure again. So I think we should start with that.

[*Commentary: The therapist validates Elena's difficulty, but makes it clear that she is not going to collude with Elena in avoiding exposure. Repeating exposure in session also should result in further within- and between-session habituation, which may make home practice easier. Finally, additional in-session practice with exposure should increase Elena's confidence about her ability to tolerate her anxiety, which should increase her willingness to do exposure at home.*]

ELENA: So you want me to do what we did last week again, now?

THERAPIST: Yes.

ELENA: (*Gives a big sigh.*) OK.

[*Commentary: Elena completed 30 minutes of exposure and reported a SUDS reduction from 90 to 30.*]

THERAPIST: So how was that for you today?

ELENA: It was easier than last week. Still awful, but my anxiety came down more and faster. I kept telling myself that if I stay with this, it will be OK.

THERAPIST: Good! So let's think about the home practice. What are your thoughts on it now that you have done a second exposure?

ELENA: I think it is going to still be hard, but easier than last week. I think I can do it.

THERAPIST: Where did you try to do the exposure last week?

ELENA: To be honest, I really didn't try. I just looked at the tape, which was in my room.

THERAPIST: So let's think a bit more on some things that might help you get it done. How hard will it be for you to set aside the time to do it?

[*Commentary: The therapist begins informal problem solving about home practice.*]

ELENA: That part is pretty easy. We're on summer break right now, so I have a fair bit of time.

THERAPIST: Do you think it would be easier or harder with other people in the house?

ELENA: Actually, I think it would be harder. Because even if I use my headphones, I will be worried the whole time that my mother or father will want to see what I am doing, and I will be worried that they will come into my room. Actually, if my sister is around, and just her, that would make it easier, because I told her a couple of weeks ago what happened and that I am in therapy.

THERAPIST: OK. Is there a time when you could practice when your sister is around and your parents will be gone?

ELENA: Yeah. They go for a walk twice a day for 45 minutes. I can ask Alisa to stay at home and be in another room. That would probably help me do it, too, because if I tell her about this, I'll feel bad not doing it.

Distractions: Life Problems and Shifting Priorities

Treatment manuals often encourage you to deliver the treatment in a set number of sessions administered in one block over consecutive weeks. Yet the reality for many patients with PTSD is that there are numerous distractions to completing treatment. As such, be prepared to assess the importance of distractions and, in some cases, modify treatment accordingly.

Distractions range from major life events, such as the death of a family member, to life problems, such as financial, legal, or marital issues. Life problems also may include practical obstacles, such as arranging transportation, child care, or being able to fit homework into a busy schedule. Finally, patients with comorbidity may be distracted when another disorder, such as drug abuse or depression, worsens.

Managing distractions entails validating their significance but not losing sight of patients' ultimate treatment goal—resolution of their PTSD. As you respond to patients' shifting needs, remember that distractions can readily serve avoidance, and avoidance often masquerades as logistical or life problems. Carefully consider the balance of priorities in your patients' lives, and how much attention you devote to life crises. Whenever possible, discuss this collaboratively with your patients. Some patients may feel a sense of obligation to you, to the treatment, or to themselves, and this may conflict with obligations to family or other needs in their lives. Open discussion of this can clarify the relevant issues.

Staying Focused on PTSD

A patient's life problems are more easily managed without PTSD. Thus, in most cases, staying the course and resolving the PTSD produces the most benefit for the patient. If you conclude that staying focused on PTSD treatment is the best course for a given patient, remember to validate the distress associated with the life problem. Failure to validate distress can harm your therapeutic relationship. Patients may become more distressed if they perceive you as being invalidating. Once effectively validated, however, most such patients will agree to a plan to continue with PTSD treatment.

Sample Dialogue

THERAPIST: I can see that your son's problems have been weighing heavily on you and causing a lot of distress. Yet, as we've discussed, there isn't much that you can do to help him at this time. I wonder if it makes sense for us to keep focused on moving you through the treatment, so that you reap its benefits and feel less stressed sooner. Also, once your PTSD is improved, you will find that you are probably better able to manage other problems.

Shifting or Modifying Treatment Focus

Sometimes life events result in shifting priorities, so that it does not make sense to proceed with PTSD treatment at that time. Many life crises are so demanding that continuing with PTSD treatment is either not possible or not a priority. Shifting focus can be a legitimate response to such situations, and shifting implicitly validates your patient's experience. When patients present with major life crises, such as learning that a spouse is having an affair or that a parent has a terminal illness, they may perceive your efforts to maintain a focus on PTSD as invalidating. In such cases, attempting to stay on course may prove fruitless.

If you conclude that a patient is no longer able to proceed with PTSD treatment, you have two options. The first option is a hiatus from treatment. This is a legitimate course of action and some patients find it helpful to take breaks in treatment. Such patients often return once the crisis has ended. In essence they complete treatment over several series of sessions rather than in a block of consecutive sessions. If your patient decides to take a break from therapy, it is wise to have a follow-up appointment planned in several months. This allows you to check in with your patient to determine his or her readiness to proceed. Without a follow-up scheduled, many patients have difficulty regaining the momentum needed to resume treatment.

Sample Dialogue

THERAPIST: It's been several sessions now that we have been addressing your mother's illness. Given the situation, I wonder if it makes sense for us to take a hiatus from treatment, until her situation is resolved.

PATIENT: Maybe. I don't think that talking about it really makes a difference at this point. But I just don't have the energy for treatment when I have to spend so much time running back and forth from the hospital. I'm afraid that if I stop coming, though, I won't come back.

THERAPIST: What if we set up a follow-up appointment to check in a few months from now? We could set up the appointment right now. That way you know you will come back, and we can determine whether you are in a better place to continue.

The second option is for you (or another therapist, if you feel you cannot competently treat the distraction) to continue treatment with a different focus, or to split the focus. For example, you may be able to shift focus for just a few sessions, then return to PTSD treatment. Judith discovered that her disability payments were about to be discontinued because of a paperwork error. She and her therapist spent several sessions on problem solving, then returned to PTSD treatment. Other problems, however, may require longer shifts. If you decide to shift focus temporarily, remember to continually assess your progress on the new problem. As noted earlier, distractions frequently serve avoidance. If you are not making progress on the distraction, it may behoove you to return to a focus on PTSD, or to split your focus. Remember that a primary goal of treatment is to help patients resolve PTSD symptoms as quickly as possible. Thus, you should return to PTSD treatment as soon as it is a viable option.

If you decide to split the treatment focus, there are two ways you can do this. First, you can divide your sessions between PTSD treatment and managing the other problem. This approach is easiest, particularly if you are able to schedule longer sessions. When you do this, begin the session with PTSD treatment and reserve sufficient time to address the life event. For example, shortly after starting imaginal exposure, Jamie found out that his 16-year-old daughter had been raped several years before and subsequently developed an addiction to cocaine. Jamie and his therapist decided to move to longer sessions (i.e., 120 minutes), which was possible because Jamie was a private pay patient. The first portion of the session was used to continue exposure. The second portion focused on problem-solving the situation with Jamie's daughter.

If longer sessions are not feasible, you may choose to alternate sessions. This option works better for patients who are able to attend therapy more frequently. For example, Lucia's eating disorder worsened after she started *in vivo* exposure. Both Lucia and her therapist believed that discontinuing exposure was not a good idea. Yet Lucia also needed help managing her eating disorder symptoms. Although Lucia could not attend treatment twice per week, she could attend twice per week every other week. Thus, sessions targeting PTSD continued on a weekly basis, while additional sessions were planned for every other week to address her most dangerous eating disorder behaviors.

Using Logistical Problems for Ongoing Assessment

Logistical problems also sometimes offer clues about additional treatment needs. For example, after her sixth session, Adrienne called to cancel her next appointment, stating that her work schedule had changed such that she could no longer make her usual appointment time. Adrienne, who lived an hour's drive away, thought she could not continue her treatment with her new work schedule. She scheduled an appointment on her day off to discuss this. In this session, the therapist initiated problem solving and they identified a possible solution. Implementing the solution required that Adrienne ask her supervisor to allow her to leave work a few hours early 1 day per week. In the course of the problem solving, it became apparent that Adrienne had some deficits in assertive communication skills. By doing a quick role play of the request for a schedule change, the therapist determined that Adrienne's deficits lay less in knowing what to say than in accepting her right to say it. The therapist suggested that Adrienne obtain a copy of *The Assertive Option* (Jakubowski & Lange, 1978) and read the chapters on assertive rights and thinking assertively. The therapist also made a mental note that Adrienne's communication difficulty might be related to patterns of thinking that evolved from her childhood abuse. She decided to target such thoughts with cognitive restructuring in future sessions.

Cancellations, No Shows, and Dropout

Cancellations and no shows happen with all forms of psychotherapy. Although a missed appointment often is not clinically relevant, missed appointments in some cases reflect life problems, distractions, or avoidance. Thus, missed appointments can be a precursor to dropping out. Obviously missed appointments also can affect the fiscal health of a clinical practice, and such concerns may be in conflict with your patients' clinical needs. As such, it is important to have a clinically sensitive plan for responding to missed appointments. If it is not already your policy to do so, we suggest following up by phone and/or letter with any patient with PTSD who is a no show or cancels an appointment without rescheduling. Phone calls are preferable, because they enable you to express your genuine concern and open a dialogue about obstacles to treatment attendance. In contrast, the intent of a letter is more easily misunderstood and may be viewed as invalidating or trigger distress.

Missed appointments during the assessment period or very early in treatment can signal ambivalence. Thus, we recommend that you respond with a brief phone call immediately, during the scheduled appointment time, even if your patient leaves a message that communicates reluctance to proceed. Use this as an opportunity to validate patients' reactions to the sessions and the difficulty of deciding to face something that has been buried for so long. Normalize any increase in intrusive symptoms that patients may be experiencing, and reiterate that these reactions are a sign of "unfinished business." At the very least, most patients find such expressions of concern comforting. It is our hope that patients will trust you enough to return when they summon the courage to move forward. It can also be helpful to ask them to come in for "just one more session" to talk about these issues in person.

A pattern of frequent cancellations also raises concerns about commitment to treatment and/or readiness for change, and needs to be addressed directly. As with patients who cancel early in treatment, we recommend that you respond to frequent cancellations with phone calls. In general, it is best to err on the side of persistence when attempting to make contact. For example, Sonja missed several appointments despite reporting a high level of commitment during psychoeducation. Sonja also was very difficult to reach on the phone. Although her therapist was somewhat frustrated, she persevered, one day leaving repeated messages on Sonja's answering machine. Sonja finally returned her call and admitted that she had been thinking about dropping out. She then noted, "I've never had someone be so persistent in reaching me. It made me think that you really care how this turns out. So, I've decided to go ahead with treatment." Sonja only missed one other session throughout her entire course of treatment. She also left a message, stating, "Don't worry, I'm not flaking out this time. I have a real conflict and will be there next week." In some cases, however, it may be necessary to come to an agreement about when treatment will be terminated or postponed if the cancellations persist.

Empirical understanding of factors that contribute to dropout from treatment is limited. Yet we do know that patients are slightly more likely to dropout of structured trauma-focused PTSD treatment than other forms of therapy for PTSD (Hembree, Foa, et al., 2003). We also have found that clinic patients who are severely depressed and evidence high levels of avoidance are more prone to drop out, and this may include those with borderline personality features, social anxiety, or generally severe PTSD symptoms (Zayfert et al., 2005). Patients who are severely depressed and/or suicidal can complete CBT for PTSD (Nishith, Hearst, Mueser, & Foa, 1995). In such cases, monitor depression and/or suicidal ideation during treatment by using assessment tools such as the Beck Depression Inventory (BDI), and/or daily ratings of mood and/or suicidal urges. This will help you to detect worsening of depression or suicidality and respond accordingly, particularly if your patient fails to attend a session. For example, if a patient misses a session because he or she is sleeping all day and has slept through the appointment time, this may be an indication that you need to focus several sessions focused on increasing activity levels and improving mood before resuming CBT for PTSD.

In summary, if your patients display irregular attendance patterns, it behooves you to examine the factors that may be influencing attendance behavior and do your best to "lure" patients back into treatment, even while recognizing that many such patients may ultimately drop out. Remember that your relationship (combined with good problem solving) often is your best tool for improving attendance.

TREATING PATIENTS WITH MULTIPLE PROBLEMS: DECIDING WHEN TO TRANSITION FROM PTSD TREATMENT

Once patients have completed exposure, decide whether and when to start treating problems other than PTSD. First and foremost, review your initial assessment. This helps you to maintain structure and focus the decision-making process. Reassessment, though it may seem burdensome, is important at this point. In our experience, most patients agree to complete the necessary assessments when you approach decision making collaboratively.

Sample Dialogue: Discussing Reassessment and Treatment Planning.

THERAPIST: So it seems that we've completed exposure to all the intrusive memories that you identified in the beginning of your treatment and a few others that you noticed were bothering you during treatment as well. You've also completed exposure to the various reminders of your assault that you had been avoiding, such as the shirt you were wearing that day, the street where it happened, and the song that you were listening to on your iPod when it happened. At this point I would like us to reassess your PTSD symptoms to see how you are doing. This will help us to decide whether any further treatment for your PTSD is needed. How does that sound?

JERRY: OK, that makes sense.

THERAPIST: (*Administers the CAPS.*) OK, so from what we have here so far, it seems like there has been quite an improvement in your PTSD symptoms. You said that you still feel a bit tense when you walk in your old neighborhood, but for the most part, you are no longer having dreams or intrusive memories of the attack. Also, you've stopped avoiding thoughts and reminders of the attack, and you've begun to regain interest in your activities. You are sleeping much better and are less irritable than you used to be.

JERRY: Yeah, I am definitely feeling a lot better.

THERAPIST: At your initial evaluation, we identified depression and panic disorder as problems that you also wanted help with. So, at this point, it makes sense for us to reassess these other problem areas to see whether these are still distressing for you.

JERRY: OK.

Assessment Strategies for Determining Additional Treatment Needs

Readministering the CAPS is the best way to find out to what extent patients' PTSD symptoms have been ameliorated. If your patient has experienced an optimal response to treatment, CAPS administration is likely to take 15 minutes or less. If, on the other hand, your patient remains fairly symptomatic, the interview will take longer. The information you glean from it, however, is informative and time well spent. During reassessment, pay particular attention to details about the content of any remaining intrusive symptoms (memories, nightmares, and flashbacks), triggers of distress or physical reactions, and thoughts, memories, images, feelings, or reminders that patients continue to avoid. These will help you to plan any further exposure exercises and/or identify target areas for cognitive restructuring. A self-report measure such as the PTSD Checklist (PCL) can also be used, but keep in mind that the concordance between self-report and interview measures is not necessarily high.

If you find that PTSD symptoms are reduced to a satisfactory degree, readminister the relevant modules of the Anxiety Disorders Interview Schedule for DSM-IV (ADIS-IV) or other diagnostic measure you used to determine comorbidity at the outset. Comorbid problems often improve to a satisfactory degree as a result of PTSD treatment. Comorbid problems do persist for some patients, and it often is necessary to plan further CBT to address them directly.

Based on your initial formulation, you may already be tracking some comorbid problems by using a questionnaire measure or daily ratings of mood or anxiety. These also can help you determine whether there is need for additional treatment targeting the comorbid problem. For example, at her initial assessment, Josephine met criteria for generalized anxiety disorder (GAD) and depression in addition to PTSD. Her therapist had included the Penn State Worry Questionnaire (PSWQ) and the BDI in her initial assessment, and had repeated them monthly during her treatment. Her scores on these measures showed a gradual decline during treatment (see Figure 10.1). After comple-

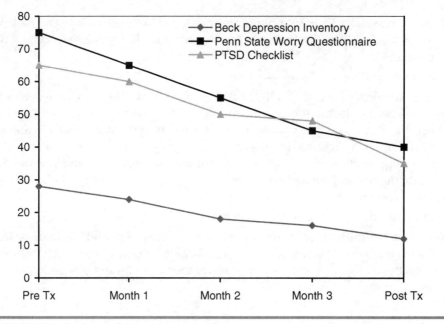

FIGURE 10.1. Josephine's treatment progression.

tion of CBT for PTSD, her therapist also readministered the GAD and depression modules of the ADIS-R, and Josephine no longer met criteria for these disorders, and her
scores on the PSWQ and BDI were now only slightly above the normal range. Therefore, her therapist did not think further treatment was necessary.

Starting CBT for Other Problems

If you and your patient decide to implement a supplemental course of treatment for
other problems, remember that you can build on your patients' knowledge base (e.g.,
about the nature of fear and anxiety, and the fight–flight reaction) and experience with
the treatment strategies. Then, you simply guide them in applying these strategies to
the comorbid problem. This often results in a shorter course of treatment. For example,
reassessment of Jerry's depression and panic disorder showed that his mood had improved substantially, and he had not had a panic attack in 2 weeks. Nonetheless, he remained fearful of physical sensations of anxiety and apprehensive about having a
panic attack in public places, even though he was less concerned about his safety. Thus,
he still met criteria for panic disorder. His therapist made a plan to conduct further education about panic attacks (i.e., learning to conceptualize them as "false alarms") and
to conduct several sessions of interoceptive exposure (see Chapter 9).

It is not always necessary to complete all elements of CBT for PTSD before deciding to make this transition, although typically most of the critical treatment tasks with
regard to the trauma will at least be under way. In some cases, when the comorbid
problems are a significant aspect of the individual's overall distress, it is prudent to
shift your attention to them as quickly as possible. For example, Adrienne met criteria
for PTSD, dysthymia, GAD, social phobia, specific phobia, and binge-eating disorder

(BED). Adrienne required only three sessions of *in vivo* exposure and two sessions of exposure to her memory of childhood sexual abuse. Subsequently, to address her feelings of shame (see Chapter 8), her therapist introduced cognitive restructuring, which was carried out in three sessions. Around this time, a visit to her primary care doctor revealed that because of her obesity, Adrienne was dangerously close to developing type II diabetes, and a visit to a dietician was recommended. This presented an ideal opportunity to incorporate a focus on her BED, while continuing to reinforce the cognitive restructuring of thoughts about low self-worth that were hypothesized to have a prominent role in her disordered eating patterns.

After learning about the physician's recommendation, Adrienne's therapist reviewed the work they had accomplished so far, targeting PTSD symptoms, fear of vomiting, and low self-esteem (dysthymia). Then, they outlined her remaining concerns. Adrienne's therapist asked her which concern she would like to address next. Adrienne identified binge eating as the next treatment target. The therapist then assessed Adrienne's binge eating using the BED module of the Structured Clinical Interview for DSM-IV (SCID), and questions about daily food consumption and the content of her binges. Finally, the therapist made a plan to reevaluate her PTSD symptoms, recognizing that these might continue to improve with further cognitive restructuring and *in vivo* exposure practice.

Mark met criteria for PTSD, social phobia, and depression. His initial treatment plan targeted PTSD. After 18 sessions consisting of psychoeducation, *in vivo* and imaginal exposure, cognitive restructuring, and activity scheduling, Mark had conducted exposure with all the memories and identifiable stimuli. He also had successfully challenged thoughts related to shame and low self-worth, and regularly engaged in pleasurable activities, such as riding his bike, fishing, and playing with his dog. His therapist readministered the CAPS and the depression and social phobia modules of the ADIS-IV. Mark's PTSD symptoms had diminished from his pretreatment CAPS total severity score of 74 to 35, yet he continued to be upset when he was reminded of the abuse. He also still met full criteria for social phobia and major depressive disorder, although his BDI score had declined from 35 to 19. Mark's therapist hypothesized that his mood remained low because he continued to be socially isolated, spending much of his free time alone. She suggested that Mark consider participating in a social anxiety treatment group that would begin the following month, and that they meet individually after completing the 12-session group treatment to evaluate the need for any further treatment.

PLANNING FOR TERMINATION

As with other treatment decisions, the decision regarding when to end treatment should be based on data indicating the degree to which your patients have attained their therapy goals. Ideally, such data will include SUDS ratings during exposure, progress through exposure hierarchies, SUDS rating during cognitive restructuring, and behavioral observation (e.g., ability to engage easily with previously frightening stimuli). In addition to these measures of therapy process, we recommend relying on valid outcome measures, such as structured interviews or psychometric questionnaires assessing PTSD or other relevant dimensions. When the outcome measures show appreciable reduction in symptoms, you will very likely begin discussing termination with your patient.

Once you recognize that you are in the end phase of treatment, you need to consider your plans for (1) tapering sessions, (2) addressing continued medication use and, (3) relapse prevention and generalization. These three issues are not independent of one another. For example, your plan for relapse prevention and generalization might typically include booster or follow-up sessions at scheduled intervals. Your plan for tapering medications may dovetail with planned follow-up sessions as well.

Planning for Generalization and Maintenance

In a nutshell, CBT for PTSD works as therapists coach patients to reverse avoidant coping and instead to confront feared stimuli and distressing memories. In doing so, CBT provides an opportunity for patients to relearn safety and to rethink what the traumatic event means with regard to their self-worth. Relapse can occur if symptoms reemerge in response to memories or situations in their lives, *and* if patients fail to apply their new coping methods. For example, some patients find that they are reminded of distressing events not addressed in therapy, or that occasionally something may retrigger aspects of a memory that was addressed in therapy in a different context. Patients who leave therapy with a mind-set such as "I've licked it; fear will never be a problem for me again" or "I've put it all behind me now, so I won't be bothered by it ever again" are likely to be caught off guard if something triggers their fear again.

Given the possibility of reemergence of fear in new contexts, consider preparing your patients for the possibility that distressing thoughts, memories, and feelings may reemerge after treatment ends, and instruct them to utilize the strategies they have learned in treatment. This kind of preparation, known as "relapse prevention," was originally developed to help those with addictive behavior maintain cessation of these behaviors (Marlatt & Gordon, 1985). It also has been shown to benefit patients with many other disorders (Fairburn et al., 1993).

By coaching your patients to expect a possible return of fear, particularly in new contexts, you prepare them to use exposure to confront the feared memory or situation rather than escape from it. Patients who entered therapy with strong feelings of guilt, shame, or low self-worth also should understand that these feelings might be triggered in the future, and that they should use cognitive restructuring to examine the thoughts underlying them.

For example, Caren successfully completed treatment for PTSD during her summer break away from college. She had been raped at a party during her first year at a rural, residential college. The local area provided few mental health resources and, as a first year student, Caren was not allowed to keep a car on campus. Given that Caren had completed treatment away from the setting in which the rape occurred, Caren's therapist warned her that she might experience a return of fear when she returned to college. Caren and her therapist spent two sessions identifying situations that might produce a return of fear. They also discussed what skills Caren should use to manage such anxiety, and scheduled a booster session during Caren's fall break. At the booster session, Caren reported that she had experienced a significant increase in anxiety prior to attending her first party. Following the plan she and her therapist developed, Caren listened to her imaginal exposure tape in her dorm room and used cognitive restructuring to convince herself to approach the party, which she viewed as *in vivo* exposure. She also took appropriate safety steps by using a buddy system when she went to the bathroom (a strategy commonly used by her sorority sisters). The therapist used the booster session to reinforce Caren for continuing to use her skills.

Similarly, in the case of Josephine, whose comorbid problems had improved with PTSD treatment, the therapist provided a session of relapse prevention in which she and Josephine anticipated potential triggers of relapse in depression or avoidance behaviors. They then reviewed application of the skills Josephine had learned in treatment to other problems.

Tapering Medications

Many patients are already taking medications when they begin treatment, and others will start medications while in treatment with you. Certain medications, particularly serotonin reuptake inhibitors (SSRIs) such as sertraline (Brady et al., 2000; Zohar et al., 2002) and fluoxetine (Connor, Sutherland, & Tupler, 1999), have demonstrated efficacy for PTSD. Other medications, such as atypical antipsychotics (e.g., olanzapine [Stein, Kline, & Matloff, 2002] and quetiapine [Hammer, Deitsch, Broderick, Ulmer, & Lorberbaum, 2003]) and antiadrenergic agents (e.g., clonidine [Harmon & Riggs, 1996] and prazosin [Raskind et al., 2003]), also are widely used based on preliminary support. Yet no studies have examined the optimal use of medications in combination with CBT for PTSD. Nonetheless, many patients who complete CBT are interested in tapering off their medications once their PTSD and other symptoms have improved. The decision to taper medications is influenced by a variety of factors, such as types of medications, side effects of medications, how long patients have taken the medications, experience with prior attempts to taper, symptom response to medications, response to CBT, types of comorbid problems, whether comorbid problems have responded to treatment, patient preferences, and the opinions and preferences of the prescriber. Limited research exists to guide decision making around duration of medication use with PTSD and the utility of tapering medication. As a result, the majority of prescribers follow recommendations that have been based on research on depression or other anxiety disorders.

Reviews of research on other anxiety disorders, however, indicate that patients who receive CBT combined with medication are at increased risk for relapse if the medication is withdrawn after termination of CBT (Otto, Smith, & Reese, 2005; Otto, Smits, & Reese, 2004). Laboratory studies also have shown that changes in internal states associated with medication use are a powerful context. As discussed earlier, if fear reduction occurs only in the drug context, and the context is later changed by discontinuation of the medication, fear reduction learning may not endure in the new (nondrug) context. If medication is withdrawn while the patient is actively doing exposure exercises, the patient has the opportunity to learn new safety associations in the nondrug context. Despite this, many patients are understandably inclined to taper medications after successfully completing CBT, most likely because they do not want to stop the medications until they feel better.

Many clinicians also feel that because PTSD is so difficult to treat, once symptom remission is achieved, it is best not to tamper with medications, because doing so might risk relapse. This is understandable. Although no data are available regarding optimal timing of discontinuation of medications for PTSD, results from other anxiety disorders may extend to PTSD. These studies indicate that the risk of relapse may be greater if a patient terminates CBT while still taking medications and then discontinues medication at a later date (Otto, Pollack, & Sabatino, 1996). As Otto et al. (2005) point out, for some patients, "the pharmacological blockade of anxiety during CBT may provide a context for learning that is too narrow for broad generalization; should episodic anxiety occur in the future, memories of the original fear learning may predominate" (p. 79).

   In contrast to studies of the drugs mentioned earlier, research has not supported the efficacy of benzodiazepines for reducing PTSD symptoms (Braun et al., 1990; Gelpin et al., 1996). Studies also have shown that patients who receive CBT for panic disorder can be successfully tapered from benzodiazepines with minimal risk of relapse. Given these findings and the earlier discussion, we believe that it makes sense to taper benzodiazepines during CBT for PTSD. Your patients' decisions regarding other medications will be influenced by their general preferences, side effects, the opinions of the prescriber, and patients' response to CBT. For example, Belinda, who had PTSD related to a sexual assault and no comorbid problems, showed a strongly positive response to CBT. She had been on paroxetine for several months prior to beginning CBT and was dissatisfied with its sexual side effects. As her therapy was winding down, Belinda raised the issue of medication and stated her clear preference to discontinue the paroxetine. In this case, her therapist agreed that it made sense to taper the medication as they entered the relapse prevention phase of treatment, and she encouraged Belinda to discuss this with the prescribing psychiatrist. She also scheduled several booster sessions and had Belinda continue home practice of both her imaginal and *in vivo* exposure assignments during and after the taper.

Case Examples: Termination and Medication Tapering

Marcus, a retired firefighter, suffered from PTSD and depression related to his work. Several years before starting CBT, he began taking sertraline and clonazepam. Marcus also experienced great difficulty sleeping, and as a result, was started on trazodone after beginning CBT. Marcus's PTSD treatment consisted of two sessions of psychoeducation, two sessions of *in vivo* exposure, 15 sessions of exposure to five memories of fires and accidents, and three sessions of cognitive restructuring that addressed guilt related to incidents in which he was unable to save victims. After completing exposure to the fifth memory, Marcus noted that the remaining memories on his list were less troublesome, and he stated that he felt like the dark cloud over him had begun to lift. His therapist readministered the CAPS and determined that Marcus's overall severity score had decreased from 95 to 42 (see Figure 10.2). Marcus had not been bothered by reexperiencing symptoms during the last several weeks, and also was no longer avoiding thoughts and feelings or reminders of the fires and accidents. He still felt emotionally numb, however, and had only regained partial interest in enjoyable activities; Marcus continued to have problems with sleeping, irritability, and concentration. His BDI score also remained elevated, with a score of 28 (Figure 10.2). As a result, his therapist implemented five additional sessions of CBT for insomnia and activity scheduling. After these sessions, Marcus demonstrated improved sleep on the Insomnia Severity Index (Bastien, Vallières, & Morin, 2001) and the CAPS sleep item. At this point, in preparation for treatment termination, his therapist recommended that Marcus discuss

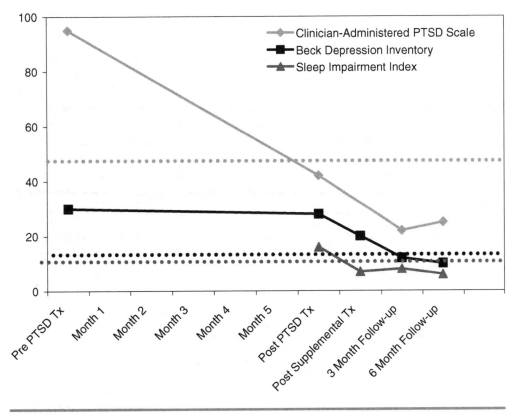

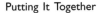

FIGURE 10.2. Marcus's treatment progression.

a gradual taper of clonazepam with his psychiatrist. During the schedule Marcus set up with his psychiatrist for a 3-month taper of clonazepam, his treatment sessions were reduced, first to bimonthly, then monthly, with a focus on relapse prevention, improving mood, and increasing breadth of emotional experience. Marcus's therapist also encouraged him to continue to expose himself to the *in vivo* stimuli used during treatment and periodically to complete imaginal exposure to make sure that his fear remained low in the new, nondrug context. During this time, cognitive restructuring practice addressed Marcus's thoughts that he would not be able to cope without clonazepam, and that he needed clonazepam to sleep. By the end of the 3-month period, Marcus had discontinued clonazepam, maintained satisfactory sleep, and showed improvement in mood, as evidenced by a reduction in BDI score from 30 to 18. In addition, readministration of the CAPS revealed further reduction in his CAPS total score to 22. Marcus expressed his preference eventually to taper off all his medications. Given Marcus's satisfaction with his sleep, his therapist discussed tapering trazodone with his psychiatrist, and a taper schedule was planned over the next several months. At 7 months post CBT for PTSD, Marcus had successfully discontinued trazodone. He decided to continue taking sertraline for the next 6 months, with a plan to schedule booster CBT sessions if he wanted to discontinue sertraline, to ensure that he did not experience a relapse of depression or anxiety symptoms.

CONCLUSION

This chapter has reviewed some final challenges involved in administering CBT for PTSD. The evidence supporting this treatment is strong, and we hope that you use it regularly with your patients. In applying CBT to your complicated PTSD cases, we encourage you to think about how to individualize the treatment to meet your patients' specific needs. Be prepared to encounter roadblocks and diversions with the majority of your patients (Zayfert & Becker, 2000). Familiarize yourself with the common decision points and obstacles. By using the principles of CBT as your road map, and the tools at your disposal to manage diversions and return the focus to the trauma as quickly as possible, you will be able to stay on course with even your most challenging PTSD patients.

> We cannot go back and make a new start, but we can start now to make a new ending.
> —ANONYMOUS